MW00577090

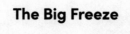

The Big Freeze

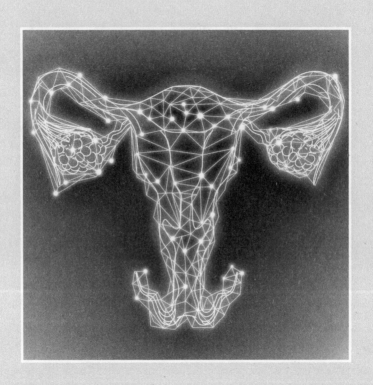

THE
Big Freeze

A Reporter's Personal Journey into
the World of Egg Freezing and
the Quest to Control
Our Fertility

NATALIE LAMPERT

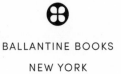

BALLANTINE BOOKS

NEW YORK

The Big Freeze is a work of nonfiction.
Some names and identifying details have been changed.

Published in the United States by Ballantine Books, an imprint of
Random House, a division of Penguin Random House LLC, New York.

BALLANTINE BOOKS and colophon are registered trademarks
of Penguin Random House LLC.

Hardback ISBN 978-1-5247-9938-0
Ebook ISBN 978-1-5247-9939-7

Printed in the United States of America on acid-free paper

randomhousebooks.com

2 4 6 8 9 7 5 3 1

FIRST EDITION

Book design by Jessica Shatan Heslin/Studio Shatan, Inc.

FOR ALL THE PEOPLE WITH OVARIES
CONFRONTING UNCERTAINTY AND THE
CONSEQUENTIAL QUESTIONS

I used to think, as a young woman, that life was something I was controlling and directing. Now I only think: What a mess we all are, with so many contradictory impulses, so many things about ourselves we'll never entirely understand.

—ZADIE SMITH, *Lenny Letter* interview, December 2017

We are all yeses. We are worthy enough, we passed inspection, we survived the great fetal oocyte extinctions. In that sense, at least—call it a mechanospiritual sense—we are meant to be. We are good eggs, every one of us.

—NATALIE ANGIER, *Woman: An Intimate Geography*

Contents

List of Abbreviations

ACOG: American College of Obstetricians and Gynecologists

AFC: antral follicle count

AMH: anti-Müllerian hormone

ART: assisted reproductive technology

ASRM: American Society for Reproductive Medicine

BBT: basal body temperature

BIPOC: Black, indigenous, (and) people of color

BMI: body mass index

BRCA: breast cancer gene

CAP: College of American Pathologists

CDC: U.S. Centers for Disease Control and Prevention

CLIA: Clinical Laboratory Improvement Amendments

CMS: Centers for Medicare and Medicaid Services

D&C: dilation and curettage

DOR: diminished ovarian reserve

FAMs: fertility awareness-based methods

FDA: U.S. Food and Drug Administration

FLE: Family Life Education

FSH: follicle-stimulating hormone

hCG: human chorionic gonadotropin

HPV: human papillomavirus

ICSI:	intracytoplasmic sperm injection
IM:	intramuscular
IUD:	intrauterine device
IUI:	intrauterine insemination
IVF:	in vitro fertilization
IVG:	in vitro gametogenesis
IVM:	in vitro maturation
LGBTQ+:	lesbian, gay, bisexual, transgender, queer, or questioning
LH:	luteinizing hormone
NYU:	New York University
OB/GYN:	obstetrician and gynecologist
OHSS:	ovarian hyperstimulation syndrome
PCOS:	polycystic ovary syndrome
PGT:	preimplantation genetic testing
RFID:	radio frequency identification
SART:	Society for Assisted Reproductive Technology
STI:	sexually transmitted infection
TSH:	thyroid-stimulating hormone
WHO:	World Health Organization

Author's Note

About the Reporting

This is a work of nonfiction. All names are real except when noted otherwise. I have indicated these instances in the footnotes and provided explanations in the Notes section at the back of the book. There are no composite characters or events, though I had to omit some people and details in the interest of book length; I did so only when an omission had no impact on either the veracity or the substance of the story.

This book relies predominantly on interviews and research I conducted. Most scenes and dialogue draw from what I saw and heard firsthand. I occasionally describe events for which I was not present and in so doing consulted with others and relied on extensive documentation. To write this book, I set out on an immersive first-person quest, and to that end, I also relied upon my journals and my medical records, as well as my own memory and the memories of others. Memory, of course, can be fallible; I have done my best.

The Notes section is intended to offer more detail on certain studies, statistics, and topic areas, as well as to guide readers to publicly available resources.

On Limited Language and Perspectives

It was my goal to present a character-driven narrative of the contemporary landscape of egg freezing. Most of the research I discuss in this book focuses on the experiences of heterosexual, white, cisgender women, because they are the people who, for now, predominantly constitute that landscape—although they are by no means the only people who use and/or require assisted reproductive technologies. LGBTQ+ people, same-sex couples, solo parents, and a wide spectrum of others plan their family-making outside the traditional male-female partnership, often relying on fertility treatment to do so.

In this book, I use the terms "female" and "woman" to refer to people with ovaries, although not everyone with internal reproductive organs identifies as a woman or a female; likewise with "man" and "male." Sex and gender exist on a spectrum, and people with ovaries include those who are transgender, nonbinary, intersex, gender-nonconforming, genderqueer, agender, and genderless.

All too often, BIPOC women struggle to access fertility treatment and technologies—a reflection of the broader, unjust ways in which reproductive healthcare's racial and ethnic inequities play out in the United States. One of the book's primary characters, Mandy, is Asian American, and I hope readers who are women of color, in particular, will see themselves in her egg freezing experience.

I recognize some of the limitations in my reporting and in the research and findings I describe here. More so, I acknowledge the fact that this book cannot capture all the complexities of the experiences of people with ovaries. However you identify, and regardless of whether you have ovaries and eggs, I hope you will find something of value here.

Introduction

This isn't the book I set out to write.

I began writing this book in my late twenties. I'm in my early thirties now, and I couldn't have imagined all that would happen in the years between. The second half of one's twenties and beginning of one's thirties is a tumultuous and tender time for many people even under normal circumstances, and this was certainly true for me, though at times the circumstances were decidedly not normal.

One unusual and unique-to-me circumstance that did *not* change during these years was the fact that I have one ovary, for reasons I'll soon explain. But I mention it now because it was my doctors' urging that I freeze my eggs and protect my ability to have biological children that turned out to dominate this roughly five-year period. And it was this dilemma that became the main impetus behind the deep dive that resulted in this book.

As I wrote, my life kept changing. And that, in turn, changed what this book was becoming. What began as a straightforward investigation into egg freezing and reproductive technologies morphed into a book about control. About what we—women, humans, all of us—try to control, why we do that, and how we ultimately have much less control than we think we do. Even as we attempt to buy it or freeze it or otherwise procure it.

Nearly half a century after the birth of the first "test-tube baby" conceived via in vitro fertilization, a third of American adults say that they or someone they know has used fertility treatment to try to have a baby. The ability to successfully freeze eggs has been among reproductive medicine's biggest achievements, resulting in the first two decades of the twenty-first century having seen egg freezing secure its place among the full range of processes by which conception begins outside the human body. What was once science fiction is now simply science: Fertility can be frozen in time. Along with in vitro fertilization, or IVF, egg freezing is on its way to becoming part of a vast demographic shift—a global trend of delaying childbirth, particularly among the affluent. (Sperm freezing is on the rise, too, with an increasing number of men eyeing fertility preservation.) We are marrying and having babies later than ever, and egg freezing lets women have biological children on a timeline that suits them. That's the idea, at least. And more women are buying into it than ever before.

For most of U.S. history, many women didn't have legal rights over their bodies, and we're still experiencing the horrible hangover. The conflict in America today over abortion is proof of how many people still believe that a woman's uterus should belong to the government. At the same time, we live in an age that prizes optimization and taking charge, and the notion that a woman should command every aspect of her future fertility—even if her reproductive rights are at present on shaky ground—has become, for many, a pillar of modern womanhood.

The pressure to take charge of one's fertility helps to explain egg freezing's rapid growth and why it has become, for a certain group of women, a mainstream, viable option, viewed as one of the best technological solutions available for women hoping to "have it all." From boardrooms to bedrooms, egg freezing is touted as an obvious and immediate way to conquer the biological clock. More and more employers cover the cost of the procedure as a workplace benefit. Celebrities sing its praises. Many of us know someone who has done it, or have seen targeted ads for it on our social media feeds, or have watched it unfold as a plotline on one of our favorite TV shows. Even if we've only heard of egg freezing in passing, we know what it purportedly offers women: More agency over their reproductive lives. More flexibility in planning a family. More options. More control.

My quest to decide whether to freeze my eggs took me to the front lines of fertility—tomorrow's final frontier for women's reproductive autonomy. I set out to learn all I could about the latest developments in assisted reproductive technology and how they affected my own future choices. I was a young journalist on a personal mission, determined to unearth information that I and so many other women were shockingly ignorant about. Along the way, I visited world-famous fertility clinics, sat in on high school sex ed classes, and peered into petri dishes inside laboratories. I attended egg freezing parties and medical conferences. I interviewed dozens of reproductive endocrinologists and fertility experts. I followed the experiences of young women who froze their eggs and a few who chose not to. I met with scientists and start-up founders, embryologists and ethicists, clinicians and corporate executives. I spoke to therapists specializing in reproductive trauma and lawyers specializing in reproductive rights. I even sat down with Louise Brown, the world's first IVF baby, who showed me every one of her twelve tattoos as we chatted about menstrual cramps, fish and chips, and giving birth.

When I decided to look into the science of egg freezing myself, I had hoped what I found would determine my choice. It did—but not in the ways I had expected. It took years to arrive at the conclusions I make in these pages. Some are clear-cut and satisfying. Others are murkier because of what we still do not know about egg freezing and won't for some time. I wrote this book to put all the information we *do* have about egg freezing in one place and to make it easy to understand.

I turned over many stones to get here, to stand up with dirt smeared across my face, brush off my hands, and say, "Okay, here's the deal." I learned what questions to ask and to whom to direct those questions. I spent a long while holding my breath, waiting to see if egg freezing—the incredible technology and the lucrative industry behind it—could and would deliver on its promises. I searched long and hard for answers. For myself. For you. My mission, I came to realize, had two objectives that were inextricably tied. I couldn't decide whether or not to freeze my eggs without first learning all the facts. And I couldn't help women identify and ask the right questions about egg freezing unless I put my skin in the game and was transparent about why making this choice—which at first I thought would be easy—became as difficult as it did. The shape of my search became a double helix, weaving journalistic objectivity with personal interest as I set about learning the truth for you and trying to make a decision for me. Ultimately, the answers I uncovered caused me to consider my questions, and all that informed them, from completely different vantage points and in an entirely new light. And that, it turns out, is often par for the course, both in journalism and in life.

The further afield I went, the deeper my reporting led into a little-understood world where medicine, politics, commerce, technology, and sex intersect in convoluted ways. It's a world that women, and those who care about them, ought to understand. And so this book is more than the result of my search for answers. It is also a tale about my journey into the future of fertility, as it unfolded against a backdrop of reproductive rights being dismantled and liberties pertaining to women being stripped away. Of all I learned, as a woman and as a journalist, the single most important truth was this: It has never been so important for a person with ovaries to understand their body, their options, and their reproductive autonomy—and the forces that threaten them.

Before all that, though, in the beginning, I set out with simple intentions, notebook in pocket and pen tucked behind one ear, a metaphorical hat labeled JOURNALIST in one hand and a hat labeled WOMAN in the other. Off I went, just me and my one ovary, giving this all we've got.

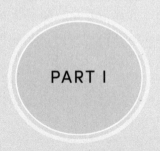

PART I

The Consultation

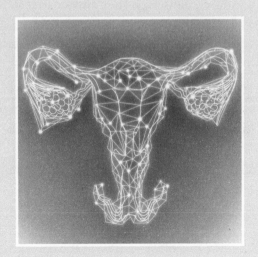

Young, Fertile, and Fabulous

~~~~~~

Walking into the Future

My official introduction to the future of fertility was courtesy of Egg-Banxx, a start-up company offering financing options to potential customers to freeze their eggs. One afternoon in early September, I read on Twitter about an informational "Let's Chill" event in Lower Manhattan, hosted by EggBanxx, where women would be gathering to learn about egg freezing while liquoring their anxieties with cute cocktails. I wasn't sure what to expect, but I registered for the event online and promptly received a confirmation email: *Forget sweating in the hot summer sun looking for Mr. Right!,* the invitation read. *It's fall now and smart women will be staying cool at the EggBanxx party tomorrow night! We hope you're as excited as we are to sip our Banxxtinis while talking about the three F's: Fun, Fertility, and Freezing!* It wasn't just idle curiosity. Fertility—and my eggs and sole ovary, in particular—had lately been very much on my mind.

The following night, I headed down to the Crosby Street Hotel to learn more.

"Ladies, you are young and fertile and fabulous!" chirped Dr. Serena Chen, a reproductive endocrinologist at the event. Her white coat and smooth dark hair emanated authority as she smiled at the attractive group of attendees. The hundred or so women around me pecked at popcorn and sipped raspberry-filled flutes of champagne. Several women sat on the edge of their seats in anticipation of . . . of what? I wasn't sure. Most appeared to be in their thirties or forties, fashionably dressed, with tan faces and flowing blow-dried hair. I noticed many sparkling diamond rings and designer handbags. It felt like a scene from a *Sex and the City* episode. I, meanwhile, wore a backpack—I'd just started graduate school at New York University—and was probably the youngest in the room by at least five years.

It was 2014, and EggBanxx, which had launched a couple of years earlier, was now attracting major attention in New York for its series of swanky cocktail parties. The company acted as a matchmaker between doctors and patients in the market for state-of-the-art fertility treatments. "We will be like Uber, but for egg freezing," said Gina Bartasi, EggBanxx's founder, in a *Washington Post* article. An early pioneer in the fertility marketing space, EggBanxx—the two *x*'s represent female chromosomes—negotiated with fertility doctors to provide lower treatment prices for patients and offered discounts and low-interest loans to women wanting to freeze their eggs. "We've learned that millennials don't like paying retail," Jennifer Palumbo, who was then director of patient care at EggBanxx, told me in an interview. Palumbo, who had struggled with infertility in her thirties, froze her eggs before taking a job at EggBanxx. Bartasi also had faced difficulties conceiving naturally; she now has twin boys, courtesy of IVF, which is when a sperm and egg are merged to become an embryo in a lab and then implanted in a woman's uterus.

Midway through the presentation, the audience was totally attentive, cocktails forgotten. As I looked around, a part of me felt profoundly out of place. And yet my uterus made me feel as if I belonged, as if it were my ticket to some sort of ladies-only club. Here we were, a bunch of women on an early fall evening in New York City, listening to a handful of fertility doctors talk about our eggs. There was something delightfully strange about it all. I scribbled phrases in my notebook I'd never heard before: *thaw data, dehydration protocols, autologous cycles.* In the margins, I made notes of things to clarify later: *embryo = fertilized egg, yes?* In between speakers, pockets of quiet chatter filled the room. I sensed a we're-all-in-this-together kind of camaraderie in the air that I hadn't felt since my college orientation session for first-year students.

Dr. Chen reached the last slide of her presentation and took questions. Someone asked if there was any sort of refund policy if a woman became pregnant naturally after freezing her eggs. Dr. Chen replied that there was not. More hands shot up. "I'm not quite sure how to put this," a woman in the back began. "What happens if your eggs become . . . poached?" The crowd erupted in cathartic laughter. I smiled, too, but the quip gave me pause. Were we really using cooking metaphors to describe our potential future children?

I raised my hand. A few minutes later—it was a big room, and a bunch of questions got answered before it was my turn—someone handed me a microphone. "Hi," I said. "I'm Natalie, I'm twenty-five, and I'm wondering what happens if I'm living in, say, the South Pacific in five or ten years and want to start a family but my frozen eggs are here in New York."

"Once you figure out where you are and what you want to do, we can ship the eggs to you," Dr. Chen replied. "They'll get sent in a container of liquid nitrogen, and, well, hopefully no one leaves them on the shipping dock alone. . . ." A few women around me giggled. Dr. Chen went on: "But if people are transporting precious things like eggs, we usually recommend you buy the eggs a ticket to take them to wherever you're going." Several women in the room nodded, seeming to find Dr. Chen's response sensible. Speechless, I sat down and passed off the microphone. As if getting shot up with thousands of dollars' worth of hormones wasn't financially crippling enough, now I had to factor in airfare for my own eggs?

I had hoped my logistical query would prompt an easy answer, something reassuring and straightforward amid all the talk of viscosity and thaw data. No wonder our questions—sometimes flippant, if well-intentioned—were laced with awkward metaphors: We didn't fully understand the slides or what these doctors were telling us. We were trying to mask our ignorance and discomfort with laughter, the same way we'd giggled at enlarged pictures of penises in elementary sex ed. Back then, we'd sat on hard classroom chairs or cross-legged on cold gymnasium floors; now, it was plush seats, high heels, and one leg crossed dutifully over the other. Being older and sophisticated didn't change the fact that many of us were as unaware of the facts now as we were then—and just as eager to hide it. The only thing separating me from these women, I realized, was a decade and a back-pack. Like them, I felt dazzled by this exciting technology and the thought of taking matters of reproductive biology into my own hands. But there was a sense of unease, too, a gnawing feeling that I—and these women—had missed the boat at some point, as if we'd ducked out of a movie and missed crucial plot information.

The PowerPoint resumed; other fertility specialists took the stage. One asked us to follow her on Twitter. ("A bit of shameless self-promotion," she said. "I'm trying to get more followers.") The presentations concluded with a "reality check" from Dr. Chen. "With the exception of the twenty-five-year-old in the back of the room," she said, wagging her finger admonishingly at the crowd, "all of your eggs are old, ladies."

Not so fertile and fabulous after all.

Afterward, audience members and doctors mingled in the lobby, fresh drinks in hand. I retreated to a corner of the bar, my brain buzzing. In the days to come, with my doctor's years-earlier recommendation that I freeze my eggs at top of mind and my questions about reproductive basics mounting, I would see this night as the official beginning of my quest for information. Near the end of the evening, I met a fertility doctor who, after hearing my story and asking my age, pushed a business card into my hand and told me to call her office to schedule an appointment. On my way out, an EggBanxx rep handed me a goodie bag. Inside, wedged between a lime-green mug and a handful of chocolate candy eggs, was a $1,000 voucher to put toward a cycle of egg freezing.

I was on my way.

Surgeries, Gold Mines, and Why I'm Telling This Story

Four years before I walked into the EggBanxx soiree, two significant events set me on a path to begin facing my fertility.

In the breezy-hot weeks of early summer, when I was twenty and home from college, my lower left abdomen began to ache one morning after breakfast. By midafternoon I was curled in the fetal position on the bathroom floor, dizzy with nausea. The pain spread from my pelvis to below my breast, sharpening and deepening. My father sat on the side of the bathtub and held a cool washcloth against my forehead. In a gentle voice, he said, "We need to go to the hospital." I braced against the tub and hoisted myself off the floor. An ambulance ride and two emergency rooms later, I lay on my back in an exam room, feet propped in metal stirrups. I was alone, except for two male doctors peering between my legs with flashlights. A gloved hand held my knees apart. The doctors took turns putting their hands inside me, trying to figure out what was wrong. Tears fell from the edges of my eyes into my ears and my hair. As the doctors dug for answers, I stared up at the harsh fluorescent lights, trying not to cry out from the excruciating ache in my side and the doctors' jabbing fingers.

Around three in the morning, they had a diagnosis: *left ovary, hemorrhagic 5 cm corpus luteum cyst, double pedicle torsion of the whole appendage.* A benign mass on my left ovary was bleeding into itself. Worse, the weight of the membranous sac had caused my ovary to become twisted around the tissues that support it. The fallopian tube twisted, too, like a kinked garden hose, blocking blood flow to nearby organs and causing severe pain. The doctors would try to untwist my ovary. If they couldn't, I would lose it.

Ovaries release eggs; eggs make babies. Normal female anatomy entails two ovaries, but I wasn't normal. Years earlier, when I was twelve, doctors had performed emergency surgery to remove my right ovary and fallopian tube: Multiple overgrown cysts—of a kind different from the one causing problems now—had caused my ovary to swell to double its size, causing it to do a full twist around the ovarian ligament, which cut off its blood supply, strangling my ovary. Nearly a decade later, for unrelated reasons, I stood to lose the left one, and with it, the remaining half of my eggs—and my ability to ever have biological children. To a twelve-year-old girl, that threat hadn't meant much. To a twenty-year-old woman lying half-naked on an operating table while a nurse shaved her pubic hair, it meant a good deal more.

There aren't many things I claim to know with absolute in-my-heart certainty, but for as long as I can remember, I've been sure I want to experience pregnancy, give birth, and raise kids. I am under no illusion that being a mother is an uncomplicated or always blissful endeavor. I get it, insofar as a person who is not yet a mother *can* get it. And yet, motherhood is the only non-negotiable on my life's to-do list. At the same time, ever since I became sexually active, my sole concern with regard to my ability to conceive has been to suppress it. "Fertility" was a word for the future. At least it had been until now.

But I wasn't thinking about babies or biology while lying in the frigid operating room. In those minutes just before surgery, I felt exposed and helpless, utterly outside of myself. My body had only recently emerged from the post-puberty teenage years, undergoing the kinds of changes that made me pay attention to it differently, and now here it was betraying me. It was a primal, raw kind of powerlessness I'd never known.

When I opened my eyes after the operation, my mother was standing next to my hospital bed. She squeezed my hand, answering my question before my brain could summon the words to ask it: The doctors had saved my ovary and fallopian tube. I could still have children.

A week in the hospital followed. The doctor said the pain I had experienced from my ovary twisting on itself was worse than that of giving birth. At this, my mother's eyes widened—she'd given birth three times, so she could relate. But for me, hearing my pain put into relative terms didn't change how agonizing it had been, or how much I still hurt. I ran my fingers along the puffy red wound above my pubic bone. The skin had begun to crust and harden. It would, over time, become a pale three-inch scar, hardly noticeable to anyone but me. In the days following the surgery, I struggled to comprehend how an organ the size of a walnut could cause so much pain and trouble. But the prognosis looked good: My remaining ovary was now in excellent condition. Once the doctors learned of my deep desire to someday have biological children, though, they urged me to consider freezing my eggs. I nodded, even though I had no idea what that meant.

A few months later, I began my senior year of college. My remaining ovary had healed well, but the doctors' recommendation that I freeze my eggs was still on my mind. I wanted a second opinion. So after class one day, I sat in the student union with my laptop and typed "egg freezing near me" into Google. A few weeks later, I skipped an economics class to go to an appointment at a fertility clinic in a nearby town. A friend who knew I didn't have a car kindly offered to drive me. At the clinic, a nurse led me to an exam room and instructed me to change into a patterned cloth gown. I lay on the table and clutched my hands while a reproductive endocrinologist looked between my legs, moving a transvaginal ultrasound wand covered in a cold gel from left to right inside me. On a screen to my left, the doctor pointed at my ovary and smiled.

"Natalie, you have a lovely ovary," she said. It was one of the best compliments I'd ever received. "Egg freezing technology is still very new and experimental," the doctor went on. "You're young. Your ovary is healthy—it's lovely," she said again, smiling when I blushed. "I don't see a need for you to take this risk right now, if ever."

Later, the clinic would send me the doctor's notes from the appointment. They read, in part: "We discussed ovarian stimulation with oocyte cryopreservation"—that is, egg freezing—"and that it is experimental and expensive, and likely not a good option for her now. In coming years, there may be more data and pregnancy rates from frozen eggs and she may want to consider this down the road." At the end of the exam, the doctor told me that the best thing I could do for my ovary and future fertility was to immediately go back on the Pill—I'd been on it two years earlier but no longer was—and stay on it until I was ready to become pregnant. (Abruptly stopping hormonal contraceptives was a bad move in my particular situation, as it turned out—more on this later.)

I was relieved to have a plan in place that protected my ovary. And I was glad to have been told I didn't need to pursue preserving my eggs. For the time being, I dismissed egg freezing and happily resumed suppressing my ability to procreate.

. . .

The second impetus behind my desire to investigate my fertility was less personal, more professional. A few months before almost losing my second ovary, I had been living in Ghana as an exchange student on a semester abroad my junior year of college. I'd arrived in West Africa in wide-eyed wonder; I left with a fierce desire to become a journalist.

In between classes at the university in Accra, I traveled by bus to a series of gold mines hours away to conduct field research for my undergraduate thesis, which explored the impact of mining industries on underdeveloped communities in western Ghana. I had immersed myself in the literature describing the so-called resource curse that plagued many African nations. Ghana's mineral-fueled growth was an important driver of the country's development, boosting its economy, and the country's recent oil boom had led the government to grant extraction rights to several international corporations. In other words, Ghana was selling concessions—legal claims on natural resources—to foreign companies to establish mining operations throughout the country's particularly resource-rich western region. Where oil and minerals originate in western Ghana is also where many Ghanaians in impoverished areas live—rural farmers unknowingly living on literal gold mines—but these poorer communities weren't seeing the benefits. I asked a Ghanaian friend to come with me to Prestea, a mining town west of Accra. My friend spoke Twi, a local language, and had grown up in the region where so much mining was taking place. Years later, I'd learn the journalistic term for this—a "fixer," a local to help arrange access and accompany a reporter—but at the time, I simply didn't want to go alone.

Seven hours and a handful of bus transfers later, we arrived in Prestea. I interviewed local men who had scrambled to dig for gold in their communities before the big companies took over, as well as some of their family members whose backyards—their source of food and livelihood—were being destroyed by the bulldozing and mining processes. I jotted down notes, photographed streams degraded by mercury pollution, and awkwardly presented gifts to village elders as a thank-you for allowing me to pepper their community members with questions.

It was my first taste of reporting, dusty and demanding. I had no idea what the rules of journalism were, and yet was fairly certain I was breaking several of them. But at the end of each long day, my brain abuzz and my limbs streaked with dirt, I felt gripped by something I couldn't quite articulate. After an interview, a bare-chested miner asked me, "Are you going to help tell my story?" And that was it; I was hooked. A breathless eagerness took hold—to probe and uncover, to tell stories that mattered. And to do justice in the retelling, as best I could.

After college, I received a Fulbright scholarship and went to live and teach in Sri Lanka. Two years later, I arrived in New York City to begin graduate school: a master's program in journalism at NYU. I dreamed of being a foreign correspondent or an investigative reporter, filing pieces from conflict zones or finding a key fact buried in a stack of newly declassified documents. That was where, I was sure, I would find the stories containing truths that were being glossed over or ignored, the narratives that transform how people understand the world.

It was during my first month of journalism school that I heard about the EggBanxx party. I had put the idea of egg freezing on the back burner since my doctors' initial urging that I consider it. But I remained curious. Here was an opportunity to learn more, enjoy a free glass of something bubbly, and maybe meet a source or two I could interview for my introductory reporting class.

It would also be the moment when my reproductive reality began to sink in.

After the swelling on my wound faded away, I kept thinking about how in the eight years between losing one ovary and almost losing the other, I had learned nearly nothing about my body, let alone my chances of giving birth. But as I got older, I found myself worrying about these things more and more. The sense I had about my fertility was that it was clearly fragile, definitely confusing, and probably something I ought to know more about. My surgeries had left me both reeling and vigilant, like a person after a car accident who no longer takes seatbelts for granted. What I'd almost lost mattered—I just wasn't exactly sure why.

By age twenty, I knew something about ovaries, condoms, and sexually transmitted infections. Add to that the rudiments of menstruation (although I still have questions) and birth control pills (I take mine in the morning). But in fact I possessed a savvy twelve-year-old's understanding of my reproductive system. As I was growing up, my parents didn't hide information about bodies or sexuality from my siblings and me, per se, but we sure never sat down to talk about how it all worked. What I learned about sexual anatomy and reproduction in school boiled down to simply this: *Do not let sperm get near your egg.* That was the message, the most important point. Until I started having sex, I understood the act to be purely mechanical. I do not remember being part of any discussions about sexual pleasure, masturbation, or firmly saying no.

In lieu of straightforward basic anatomy lessons or frank conversations about gender identity and sexual orientation, I took my cues from the media, culture, and my own experience. I learned—and learn still—about my body and sex from my friends; from glossy women's magazines; from apps on my iPhone; from porn; from movies; and, most fundamentally when I was younger, from my childhood copy of *The Care and Keeping of You,* the American Girl book about changing bodies. (My copy is inscribed: *Easter, 2000. To Natalie, as your body grows and changes. Love, Mom.*) In my teens and twenties, I never learned about endometriosis, uterine fibroids, or polycystic ovary syndrome, despite how prevalent these conditions are. No one educated me about hormones or the quality of my eggs. No one explained that a woman's ability to become pregnant declines considerably in her mid- to late thirties, and that by the time she's forty-five, fertility is close to zero. No one talked to me about how a woman can ask a doctor to perform diagnostic tests—to check things like her ovarian reserve, the number and quality of her eggs—that may offer a snapshot of her current fertility and possibly a preview of what may or may not be coming down the pipeline.

Maybe it's silly of me to think that the adults in my life—parents, teachers, others—would have had some idea about these things.

Maybe most of us are pretty much in the dark. It was only because of my emergency surgery at age twenty that I was forced to confront reproductive health issues earlier than most of my peers did. And while my sole ovary makes me physiologically different from them, I am otherwise quite similar; the unrelated ovarian cysts I developed at age twelve and age twenty can happen to anyone. I have one healthy ovary with eggs inside it, and that's all I should need. Ovaries and kidneys are similar in this way: You can get by with just one. Now, my twenties barely behind me, I've learned so much at this point in my research that I only now realize how much there is to know.

What has finally dawned on me is that until I started investigating fertility—my own and everyone else's—I had been living in a vast bubble of ignorance and silence. So had almost all of my friends; so had millions of young women in the United States and across the world. It's a bubble in which too many women simply deal with their bodies instead of understanding them. This is true regardless of race, class, or education level. We lack essential information regarding our inner workings. We take our reproductive health and fertility for granted—because no one has taught us that we shouldn't. Putting off getting pregnant is an article of faith, a badge of honor for nearly all the young, ambitious women I know. For many of us, from when our periods first begin until our thirties or even forties, pregnancy is something to avoid. We will not be solely defined by our ability to bear children, we declare. As women of a certain generation, we grew up knowing we can have careers *and* families. We can marry our true loves. We can play just as hard as the boys. To do so means many of us decide we won't get pregnant and settle down at twenty-five, or thirty-two, or thirty-eight. Children can wait—until we're ready.

Control on Ice

I became a journalist thinking I would find the stories that most needed telling in remote, shadowy corners of the world. Instead, much to my surprise, I realized there was a big story right under my nose—and inside me, as well as many other women. Turns out eggs have stories that need to be told, too.

The more I realized how ignorant I was about my fertility, the more determined I became to investigate it. In the days following the EggBanxx party, I kept thinking about all those women a decade or two older than me who were still seeking answers to fundamental questions. I kept thinking about my remaining ovary, too, and it dawned on me that almost losing it was a wake-up call I didn't know I needed. It set me on a path to educate myself about the particulars of my body and the basics, and to get real about my possibly diminished odds of having biological children. That I wanted kids—had always known I did, cannot remember not having this fierce desire—was another reason I became so invested in learning more about fertility. As a young woman with one ovary, and all this on my mind, I came to realize that I had a monumental personal decision to make: *Should I freeze my eggs?* How did it work—and did it *always* work? Was it safe, not just for me but for women around the world, allowing us to give birth later than we'd ever imagined? Or was it a half-assured medical treatment, marketed like a cosmetic surgery or the newest fancy tech product, shiny with ease and convenience but with little regard to potential downsides?

As a journalist, I was intrigued by egg freezing's rapid growth. By all accounts, official and empirical, more women than ever are freezing their eggs. In 2009, a mere 482 healthy women in the United States froze their eggs. In 2022,[*] 22,967 did. That's more than a 4,000 percent increase in just over a decade.[†] Today, the International Federation of Fertility Societies calls cryopreservation "one of the most significant recent advancements in assisted reproduction technology." And yet, ten years ago, it was a phrase about which most people furrowed their brows, maybe for sounding like a dystopian movie; if it was talked about at all, it was in a doctor's office or in low murmurs with a friend over coffee, not at happy hour with co-workers or across the internet,

---

[*] This is the latest year for which official data is available as of this writing. Preliminary 2022 egg freezing data came out in 2024. There's typically a two-year lag when it comes to compiling assisted reproductive technology statistics. For further explanation, see the Notes section at the back of this book.

[†] And that's just in the United States. The United Kingdom has also seen record numbers of women freezing their eggs in recent years.

as it's being discussed today. Now, having shed almost all of the stigma it once had, egg freezing has exploded into our vernacular.

Across social media, in magazines, on the subway, it's difficult to escape the feminist-friendly, direct-to-consumer marketing of the fertility tech industry, from Instagram ads recruiting egg donors to group discounts encouraging "freezing with friends" to the wildly popular #EggFreezing on TikTok, where many young users extol the virtues of freezing their eggs while in their biological "prime." Fertility technology has provided plot points for television shows, documentaries, podcast episodes, and special reports from nearly every major streaming service and media outlet. And it's next to impossible these days to read the news or scroll a screen without seeing a headline or post related to reproduction, parenthood, or babies.

Celebrities like Rebel Wilson, Priyanka Chopra, and Chrissy Teigen have spoken openly, and enthusiastically, about their decisions to freeze eggs. Others, such as Jennifer Aniston, lament not doing so: "I would've given anything if someone had said to me, 'Freeze your eggs. Do yourself a favor,'" the actor told *Allure,* speaking publicly for the first time about her fertility struggles and years spent trying to get pregnant. Teigen and husband, John Legend, have four children who were conceived with her frozen eggs, one of whom was born from a surrogate pregnancy. Barbara Bush, daughter of George W. Bush and Laura Bush, froze her eggs and was prepared to become a single mother before meeting and marrying her husband. Amy Schumer shared a picture of her bruised stomach as she took hormone shots before freezing her eggs. Kourtney Kardashian went so far as to film her egg freezing preparation on *Keeping Up with the Kardashians.* The singer Halsey froze her eggs at age twenty-three after undergoing multiple surgeries to treat endometriosis. Actor Olivia Munn revealed on Anna Faris's podcast that she'd frozen her eggs before she turned thirty-five. "Every girl should do it," she said confidently. When Céline Dion was forty-two, she gave birth to twin sons using embryos she had kept frozen for eight years.

Advances in reproductive medicine have fundamentally altered how people approach partnership and if, when, and how to start families. The changed way of thinking is at once personal—young women today use our phone apps to date, to track our periods, to order our birth control—and cultural. A slew of social, economic, legal, and political forces together form the larger environment within which fertility technologies such as egg freezing are developed and used. Then there are people like Stanford bioethicist Henry Greely, who predicts that in the next twenty to forty years, people with good healthcare coverage will no longer rely on sex to have babies; instead, most children will be conceived in labs. How and why that world will arrive is a broader and different conversation, but the technological innovations—particularly concerning stem cell therapies—matter in consequential ways, too. They may not dictate our behavior, but they do influence it. Like egg freezing, they can't be ignored.

To talk about egg freezing, I learned, is to talk about a woman's place in the world, her hopes and values, her grappling with her body, age, relationships. When it comes down to it, egg freezing is an incredibly personal decision. You have your own perspectives, goals, and limited timeframe. Your fertility is affected by so many variables, a few of which are unique to you, others not. And so it is for the scores of individuals who graciously shared their stories with me about their fertility, sexual health, and reproductive lives, who most inform these pages. Among them were dozens of women—three of whom I'll focus on in detail—struggling to make important decisions about their fertility. Their experiences, along with my own, I discovered, are the best way to tell this story.

Remy,* in her mid-thirties, is an anesthesia resident in Nashville. Remy is determined to take charge of her fertility, despite having considerable medical school loans, credit card debt, and a love life that's not gone according to plan. Egg freezing is her answer to ensure that nothing gets in the way of her carefully designed future.

Mandy, in her early thirties, is a recently married young professional in the San Francisco Bay Area who, like me, is considering freezing her eggs for medical reasons. She's frustrated by the lack of quality information she can find on the topic. This big, costly decision is beginning to feel to her like a ticking time bomb, and while

* Name has been changed.

she isn't sure if she wants to be a mother someday, she knows she wants to preserve the option of having biological kids if she can.

And Lauren, an entrepreneur living in Houston, froze her eggs two days before her thirty-ninth birthday. After her efforts to preserve her fertility take a scary turn, freezing her eggs ends up changing her life in a way she never could have imagined.

What I did not expect: that my quest to decide whether or not to freeze my own eggs would grow into a reckoning about trying to control virtually every component of my life. I realize now that the constant pressure to manage my body and my potential to have babies is deeply intertwined with society's expectations, and my experience, of being a woman. So is the inclination to worry and try to have it all figured out. As I contended with big decisions about love and work, about my body and my reproductive future, I considered the fact that my generation has many opportunities that our parents and older generations didn't have. That's a blessing and a curse. For all the choices many of us are so fortunate to have, we are overwhelmed by too much information, often of the wrong sort. Our lack of basic knowledge about our reproductive health and the realities of fertility is just one example, but it's a big one. It doesn't help that most of the quality information out there is reserved for older women struggling with infertility and couples having trouble conceiving naturally.

The problem here is the overwhelming absence of resources for the young woman who has no known fertility issues—at least, not yet—but who, as we'll see, is part of a global trend of women having children later in life and, as a result, increasingly struggling with age-related fertility decline; for the young woman who wants to understand the options, technologies, and paths available to her *before* her long-term partner informs her they never want kids, or a preexisting medical issue compromises her fecundity, or she's (all of a sudden, it feels like) in her mid-thirties, when doctors start applying terms like "geriatric pregnancy" and "advanced maternal age"; for the young woman who realizes that the rudimentary education she's received about her reproductive system isn't going to cut it. I set out to write a book for that young woman—in part because I *was* that young woman. I wanted to write the book I wish I'd had when that scar was still fresh, back when I was twenty.

If I was going to face tough choices concerning my fertility and potential parenthood, I'd better try to understand what lay in my future, as best I could. If I was to be informed about my body, I needed to figure out what essentials I'd missed en route. If I was to be prepared to make smart decisions about the fundamentals, I had to identify the gatekeepers who were coming between me and my uterus. And along the way, I wanted to get to the bottom of why I had learned so little—and how to make up for it.

To start, though: What to do about my eggs? If my doctors suggested I think about freezing them, then the first thing I needed to do was get the image of a carton of brown, farm-fresh eggs out of my mind.

2

An Intimate Geography

~~~~~~

"What's a Cervix?"

Vera Lloyd stood before several dozen ninth-graders in a small high school gymnasium in northern Virginia. A petite woman with gray-streaked short black hair, Vera, a public health nurse, was wearing a pastel-colored blouse and summery sandals. She'd be turning sixty soon, and had worked in and around Stafford County for almost twenty years. A few feet away, Vera's longtime colleague Vanessa Akin arranged condoms and packs of birth control pills on a folding table.

A Monday morning in May. First period. In the wrestling room next to the gymnasium at a high school about forty miles south of Washington, D.C., boys and girls sprawled across blue mats. Under the fluorescent lights, several of the teenagers stifled yawns, still waking up; one boy, wearing athletic shorts and bright white sneakers, was fully asleep, his limbs stretched out on the ground not far from where Vera stood. The students sat in small clumps or alone; a few had their backs against the walls and arms crossed over their chests, cool-kid style. I was sitting in on Vera and Vanessa's presentations because I'd wanted to observe a modern-day sex ed class, theoretically one of the places we begin to learn about our bodies. Today was the first day of the school's two-week curriculum on the subject. At the moment, Vera was holding a plastic speculum and talking about pap smears. There was a *click, click* as the speculum widened. Several girls gasped, horrified that the object in Vera's hands—or any object, for that matter—functioned to hold open a vagina. "Oh my God," a girl with French braids whispered, covering her face with a lime-green folder. Raising her voice over the sound of bouncing basketballs from gym class next door, Vera asked if there were any questions. A student wearing a yellow shirt that read GIRLS DO IT BETTER raised her hand. "What should you do if you think a tampon has gotten lost in your cervix?" Several students giggled. A girl sitting near me turned to her friend and murmured, "What's a cervix?"

The nurses delivered their presentation in two parts, as they had for every year they'd taught together. Vanessa kicked things off with methods of birth control; Vera followed with a graphic slide presentation about sexually transmitted infections, or STIs. They'd brought their usual props, which were always a hit. When Vera described bacterial vaginosis, a condition that occurs when there is too much of certain bacteria in the vagina, she held up a pink thong—"Ladies," she said, in a well-practiced presentation voice, "this is *not* underwear"—and explained how its narrow piece of fabric acts as a connector of microbes, making it easy for bacteria to travel from the wearer's rear to her vagina. During her bit about the vagina being more or less a self-cleaning oven, Vera motioned disapprovingly to a pack of scented Summer's Eve feminine cleansing wipes on the nearby table, emphasizing that vaginas should not smell like peaches and cream. She sounded a bit exasperated, and I wondered if all her presentations began this way, with subtle myth-busting about thongs, fragrant wipes, and other items familiar to high school girls.

Vanessa's visual aids were funny-looking—a few looked like products one might find at Target, others not—and almost all pink. Students craned their necks to see better. "Sperm poison," Vanessa announced, holding up tubes and containers of foams, creams, and jellies. Next, a female diaphragm and a pack of birth control pills. When Vanessa held up a female condom, no one—including me—seemed to know what it was.

"Now, guys," Vanessa said, picking up a familiar-looking box of Durex male condoms, "what's your complaint about wearing one of these?" Several students snickered. Vanessa didn't wait for an answer before addressing the girls. "Don't listen to any boy who tells you the condom won't fit," she said. She removed a condom from its wrapper and, arms above her head, stretched the latex between her hands until it was longer than a ruler. The students roared with laughter. "If he wants to feel better about himself and go buy a big-man giant-size condom, he can," she said, stretching the condom wider, "but regular ones like this will fit him, I promise."

Vera, sitting on a folding chair next to me, looked up from the *Getting Ready to Retire* pamphlet she was reading. "The things you have to say," she sighed, shaking her head.

The way sex education is taught in schools in modern-day America is, in short, a mess. The reasons for this are more or less the same as they were a century ago, when sex ed started: Whose values are the right ones to teach to adolescents, and who should make that decision? In his book *Too Hot to Handle: A Global History of Sex Education,* Jonathan Zimmerman, an NYU history and education professor, explains that since sex ed was introduced in schools in the first few decades of the twentieth century, critics have condemned it for fostering the same promiscuity it purported to control. Predictably, the debate rages on in an ideologically divided America, where fights about parental, local, and federal control over education dominate public discourse. Across the country, local politics and beliefs dictate the substance and style of a school district's sex ed curriculum. The vast majority of such programs in the United States are abstinence-based or abstinence-only, as opposed to evidence-based and comprehensive. Abstinence-based programs, sometimes called "sexual risk avoidance" programs, promote abstinence until marriage and belabor contraception failure rates—if they cover contraception at all. In more than half the country, school districts aren't required to go over methods of birth control. But the fact is, there is little evidence that providing accurate information in an appropriate context increases sexual activity. On the contrary: Research shows that comprehensive sex education reduces rates of teen births and risky sexual behaviors, as well as a child's risk of being sexually abused.

After my first surgery at age twelve, I partially listened when a doctor explained why he had removed my ovary and fallopian tube, body parts I vaguely remembered from fifth-grade health class. (It was sex ed but had an innocuous name: Family Life Education, or FLE.) Later, after the doctor left the room, I asked my mother what those organs did. It was out of embarrassment, and not because I already knew, that I didn't ask her the same question when I almost lost my second ovary at the age of twenty. Was I exceptionally ignorant? Young women are generally expected to know how to handle menstruation, prevent pregnancy, perform breast self-exams—but do they actually know anything about fertility? If they, like me, hadn't received much or adequate sex ed in the many more school years that followed fifth-grade FLE class, the answer was probably not. As it turns out, my experience was completely typical. As of 2023, only twenty-five states and the District of Columbia mandate that schools teach both sex education and HIV education. Most states allow parents to opt out on behalf of their children. And I was shocked to learn that only seventeen states require information presented in sex education classes to be medically accurate.

So, what does sex ed cover in the states where it *is* taught? Many of the classes taught in middle and high schools limit discussions of puberty to the bare-bones basics: periods and unwanted pregnancy, erections and ejaculation. The classes require students to identify the parts of the female and male reproductive systems, but they tend to stick with a woman's internal parts—uterus, ovaries, vagina—while skipping the external parts, as if the vulva,* labia,† and clitoris‡ don't

---

* Many people say "vagina" when they mean "vulva" and mistakenly use the terms interchangeably. The vagina is the muscular canal-like tube inside the body that connects the uterus to the vulva. "Vulva" refers to the outer genitals that you can see (including the pubic mound, the labia, the clitoris, the vaginal opening, and the opening to the urethra).

† Labia are the inner and outer fleshy folds of skin of the vulva, found at the opening of the vagina.

‡ A major (for many, the main) area of sexual sensation, the clitoris is a complex network of erectile tissues and nerves located above the vaginal opening. The

exist. Important topics such as fertility fundamentals and how to resist unwanted sexual pressure are rarely covered. Female pleasure or any indication of it is almost always a taboo subject. And when it comes to birth control, well, the research shows that young people are less likely to receive information about birth control now than they were twenty-five years ago. This should have shocked me, but by that point I'd already learned too much about the dismal state of sex ed in the United States for it to be surprising.

"It was as if we were being given documents about our bodies but with all the important info redacted," writes Katie Wheeler, reflecting on her sex ed experiences in *The Lily*, a publication for millennial women put out by *The Washington Post*. States differ when it comes to mandating what is to be taught in public school sex ed classes and when, and many high schools and middle schools don't teach the sexual health topics that the U.S. Centers for Disease Control and Prevention (CDC) considers essential for healthy young people. Fewer than half of adolescents receive sex education that meets the minimum standards articulated by national standards.

It's worse for teens in rural areas than for those in more urban communities. For example, sex ed teachers at schools in Mississippi are barred from demonstrating the proper use of condoms and other contraceptives. Texas requires that education materials for students under the age of eighteen must state that "homosexual conduct is not an acceptable lifestyle and is a criminal offense." In Tennessee, a bill known as the "Gateway Law"—added years ago to the state's abstinence-only curriculum—prohibits sex ed courses from including instruction on "gateway sexual activity" that encourages youth to engage in "non-abstinent behavior"; educators who fail to comply can face punitive measures. "Kissing and hugging are the last stop before reaching Groin Central Station, so it's important to ban all the things that lead to the things that lead to sex," former Tennessee governor Bill Haslam, who signed the bill, said on the TV show *The Colbert Report*.

---

clitoral hood, about the size of a pea, is the only part that's visible, but the whole clitoris is much bigger. The majority of the clitoris is internal, is about 3.5 to 4.5 inches long, and stretches down either side of the vagina in a wishbone shape.

The kicker is that in most states, school districts have the power to adopt and censor aspects of sex ed as they see fit. Only ten states require that sex ed curricula provide instruction that isn't biased against any race, sex, or ethnicity, while a handful of states explicitly require instruction that discriminates *against* LGBTQ+ people. In many states, such as Virginia, local control over sex education makes it easy for schools to demand that nurses like Vera stick to a restrictive and harmful sex ed curriculum—which is particularly detrimental to sexual and gender minority youth. "They won't let us talk about homosexuality," Vera told me. "They won't let us talk about abortion." If the students bring up these topics in a group setting, she added, "we have to deflect."

Back in the high school wrestling room, Vera's STI curriculum amounted to a slide show consisting of pictures of diseased genitals. I reacted the same way the students did—the images were horrifying. Upon seeing a chlamydia-infected penis on the screen, one boy yelped and yanked the hood of his sweatshirt over his face. "Pushing pus out of a penis is very painful," Vera said matter-of-factly, clicking to the next slide, a picture of a baby born with gonorrhea-infected eyes. The entire room, including the P.E. teachers sitting against the back wall, gasped. I waited for Vera to pair some of the graphic photos with a few of the equally alarming statistics about STIs in the United States—that people ages fifteen to twenty-four account for nearly half of the twenty-six million new cases of STIs each year, for example, or that on any given day one in five people in the United States has an STI—but they went unmentioned.

"When you have sex," Vera said at one point, "you either get a baby, a disease, or both." Several students giggled, but I raised my eyebrows. It didn't sound as if she were making a joke. I thought of Coach Carr's infamous line in the movie *Mean Girls:* "Don't have sex. Because you *will* get pregnant. AND DIE." As in the movie, the shock-and-awe effect aimed at the students around me was clearly intentional. While Vera and Vanessa at times quite rightly leaned on humor to communicate their sex ed points effectively, their message was heavy on warnings and scare tactics. The terrified looks on the students' faces spoke volumes. I couldn't help but feel that that morning's presentation, despite Vera and Vanessa's best intentions—and the maddening fact that they weren't allowed to say more on certain topics—might leave these teenagers feeling insecure and confused about their bodies and sex instead of informed and empowered.

"There still seems to be a combination of prudishness and ignorance around the unique, and sometimes idiosyncratic, functions of the female body—which is shocking, considering half the world is born with one," writes Jenna Wortham in *The New York Times Magazine*. The opacity surrounding women's health is not a modern malady. Nor is the prudishness. The history of neglecting to teach women the basic scientific principles of their reproductive biology and sex anatomy is a problem rooted in earlier times and still hanging on. In most sex ed lessons decades ago, and still today, young women are taught that their bodies can and will create life. "Your body is a miracle," the refrain goes, a comforting platitude offered as a balm to the scary STI stories and rushed reproduction overview. It sounds nice, but the fact is that our collective, modern-day ignorance is partly due to the religious underpinnings of sex ed policies. The two seemingly can't be untangled. And appropriate separation between church and state as it applies to sex ed is definitely not around the corner.

Why do I believe that this sex education problem isn't likely to change anytime soon? Because regardless of the science, sex ed is political. In the United States, it is extremely difficult to pass legislation to improve states' sex ed curricula; many have tried and failed. But if we can't teach young women and men about their bodies and sex—comprehensively and transparently—in school, then where? There is no forum for teenagers to talk about sexual development, self-exploration, or how bodies actually work. No place, really, to learn about masturbation or the female orgasm. No safe space in which to shake the shame that society promotes by using euphemisms for genitals.★

One girl I spoke with told me she thought she was dying when she first got her period. Another said the first person to touch her clitoris

---

★ The Latin word given to the female genitalia, pudendum, literally translates as "part for which you should be ashamed."

was somebody else. Yet another believed something else Coach Carr said in *Mean Girls* to be true—"If you do touch each other, you will get chlamydia and die"—until she contracted chlamydia in her late teens and did not, in fact, die.

I thought about these anecdotes and the myriad forces shaping sex ed policies while I sat inside the gym that morning, scanning the roomful of fresh-faced teenagers. I couldn't get over how young they looked. I thought about all that they were *not* learning that day. Boys clueless about condoms. Girls thinking STIs could kill them.* I worried about how misguided our priorities are when it comes to educating young people about their bodies and shaping their ideas and attitudes about sex, and how the patchwork quilt of sex ed laws across the country means that many, many kids receive either abstinence-only lectures or nothing at all. The truth is, if the goal of sex ed is to prepare young people for real-world activities and decisions, it seemed pretty clear that we were failing.

Eggs and Female Gonads: A Primer

It's not rocket science to figure out that there is a direct connection between understanding our bodies and understanding our reproductive choices. The disturbing thing is that the fuzziness with which we stumble around, sorting out a few of the basics early on, here and there—"What's a cervix?" the girl had whispered—sticks around, like a layer of dust on an out-of-reach shelf, well into adulthood. Our practice of more or less ignoring sex education in schools has resulted in a nation of young people who aren't adequately informed about reproduction and fertility, and then as adults they are making choices about their lives—in particular, putting off having children while they pursue careers, degrees, relationships—without understanding the limits of their biology. Meanwhile, reproductive technologies that young people may or may not want to avail themselves of, now or in the future, continue to evolve and change. As Jess, a young woman I

---

* Which sounds dramatic, but it's true: Some STIs, such as HIV and syphilis, can be fatal if left untreated.

interviewed soon after she graduated from college, put it: "Knowing reproductive options leads to big decisions. And if we aren't educated about these options, then how can our big decisions be truly informed?"

Numerous studies over the past two decades have determined that many young women know very little about the limits of their reproductive systems. One, a 2020 U.S. Department of Health and Human Services report that summarized findings from a survey of three thousand people between the ages of eighteen and twenty-nine found that fewer than half of the women respondents knew that the ovaries do not keep producing new eggs until menopause, and only 65 percent were aware that women's fertility declines sharply after their mid-thirties. The authors noted that the respondents' lack of knowledge "may have grave implications for their ability to plan their fertility" and that some of the topics about which the respondents were mistaken "may lead women to delay getting pregnant to a time when they may be at high risk of infertility and possibly involuntary childlessness."

Other research focused on fertility awareness has borne out the argument that young adults of reproductive age want to have children but are not sufficiently informed about age-related fertility decline and infertility risk factors. They also tend to seriously overestimate fertility potential and chances of conceiving, both naturally and through assisted reproductive technologies; on top of the misconceptions they have about age and fertility, many women also believe that medical treatments can dependably extend the biological clock into a woman's forties and fifties. That, as we'll see, is hardly the case.

The reason researchers are beginning to look closely at how young people think about fertility is, in part, because of another trend: Women don't tend to seek help for infertility until they're in their late thirties, by which point their chances of getting pregnant and having a healthy baby are already diminishing. And this translates into the fact that women know very little about a crucial component of female fertility: their eggs.

.   .   .

"If you have never had trouble with your eggs," writes Natalie Angier
in *Woman: An Intimate Geography,* "if you have never had to worry
about your fecundity, you probably haven't given your eggs much
thought, or dwelled on their dimensions." Tiny but fierce, human
eggs are powerful pieces of biological tissue. An egg, or ovum, to use
its more scientific name, is the female reproductive cell. It's the largest
cell in the human body, even though it's barely a tenth of a millimeter
across—roughly the size of a grain of sand. An egg is also about
thirty-five times the width, and ten million times the volume, of a
sperm cell (a fact that I think women ought to brag about more
often, considering how many men take great pride in their—eye
roll—"seed" and strong and agile "swimmers"). Boys don't make
sperm until they reach puberty, at which point they begin producing
fresh sperm every few months; most men create around two trillion
sperm cells in the course of their lives. Contrast that with baby girls,
born with one million to two million egg cells in their ovaries—but
that's all they get.*

Human egg cells, or oogonia, as they're called when they start to
develop, begin their formation while the fetus is still in the uterus—
specifically, in the ovaries of the female fetus, at about seven weeks'
gestation—and start maturing individually in adolescence. By puberty, a young woman has about 25 percent of egg cells remaining of
the couple million or so she was born with.† Over her reproductive
lifetime, beginning with puberty and ending with menopause, she'll
release one egg per month for some five hundred months.‡ Her eggs
are kept within a vault in her ovaries, where they grow inside little
fluid-filled pouches called follicles, one egg per follicle. Every month

---

* Ovaries, by the way, are the female gonads. Gonads, or sex glands, are the male
and female primary reproductive organs. (The male gonads are the testes.)

† When I asked a fertility doctor about why this range was so wide, she explained
that we don't really know, but that this is in part why egg count fluctuates based
on the individual. If a woman has a lower egg supply than expected for her age,
she was perhaps born with fewer eggs or went through them more quickly.

‡ Some women can release two egg cells per cycle, which can result in the conception of fraternal twins. Identical twins—genetically the same, unlike fraternal
twins—are made when the fertilized egg cell divides in two.

or so, an exquisite scientific selection takes place deep inside her body. In one of her ovaries, a single dominant follicle begins to develop, and the immature egg cell—an oocyte—growing inside it is anointed The One. As the follicle gets bigger, the oocyte nestled within transforms into a full-fledged mature egg—or ovum—and, through a complex hormonal chain of events, is solicited for ovulation, which is when the follicle bursts and the egg is released.

But what about all those potential eggs that are *not* chosen as The One? Throughout a woman's youth and early middle age, a proportion of her oocytes are neatly destroyed through a process of programmed cell death called apoptosis. With the start of her menstrual cycle and until menopause, approximately one thousand oocytes die every month—with only one of those thousand destined to ovulate. The average woman has between three and five hundred thousand oocytes remaining when she reaches puberty. By age thirty-seven, she has approximately twenty-five thousand, and as she approaches menopause, very few oocytes remain. Of all these immature eggs, however, just five hundred or so become mature eggs—normally one egg per month that's released through ovulation, as I mentioned—with baby-making potential.

So, women are overbudgeted with eggs; they are born with a huge surplus and most eggs just sit there in the ovaries, aging. Nonetheless, eggs are finite, and as a woman gets older, she starts running out of functioning ones. There isn't any rollover; at the end of the fiscal period, management says *buh-bye* to assets that don't get used. This phenomenon, the degrading and dying, is completely natural, and independent of any hormone production, birth control pills, pregnancies, nutritional supplements, or health or lifestyle components. It's just what happens when Nature does her thing. "The eggs do not simply die—they commit suicide," Angier writes. "Their membranes ruffle up like petticoats whipped by the wind and they break into pieces, thence to be absorbed bit by bit into the hearts of neighboring cells. By graciously if melodramatically getting out of the way, the sacrificial eggs leave their sisters plenty of hatching room." By the thousands, the eggs make their graceful exit. It is a choreographed dance of coming into and out of being. A ritual as old as time.

. . .

Eggs were on my mind when, not long after I'd sat in on the sex ed class, I met a friend for happy hour. She was twenty-eight, had a master's degree from an Ivy League university, and worked in the publishing industry. We ordered appetizers and got to talking about some of my recent research and reporting. "Wait," my friend said, putting her glass of wine down sharply in surprise. "You're telling me I have thousands of potential eggs? Like, right now, in my body?"

"Yep," I said, reaching for a Parmesan crisp.

She stared at me, eyebrows raised in shock. "I honestly thought I had four or five—total," she said.

"Hmm," I replied. "I think you're thinking about ovaries? Most women have two of those."

"No, I know about ovaries," she said. Her face brightened. "Whoa. I can't believe I have thousands of eggs. This is exciting!" She picked up her wineglass and took a big swallow.

As empowering as it feels to be born with so much potential life nestling in our bodies, women should keep in mind that the ovary is the first organ to age in such a profound, literally life-changing way—at least twice as fast as other organs in the body. And while that fact spurs a wide range of emotions for many women, it's simply an objective biological truth. Here's another: A woman's fertility is determined by the quantity and quality of her eggs. As she gets older, her reproductive system slows down and both her egg quantity and egg quality diminish, as the number of egg-containing follicles in her ovaries undergoes a steady decline. Fewer eggs means fewer chances to conceive each month. And older eggs have more chromosomal abnormalities, making it increasingly difficult to become pregnant. So, a woman's age is the most important predictor of her ability to get pregnant. By her mid-forties, her chances of having a pregnancy without assisted reproductive technology are exceedingly low.*

---

* While it's a biological reality that fertility in human females declines over time, most female mammals, including chimpanzees, maintain the ability to get pregnant for most of their lives.

While all that may sound alarming, fertility decline over time is less of a cliff than it is a hilly terrain—with a few peaks and valleys, fluctuating periods of fertility and infertility—that gradually gets steeper, particularly in a woman's mid- to late thirties. "There's no one age where a woman turns into a pumpkin," said Dr. Anne Z. Steiner, a reproductive medicine specialist and professor of obstetrics and gynecology, in an interview with *The New York Times* about a study she published on measuring female fertility decline. "The difference between 30 and 33 is negligible. But the difference between 37 and 40 is going to be pretty drastic."

You can see why it's a problem, then, that many women postpone childbearing in their most fertile years, and then expect to be able to successfully conceive as soon as they try—and, if they can't, that fertility treatment will be a cure-all. When I asked Arthur Caplan, a bioethicist at NYU Langone Medical Center, about this, he said as much: "There is this notion that you can get pregnant whenever you want—the technology is here, we've got the answers, it's in your control. But spending your twenties thinking just about not getting pregnant is not consistent with how your eggs work."

Preventing pregnancy is fear-based dissuasion, as we've seen, rooted in our school health classes. The messaging we experience as we grow up directs us toward other worthwhile pursuits: education, work, travel. Starting a family is an undertaking for *later.* And then all of a sudden—at least that's how it feels—we're in our late twenties and early thirties and besieged with warnings about our fading fertility. There's very little breathing room between these polar opposite messages of "prevent pregnancy" and "preserve fertility." As a modern American woman in the heart of this demographic, I can't help but feel confused. And frustrated. I see mixed messages everywhere. I'm told to lean in. I'm told to quiet down. I'm told I should want to have it all. I'm told I can't. I grew up using various forms of contraception, spending the majority of my fertile years avoiding pregnancy, and then, after I am "launched" into a fledgling career and relationships, I learn that my eggs have a shelf life, may even be nearing their expiration date, and I should seriously consider freezing them—yesterday.

Egg Freezing Appointment #1

EggBanxx had made an effective pitch. Only two weeks after their egg freezing party, I was sitting in the waiting room of a New York City fertility clinic, filling out a long questionnaire. The morning of the appointment, I woke early. In the shower, I rehearsed my answers—and explanations for not having answers—for questions I knew I'd be asked: *Date of your last period? Why are you interested in egg freezing? Ah, you only have one ovary? Tell me about that.* I shampooed my hair, already feeling mildly exasperated about telling yet another doctor the serpentine story about my ovaries.

I took the subway to Grand Central and walked several blocks northeast to NYU Langone Fertility Center. On a corner near the clinic's entrance, I paused. It was a crisp, sunlight-streaked morning, the kind that lifts the mood of the whole city—and mine, too. I took a deep breath.

In the waiting room, I completed the new-patient paperwork and signed my name what felt like a dozen times. I expected to be taken to an exam room when my name was called, but the nurse led me to a fancy office and instructed me to wait. I sank into an overstuffed chair and looked around. Taped to the wall above the desk was a piece of pink construction paper with purple flowers drawn as tall as trees. "Dear Nicole," it read, in a child's scribble. "Thank you for helping me be born." Next to the drawing was a plaque announcing Dr. Nicole Noyes as *New York* magazine's Doctor of the Year. This was the fertility doctor who had handed me her business card at the Egg-Banxx party. When I made the decision to make an appointment to discuss egg freezing, I'd dug up her card from the goodie bag I'd stashed in my closet. This initial consultation, at least, would be covered by my graduate student health insurance plan.

NYU Langone's was one of the first egg freezing programs in the country—it began offering the procedure for non-medical reasons*

---

* There are a few different terms used to describe freezing eggs for non-medical reasons: "elective egg freezing" (has insurance implications, best to avoid), "social egg freezing" (makes it sound more fun than it is), and "planned egg freezing" (better than the other two terms, the idea being you're preserving your fertility

in 2004—and Dr. Noyes was one of its pioneers. After this appointment, I'll hear and see Dr. Noyes's name everywhere—in newspaper
articles, on panels at reproductive technology conferences, in conversation with other fertility doctors, from women whose eggs she had
frozen. That morning, though, all I knew was that she was kind of a
big deal.

Dr. Noyes walked into the office, having just finished a conversation with a nurse in the hall. "Hello, hello," she said, holding out her
hand for me to shake. She had short brown hair, bangs, fashionable
glasses, a white coat. In her fifties, if I had to guess. I was immediately
struck by how hip and smart she seemed, fiery and cool at the same
time. She sat at her large desk and began peppering me with questions
about my life—my education, my writing, my aspirations. She made
a few nice comments about my accomplishments and told me I was
impressive. We discussed aspects of my medical history in detail. The
surgeries, all the scares. She asked me if I wanted biological children
someday. "More than anything," I replied. My voice came out soft
and I suddenly felt self-conscious. That feeling of high stakes was
back. "But after I lost my ovary—after the unilateral salpingo-
oophorectomy . . . ," I said, the o's rolling off my tongue before I realized I was trying to sound smart. What was I trying to prove?

"Are you nervous?" Dr. Noyes said abruptly.

"No! I mean—well—" I stammered. I tried to explain that I'd
come to believe my two unrelated ovary emergencies happened for a
reason. That I thought it was perhaps not a coincidence I was sitting
in her office. If there was a silver lining to my surgeries, I said, it was
that I'd been forced to confront my fertility before it was Too Late.
Dr. Noyes pushed her glasses to the top of her head and studied me.
The all-business, no-nonsense demeanor from the EggBanxx event
had faded some; something in the way she was asking so much about
my life, and not just my reproductive system, felt . . . human. "It's rare
for someone your age to have had two major surgeries like the ones
you've had," she said. "It's pretty hard for an ovary to do a full twist.

_____
now because you plan to have children later). The qualifier isn't really needed,
though, and most people refer to it simply as "egg freezing."

And torsion—that's a real fierce pain." I nodded. I thought about how, in the days before my first surgery, when I was twelve and the pain was most acute, I'd get down on my hands and knees, pounding the floor as I cried.

Dr. Noyes and I started talking about birth control and women postponing motherhood. "We're basically blocking our biology," Dr. Noyes said. "We get this big message like it's wrong to have a baby when you're most fertile—and what women do with that information, I think, is critical. You can't just turn a blind eye and say, 'I'll just deal with it when I'm ready.' The fact is, you're fertile from, like, sixteen to thirty-eight. Everything after forty is a gift."

She flipped through pages of health records I'd brought along. When she got to my visit with the fertility doctor who told me I had a "lovely" ovary, she furrowed her brow. " 'Lovely'?" she said, glancing up at me. "That's not a medical term." I half-shrugged, feigning ignorance, choosing not to gush to this cool doctor about just how much that comment regarding my ovary had meant to me back then—and still did now.

We talked about my irregular periods. "It just bleeds, gets confused," said Dr. Noyes, referring to my ovary. "You're probably not ovulating, not releasing eggs. That's good—more for me." She wet her finger and continued turning the pages of my chart. Almost to herself, she murmured: "We can also sew it to the wall to stop it from moving." I had no idea if she was joking or not.

"I'm not concerned you're going to lose the ovary," she said, looking up at me again. "I don't want to understimulate you and only get, like, five eggs. I want to get at least ten." I blinked. Another sharp turn; we'd arrived at egg freezing. Dr. Noyes continued: "And you're at such a good age. You have so much ahead of you." She took her elbows off the desk and for a moment I thought she was about to clap. "It's gonna be awesome," she said. "Just awesome."

Dr. Noyes didn't explain egg freezing in detail to me that day. I took notes while she glossed over the basics, and I filled in the holes with my own research later. The procedure has multiple steps: ovarian stimulation, egg retrieval, and freezing. A woman getting ready to have her eggs retrieved must first give herself shots of hormones to ramp up her ovaries, coaxing them to grow more eggs to maturity than the usual one per month. More on the specifics of fertility drugs later, but here's the gist: In a normal menstrual cycle, remember, a single follicle containing a single egg bursts at ovulation and releases the egg. With egg freezing, the self-injected drugs hyperstimulate the follicles in the ovaries so that a couple of *years'* worth of immature eggs—upward of a dozen or more—mature in a single month, with the hope that all or most that are extracted will be frozen.

A woman injects herself daily in the comfort of her home—or vacant conference room at work, or restaurant bathroom, or wherever—over the course of ten to fourteen days. Throughout the days of shots, she returns to the fertility clinic every few days to have the size of her follicles monitored and for blood work to check her hormone levels. Then, when her ovaries are plump and ripe, teeming with what the doctors hope are dozens of eggs, she is put under sedation in a private room at the clinic and her eggs are surgically removed, in a "no scar, no stitches" procedure that takes less than half an hour. During the egg retrieval, a doctor, guided by ultrasound technology, pierces the vaginal wall with a long, thin needle and pushes through to the ovary, maneuvering the needle to puncture one follicle after another. One by one, the doctor draws the follicular fluid into a test tube using light suction. Floating within the fluid are the eggs. Once extracted, the eggs can be frozen unfertilized, or they can be injected with sperm and made into embryos, which can then be either frozen and put in cryogenic storage or else transferred to the uterus right away.

Learning about the procedure from start to finish reassured me. I was already beginning to be swayed by egg freezing's hope, by how well it seemed to fit into my plans for organizing my life and planning for the future. Also, though, I suspected the process was expensive—possibly prohibitively so—as well as unpleasant, and not without its risks.

Dr. Noyes said she wanted to run blood work and a few tests. Amazingly, once I was in the exam room, I relaxed a little. These uncomfortable surroundings, at least, were familiar. The stirrups, the overhead lights, the flimsy gown. I climbed onto the padded table, the tissue paper crinkling beneath me, and let my knees fall to either side.

As she nosed the ultrasound wand inside me, Dr. Noyes peered between my legs and motioned to the screen to my left. "Your left ovary is quite active," she announced. I smiled. Medical term or not, I felt proud. It *was* lovely, my active ovary. *Good job, you.* I left the clinic with an ultrasound image of my ovary and a strong recommendation to freeze my eggs. I stepped out onto East 53rd Street, clutching the small picture in my hand as I made my way to the subway. The sun warmed my cheeks. Nearby, the East River glistened under the vivid blue sky. I straightened my posture and tightened my backpack straps around my shoulders, walking a little taller. I realized I was grinning, for no particular reason except I felt pleased that a renowned doctor thought I was a good candidate for egg freezing. I knew more about my fertility than when I'd woken up that morning, and this struck me as significant.

Back at my apartment, I taped the black-and-white picture of my ovary and follicles to the fridge. There it stayed, an image that came to be the Rorschach inkblot it resembles. I could feel its significance gathering inside of me, this Polaroid-sized printout—and, later, ones just like it—that represented what fertility and motherhood had come to mean to me: all that I'd lost, or almost lost, and all that I had to look forward to.

Egg Freezing's Rise

~~~~~~

Mistress of Her Own Body

Brooklyn, 1916. On a bright mid-October day in Brownsville, then a poor and densely populated area of Brooklyn, the country's first birth control clinic opened its doors at 46 Amboy Street. Margaret Sanger wasn't sure what to expect and was taken aback when well over a hundred visitors came that opening day.* The pamphlets advertising the clinic were printed in English, Yiddish, and Italian. They read: "MOTHERS! Can you afford to have a large family? Do you want any more children? If not, why do you have them? DO NOT KILL, DO NOT TAKE LIFE, BUT PREVENT. Safe, Harmless Information can be obtained of trained Nurses at 46 AMBOY STREET." For the next several days, Sanger worked with her sister Ethel, a nurse, and their friend, an interpreter, distributing information about birth control to more than 450 visitors in all.

Ten days after it opened, local authorities shut the clinic down.

---

* Before I tell you more about this part of Sanger's story, it must be acknowledged that Sanger believed in eugenics—an inherently racist and ableist ideology that labeled certain people unfit to have children—which undermined her movement for reproductive freedom and caused harm to many people. It's one of many awful examples of how the fight for reproductive rights in the United States has also been marked by an ugly alliance with the eugenics movement.

Sanger was arrested, charged with disseminating information relating to contraception, and later served thirty days in the Queens County Penitentiary. But her mark had been made, a century-long process begun. The clinic pushed the topic of birth control into public debate, marking a seminal moment for the women's rights movement and igniting a series of changes in how people regarded contraceptives. Sanger would go on to establish what became the precursor to today's Planned Parenthood Federation of America.

"Woman can never call herself free until she is mistress of her own body," Sanger wrote in an essay titled "Morality and Birth Control." She was one of her generation's leading female revolutionaries and activists, pushing for structural change and fighting back against repressive policies on contraception and abortion. In a deft show of marketing prowess, Sanger used the term "birth control" instead of "contraception," to make it sound less draconian. Separating sex from reproduction was a key first step, but there was more to the movement than that. The new term didn't invoke sexual connotations, declarations of independence, or threats. "Birth" was fine; without birth there could be no life, everyone accepted that. For Sanger, Jonathan Eig writes in his book *The Birth of the Pill,* "the key word was 'control.' If women truly got to control when and how often they gave birth, if they got to control their own bodies, they would hold a kind of power never before imagined."

For much of history, women had very little say when it came to their bodies—especially in the bedroom. Married women were typically barred from employment, spending countless hours raising children, confined inside houses under the direction of their husbands. Saddled with childbirth and childcare, they had little power or self-determination. Sanger made it her life's work to see to it that this changed, that women gained autonomy at least over their reproductive lives. But with no reliable methods of birth control available, many women found it difficult to free themselves from being trapped by multiple pregnancies.

They did try. One of the worst examples of the lengths women went to avoid getting pregnant was using Lysol, the harsh cleanser for mopping dirty floors and scrubbing toilets. Women would use it as a douche, and Lysol's advertisements actually *encouraged* women to employ the disinfectant as birth control. At one point during the Great Depression, it was the bestselling method of contraception. (*No,* Lysol is not effective at preventing pregnancy; *yes,* it is dangerous to use Lysol in this way.) Women experimented with a few other means of contraception, but the big shift didn't come until the late 1950s, when oral contraceptive pills were first introduced.*

The U.S. Food and Drug Administration (FDA) approved Enovid, the first birth control pill, in 1960.† Since then, hormonal birth control has allowed millions of women to exert control over their fecundity. Still, it was a rocky start. Even though the Pill was available, doctors in many states could not legally prescribe it. The federal government and many states had anti–birth-control laws in place. Before laws were on the books allowing for birth control services, whether or not a woman could legally take birth control was largely determined by her relationship status. In 1965, the Supreme Court deemed the Pill legal for married women. It wasn't until 1972 that it was ruled legal for all women, regardless of their marital status. Meanwhile, companies had begun to develop and sell various types of IUDs, or intrauterine devices, inserted into the uterus; today's IUDs are T-shaped devices about the length of a large paper clip, made from flexible plastic and sometimes copper. By the early 1970s, nearly 10 percent of women in the United States using contraception relied on the IUD.

Then came the Dalkon Shield.

During the first few years of the IUDs' heyday, over two million American women were fitted with this particular IUD—advertised as a safer alternative to the Pill—and it quickly became the most

---

* Prior to FDA approval, when promoting birth control was still illegal in many states, oral contraceptives were prescribed to treat menstrual issues.

† In the mid-1950s, Enovid clinical trials were conducted on more than two hundred women living in a housing project in Puerto Rico. The women were not told that the Pill was experimental or that there was a chance of potentially dangerous side effects. Nor were they told that they were taking part in a clinical trial, which was being run by biologist Gregory Pincus and gynecologist John Rock. Three women died, and their deaths were not investigated.

popular one on the market. Then women started getting sick. The Dalkon Shield, it turned out, was defective in detrimental, life-changing ways. Created by a doctor and an engineer, this new IUD—called a shield because it resembled a police officer's badge—was nearly circular, with five small plastic fins along two opposite sides that secured the device in place in the endometrium (the tissue that lines the uterus). The device's larger surface area necessitated a more durable tail string compared to the tail strings of other IUDs. The doctor and the engineer identified a string they thought would work well called Supramid, a cable-type suture material made of hundreds of small fibers wrapped by a single sheath. It was the device's multifilament string that caused bacteria to get trapped in the string and therefore the uterus. Thousands of patients suffered infections, miscarriages, and a host of other significant problems. More than three hundred thousand claims were filed against A. H. Robins Company, the firm that sold the device. After paying billions of dollars in damages, the company filed for bankruptcy protection, and the whole thing became one of the most famous mass personal injury cases on record.

All this resulted in the 1976 mandate that the FDA regulate and approve medical devices, including IUDs. The Dalkon Shield's serious design flaw was corrected; modern IUDs use monofilament strings, which pose less risk of bacteria traveling into the uterus. But the Dalkon Shield dented the legitimacy and popularity of IUDs in the United States, and its legacy is one reason the Pill has remained so popular for so long. The Pill was incredibly important for women on a personal, day-to-day level, but it was also crucial in changing society. In a word, the Pill offered women *agency*. It had far-reaching implications for women's social mobility, marriage choices, and economic independence. It paved the way for droves of them to enter the workforce. It helped make it possible for women to get degrees and climb the corporate ladder without getting fired because of unintended pregnancy. It was effective, it was inexpensive, and it offered women a say over their reproductive capabilities in ways they'd never had before. For that reason in particular, the Pill took the notion of controlling one's fertility to a whole new level.

. . .

More and more people are attempting to have children later in life. Across the globe, women and men are increasingly waiting until their mid- to late thirties, and even forties, to start families. One reason we're putting off having children is that we're marrying later. From the early 1940s through the early 1970s in the United States, women's median age at marriage was twenty. Now it's twenty-eight. Another reason is that women are getting more education and work experience before having children. Women with college degrees are more likely to have a child at age thirty or later than women with lower levels of education. They have children roughly seven years later than women without college degrees, using those years in between to finish school and focus on career goals.

The median age of U.S. women giving birth is now thirty, the highest on record. The average age of first-time mothers has gone up considerably in the past fifty years. In 1972, it was twenty-one. Now it's twenty-seven. This may seem young, but it's actually not. And in part because women are waiting longer to have their first child, they're having fewer children overall. This isn't a new phenomenon; the number of women who are still childless after age thirty has been steadily trending up since the mid-1970s. Since 1976—around the time IUDs improved and the Pill was deemed legal for all women—the number of women ages thirty to thirty-four who have not yet had a child actually doubled, from about 15 percent to 30 percent of all women in that age group. None of this necessarily means women aren't choosing to be mothers; in fact, 86 percent of American women are, according to a Pew Research Center analysis of U.S. Census Bureau data.* What it points to is that women are simply having children later. The phenomenon of deferring motherhood has become increasingly common in the United States over the past three decades, as birth rates have de-

* I was glad to see that the Pew report notes that its use of the term "mother" "refers to any woman who has ever given birth, even though many women who do not bear their own children are indeed mothers."

clined for women in their twenties and jumped for women in their late thirties and early forties.

The takeaway from all these statistics is that these trends—marrying later and waiting longer to have children—won't change anytime soon. Money is one reason why: Many women delay pregnancy to hold out for a higher salary. Data compiled by a Census Bureau working paper points to an interesting fact: If women have a baby between ages twenty-five and thirty-five, their earnings take a significant hit. This ten-year window is a significant chunk of a woman's fertile years. It's also, of course, prime time to build a career. According to the paper, giving birth during this ten-year span—when a woman's prime window of fertility largely overlaps with her salary-building years— exacerbates the gender pay gap. American women already earn, on average, only 83 percent of what men earn, and for Black and Hispanic women, this inequity is even greater. If biology had its way, that ten-year window—ending at thirty-five—is the age when all the women who hadn't started having babies in the previous decade would begin. Yet it makes sense that women want to avoid getting pregnant in this period of their lives, now that they have become a permanent fixture in the workforce. And so they spend this decade leaning into their careers, breaking glass ceilings rather than breaking bread with children they don't yet want.

Women in professional careers want to delay childbearing but are no less keen to have a child than women who opted not to delay. They delay, in part, because they want a better economic platform from which to launch their families. They wait to have children because they want to avoid what's been called the "motherhood penalty," the decline in earnings that I've just described that women can expect with each child they have, often locking them into lower incomes throughout the rest of their careers.* Women don't want to have to choose between a career and children. And so, many don't.

These overlapping—and to some degree, competing—desires are

---

* As a 2023 CDC report noted, "Having a first child at older ages has been associated with a positive impact on women's wages and career paths, in addition to having a positive impact on their children because they are more likely to have parents with greater family and economic stability."

music to the fertility industry's ears. Because while American society has been hugely changed by modern contraceptives, the number of years during which a woman's body can reliably bear children has remained fixed for millennia. It's all about the eggs, remember? We cannot escape the inconvenient truth: Fertility wanes as a woman gets older. And yet. In 2021, about one in five babies were born to women aged thirty-five and older, and nearly 20 percent of women in the United States today have their first child after age thirty. Also, for nearly forty years, the proportion of American women giving birth in their forties has been on a steady rise.* This, as we've established, is not exactly when our bodies would like to be having babies.

On the one hand: a dramatic historical shift when it comes to women having children later in life, coupled with the power of contraception. On the other: the fixed window of time a woman's body can bear children. So how do we solve this insoluble equation? By finding ways to extend the fertility window with new technology. In the face of these demographic changes, women and men are turning in increasing numbers to assisted reproductive technology (often abbreviated as ART) to help them overcome fertility issues stemming from age and medical conditions. ART is an umbrella term for techniques that involve the handling of eggs and embryos outside a woman's body to help her become pregnant. Hence the rising demand for medical intervention and fertility treatments for more people than ever before, and the industry that has rushed to meet it, eager to capitalize on a very real biological conundrum: As more aspiring mothers delay childbirth to climb the career ladder or find the right partner, it makes a whole lot of sense that they would also be eager to buy into what egg freezing companies are offering.

For those with sufficient means, ART helps millions of people have biological children who otherwise could not. More than nine million babies have been born from IVF since 1978. The most common ART and one of those most widely available, IVF is now con-

---

* *The New York Times* noted that the rise "subsided in 2020 with the pandemic, when the overall birth rate in the U.S. dipped, but the rate among women in their late forties grew."

sidered mainstream medicine in many countries; in the United States, the number of ART procedures—mostly IVF—has jumped nearly 80 percent since 2015. The technique to unite sperm and eggs outside the body and implant them directly into the womb has been heralded, for good reason, as the most remarkable achievement in ·fertility to date. On IVF's heels came egg and embryo freezing, another extraordinary advance in fertility science. As a technology focused on preserving pregnancy potential and being proactive, egg freezing, in particular, is part of this same continuum, revolutionizing how women think about not just their fertility but also their agency and reproductive autonomy.

"If women had the power to control their own bodies, if they had the ability to choose when and whether they got pregnant, what would they want next?" Jonathan Eig writes. In a culture where the optimal time to advance a career and find a life partner coincides directly with the period in which the body is best suited for reproduction, the "what next" may well be the ability to not have to sacrifice one for the other. This is what makes the idea of conquering the biological clock so powerful: that doing so is what will make it possible for women to build their careers and their personal lives when they choose to—as opposed to when their biology dictates. And so as it changes the face of reproductive decision-making, ART is ushering in the second phase of trying to have it all.

I kept thinking about Eig's provocative question. That clause, *the ability to choose when and whether to get pregnant:* check. We're all good there; bless you, birth control. It was the first bit of his question I couldn't shake: *the power to control their own bodies.* A sense of foreboding lurks beneath Eig's premise. To control their own fates, women first needed to keep from getting pregnant; then they needed to be able to preserve their fertility.

Enter Egg Freezing

In medical parlance, egg freezing is known as oocyte cryopreservation. Eggs from a woman's ovaries are extracted, frozen, and stored on ice. Once extracted, or retrieved, the eggs are exposed to cryoprotectants—

a concentrated solution of chemicals that prevents damage to the eggs when they're being frozen—and then immersed in liquid nitrogen, where they freeze almost instantly. Cryopreservation, the freezing part, halts an egg's processes of metabolic and genetic deterioration. Using her young eggs, a woman can theoretically carry a baby to term decades beyond the traditional childbearing years. If, after her eggs are retrieved, a woman is ready to get pregnant, her eggs are fertilized with a man's sperm to make an embryo that's then implanted in her uterus. That's IVF. But if she's not ready to get pregnant, putting her extracted, unfertilized eggs on ice affords her the option to use them if she needs to go through IVF later. Ideally, she freezes in her twenties or early thirties, although most women who freeze their eggs are in their mid- to late thirties.*

The power of egg freezing lies in its potential to change the temporal limits to female fertility and buy time: time for a woman to find the right partner rather than "settle" for someone in order to meet a biological deadline, to pursue a demanding career without having to rule out motherhood later on, to figure out the family structure she wants rather than being at the mercy of fate. These aren't the only reasons people freeze eggs (more on that in chapter 5), but for the typical young, healthy woman hoping to preserve her fertility, retrieving and storing her eggs will give her some breathing room, as well as a better shot at conceiving with her own eggs—as opposed to donor eggs—when she's older, if and when she decides to become pregnant. Buying time is the *idea,* at least; I'll go into detail about egg freezing success rates in chapter 8. First, though, let's talk briefly about how egg freezing came to be.

In 1965, after seeing promising results freezing rabbit eggs, University of Chicago gynecologist Dr. James Burks managed to cryopreserve ten human eggs in liquid nitrogen, nine of which survived when he thawed them. While this was technically (and most likely) the first time human eggs were successfully frozen, Dr. Burks is rarely men-

---

* Also, though, increasing numbers of young women under the age of twenty-five—Gen Z women—are opting to freeze their eggs. "The average age of my egg freezing patients is rapidly declining every year," Dr. Serena Chen, the fertility doctor who spoke at the first EggBanxx party I attended, told *Vice* in 2023.

tioned in what little literature exists on egg freezing's history. The real story begins in the 1980s, when scientists began experimenting with different methods of freezing and thawing human eggs. In 1986, in Australia, Dr. Christopher Chen reported the world's first pregnancy—resulting in twins—that used previously frozen human eggs. The birth came on the heels of the first baby born from a frozen embryo two years earlier, in 1984. Different sources say different things about Dr. Chen and his methods, however, and most regard his two successful cases as impressive flukes. His methods were never repeated. Meanwhile, inside a laboratory at the University of Bologna, two female Italian doctors had been quietly working to develop reliable egg freezing technology.

In the late 1980s, Dr. Raffaella Fabbri, a biologist, and Dr. Eleonora Porcu, a fertility doctor, began working together at the university's Department of Obstetrics and Gynecology. They saw the possibility of freezing eggs as a way around freezing embryos, which troubled the Italian public—and, more importantly, the Roman Catholic Church. An embryo is a fertilized egg, and when all of a woman's harvested eggs are fertilized in a petri dish, doctors intentionally create more embryos than can be used, to maximize the chances that an embryo made this way will successfully implant in a mother's uterus (more on embryo attrition rates later on). There are various ethical and personal concerns when it comes to freezing leftover embryos, which often end up getting destroyed. In Italy, Spain, and other parts of Europe, religious belief made many IVF patients uncomfortable about keeping their excess embryos in a freezer indefinitely. The Church had long deemed the practice of freezing embryos immoral. Searching for an alternative, fertility doctors saw egg freezing as a way to avoid flouting the Church's denunciation of embryo freezing. If IVF patients could freeze their leftover unfertilized eggs, they wouldn't be forced to waste them; plus, it would be easier to discard unfertilized eggs later on, if necessary.

Fertilizing and freezing gametes (sperm or egg cells) involves fragile and difficult-to-get-right practices. Egg cells, in particular, are extremely delicate. Sperm cells have been successfully frozen since the 1950s, and human embryos since the early 1980s. But eggs, which, tiny as they are, are full of water, proved far trickier. And so despite the few favorable results early on, egg freezing remained a finicky, understudied process with meager survival and fertilization rates. Another challenge in the beginning was that other researchers at the time—and Dr. Chen, specifically—had attempted to reconstruct and reproduce egg freezing experiments but had failed to repeat their initial success.

Seeing an opportunity, the chief of Dr. Porcu and Dr. Fabbri's lab asked them to keep working on preserving eggs. With his blessing, and without defying the Church's anti-embryo-freezing stance, the doctors continued their experiments. Vitrification (which I'll explain in a moment) hadn't been developed yet, so the two women were figuring out how to improve the slow-freeze method, which relies on the balance between the formation rate of ice crystals and the dehydration rate of cells to prevent ice crystals from forming. The water contained in a human egg is difficult to expel. And egg cells must be sufficiently dehydrated before they're frozen; otherwise, too much water will cause ice crystals to form, which can rupture cell walls, thereby resulting in genetic damage and making the eggs unusable. The Italian doctors needed to figure out a way to better dehydrate the cell before freezing it. Dr. Fabbri tried adjusting the sucrose concentration in the cryoprotectant—the substance that prevents the formation of ice crystals during the freezing process—and found that increasing the sucrose, which helps draw water out of the cell, as well as exposing the eggs to the cryoprotectant for longer, meant that more frozen eggs made it through the thawing process. Incredibly, survival rates went up to 90 percent.

Another egg freezing obstacle that had stymied scientists was that sperm ordinarily cannot penetrate an egg that has been frozen and thawed. But a new method, called intracytoplasmic sperm injection, or ICSI, in which sperm is injected directly into eggs, had recently been introduced. ICSI is similar to conventional IVF insemination in that, after eggs and sperm are collected from each partner, the eggs are fertilized and, hopefully, become embryos that are transferred to a woman's uterus and develop into a fetus. But the method of achieving fertilization is different. Conventional insemination entails placing the eggs in direct contact with sperm—mixing them in a petri dish in the laboratory—so that large numbers of sperm can swim around and ultimately one fertilizes the egg; basically the "best sperm wins" dynamic of natural conception. ICSI takes a more hands-on approach: An embryologist uses a needle to inject a single sperm into each egg. Dr. Porcu began experimenting with injecting sperm directly into frozen-then-thawed eggs. In 1997, just a few years after ICSI was developed and after the Italian doctors had been working together for a decade, Dr. Fabbri and Dr. Porcu were the first to report a baby born from a frozen egg using ICSI.

By building on the techniques of other doctors and their own discoveries, the Italian doctors had changed the destiny of egg freezing. The altered cryoprotectant solution and the use of ICSI together had made all the difference, resulting in the first pregnancy of its kind in the world. In 2001, Dr. Fabbri received a worldwide patent for her novel method and solution for cryopreserving human eggs. On the heels of her team's breakthrough, three further significant developments would kick off the egg freezing revolution.

Game Changer #1: Vitrification

By the early 2000s, scientists managed to conquer the cryoprotectant solution problem, paving the way for bettering the method the Italians had developed that had improved frozen egg survival rates. Technological advances now gave scientists the ability to flash-freeze eggs using vitrification, which made the freezing process more reliable. Until 2003, when it was proven that vitrified eggs could successfully yield live births, the only way to freeze eggs was through slow-freezing, a method that often produced the harmful ice crystals I mentioned earlier. Vitrification, on the other hand, chills the eggs to −196 degrees Celsius in a fraction of a second. The ultra-rapid cooling technique prevents ice crystals from forming more reliably than the Italian doctors' novel cryoprotectant discovery had. Vitrification significantly improved egg survival and pregnancy rates: Flash-frozen eggs have an 85 to 95 percent survival rate, compared to a 60 to 80 percent survival rate for slow-frozen eggs. The improved technique quickly became a firmly established technology, and is the current cryopreservation method the vast majority of fertility clinics rely on.

Initially, egg freezing was done only for reasons of medical necessity. The first women to take advantage of the Italian doctors' promising flash-freezing method were cancer patients who froze their eggs as a way to save their fertility before undergoing treatments known to harm reproductive organs and fecundity. Some chemotherapy medications destroy eggs, and eggs are exceedingly sensitive to radiation; both treatments can leave a woman sterile. For a young woman diagnosed with an aggressive form of cancer, the ability to preserve her healthy eggs outside of her body can mean everything. But it didn't take long for egg freezing to move beyond the "for medical reasons" realm. The possibility of extending the shelf life of one's eggs was enticing, and before long, healthy women began raising their hands to freeze their eggs.

Game Changer #2: No Longer Experimental

In 2012, the American Society of Reproductive Medicine (ASRM), the fertility industry's principal professional organization, lifted the "experimental" label on egg freezing. This was a big deal. A big-tent membership organization covering all areas of reproductive biology, ASRM was founded in 1944 by a small group of fertility experts to address the need for more research into infertility and more widely disseminated information on the subject. When the ASRM decided egg freezing should no longer be considered experimental—despite the lack of quality research on the procedure—their declaration raised eyebrows.

ASRM is governed by a rotating board of directors, a group of about twenty MDs and PhDs. Like other multidisciplinary professional associations, ASRM is a long-standing unified forum for debate within its field and wields a lot of influence. Fertility doctors and clinics pay close attention to what it does and does not advise when it comes to the ethics and efficacies of reproductive technologies. So when the organization changed its stance on egg freezing and issued a report to practicing clinicians across the country, the U.S. fertility industry leaned in with perked ears.

More than nine hundred babies had been born from frozen eggs by 2008, the year ASRM labeled the procedure as experimental. With that designation, ASRM approved the use of egg freezing only in clinical trials overseen by an institutional review board. Despite the society's recommendation, many clinics offered egg freezing outside of this framework, as a clinical service for a fee, without securing informed research consent from patients, which is required for any experimental procedure. Ethically problematic, to be sure, but for at least one subset of egg freezing patients—women with cancer, desperate to preserve their fertility before undergoing chemotherapy or radiation—there wasn't time for long clinical trials. One reason ASRM wanted to take a fresh look at the process was to make it easier for doctors to freeze the eggs of these cancer patients without the obstacles of informed research consent.

That was all well and fine, but after reviewing nearly one thousand egg freezing studies, the ASRM committee stopped short of giving egg freezing for non-medical reasons the green light. "There are not yet sufficient data to recommend oocyte cryopreservation for the sole purpose of circumventing reproductive aging in healthy women," the report stated. While early studies on egg freezing proved reassuring—largely due to the improved freezing and thawing techniques—there wasn't yet enough to go on for women who wanted to freeze their eggs simply to delay childbearing. So ASRM lifted the experimental label, but with a caveat, concluding there were still too many questions about the procedure to warrant its use in women beyond those with cancer and other fertility-threatening medical conditions. Other prominent associations agreed. The American College of Obstetricians and Gynecologists (ACOG) joined ASRM in discouraging egg freezing for non-medical reasons because, in addition to the lack of data and research, too little was known about its personal, social, and scientific ramifications.

When the 2012 report was published, Dr. Samantha Pfeifer, ASRM committee chair at the time, reiterated the committee's decision: "While a careful review of the literature indicates egg freezing is a valid technique for young women for whom it is medically indicated, we cannot at this time endorse its widespread elective use to delay childbearing," she said. "This technology may not be appropriate for the older woman who desires to postpone reproduction." ASRM's position was clear. But the caveat was quickly downplayed by clinics eager to market this new offering. In the end, removing the experimental label opened the door to a much wider audience.

To some degree at least, ASRM understood the impact that upgrading non-medical egg freezing from experimental to standard would likely have. It certainly knew that many women were interested in this emerging technology, because the association had actually said so in its 2008 report maintaining that egg freezing was not an established medical treatment. The 2012 report, in which ASRM reversed its stance—egg freezing *was* now an established medical treatment—took its cautionary tone regarding egg freezing's potential widespread use up a notch, then up again. Scientific advancements such as egg freezing may allow women the opportunity to have biological children later in life, the report said, but "while this technology may appear to be an attractive strategy for this purpose, there are no data on the efficacy of oocyte cryopreservation in this population and for this indication." And then the committee took it even further with a warning: "Marketing this technology for the purpose of deferring childbearing may give women false hope and encourage women to delay childbearing."

Game Changer #3: Apple and Facebook

Yet two years after the ASRM decision, in October 2014, Apple and Facebook announced they would help cover the cost of egg freezing for female employees, offering up to $20,000 per person. The news that some of the biggest companies in Silicon Valley were now subsidizing the procedure for women with no known fertility issues as part of their benefits packages immediately set off a controversy, and debate ensued. Employers paying for non-medical egg freezing applies even more pressure on women to keep working while putting their personal lives on the back burner, went one argument. This levels the playing field for women, went another. I followed and joined the debate along with my feminist friends, and considered what such a benefit said about how companies regard young female employees and how we as a country treat mothers. That was a larger and ongoing conversation, I knew, one I was becoming increasingly attuned to as my thirties loomed. But, frankly, I was more interested in the practical, achievable aspects of this new technology, especially since now I no longer felt like such an oddball for seriously considering undergoing egg freezing myself.

While IVF has been around for decades, it was only since the mid-2010s that egg freezing really took off. Of the five hundred or so fertility clinics in the United States, almost all offer egg freezing. At these clinics, between 2009 and 2022, nearly 115,000 women opted to freeze their eggs,* and the number of procedures to freeze eggs quadrupled between 2015 and 2022. That growth was spurred in part by Apple and Facebook's announcements, which in turn ushered in the benefit at an increasing number of large companies (more on that in chapter 9).

The night the news broke—spokespeople for both Apple and Facebook told an NBC News reporter about their companies' new perk—I happened to be at another egg freezing event in New York City. Now that I knew more, and had learned I was a good candidate, I wanted to see how I'd feel about it when I heard the pitch again. It was a cool autumn evening, and inside the Harvard Club, the mood was light and full of intrigue. Women sipped wine and crunched on veggies they'd piled onto cocktail napkins. Again I was several years younger than most of the women in the room. Again I couldn't help but think of Carrie Bradshaw. I wore my blue-light glasses so that I would look older and not attract as many stares as I had at that first EggBanxx event, the looks that said, *You and your young eggs don't belong here.* Drinks in hand, we took our seats under

---

* As of this writing, the actual number to date of women in the United States who have electively undergone egg freezing is likely closer to 150,000. More on this in chapter 8.

a glistening glass chandelier and listened to doctors sing the praises of egg freezing.

A few days later, I saw my first egg freezing ad on the subway. "To Emma (Age 42). Love Emma (Age 30)," the blue-and-pink poster on the Q train read. "If you are not ready to have a baby, freeze your eggs now and give yourself the gift of time."* And then I began to notice targeted ads on my social media feeds. One, sponsored by a boutique fertility clinic in Manhattan, featured a pink illustration of a sperm wiggling its way into an ovum. "When you freeze your eggs, you #freezetime," the ad read. "How often do you get to do that?" The ads, in combination with the celebrity endorsements and new employer-covered fertility preservation perk, shimmered with the illusion of control. That powerful idea: *control.* Until I saw egg freezing ads on the subway and my Instagram, I wasn't aware that my fertility—present, future, or otherwise—*needed* to be controlled. Or that it was something I was supposed to be controlling. And control doesn't come cheap. The answer to "How much does egg freezing cost?" requires an involved discussion we'll get to in chapter 9, but the average cost of one egg freezing cycle in the United States is roughly $16,000, which includes the doctor visits, the medications, and the average number of years of egg storage—and most women do more than one cycle. Insurance rarely covers it. Some employers do, as I said, but most women pay for it themselves.[†]

The Apple and Facebook announcements would prove to be a watershed moment, helping to mainstream both the concept of egg freezing and the conversation around it. Egg freezing, it seemed, was suddenly everywhere. Meanwhile, the confluence of two trends—older parents and increased insurance coverage for IVF—meant that demand for fertility services continued to rise. But questions lurked. What do fertility preservation technologies actually offer women, and what are our fantasies surrounding them? Is egg freezing a genuine

---

* These newer, more upbeat ads have replaced those plastered on buses in major U.S. cities since the early 2000s, like the one featuring an image of a baby bottle shaped like an hourglass, running out of milk.

[†] This is a huge health equity issue. More on this in chapter 9.

help and good investment, or is it merely a bad bet laced with hope? And: how to judge whether or not the potential future upsides are worth the expense, yes, but also the consequential risks—of which there are several, I'd come to learn.

One thing I was crystal clear on after this second egg freezing event was that the pressure to procreate has a timeline and echoes warnings: "Before it's too late" and the *tick-tock, tick-tock* of our uteruses. A week or so after the event, I called Barbara Collura, executive director of RESOLVE: The National Infertility Association, a non-profit advocacy organization, to seek her advice about where to start in my quest to find objective answers about egg freezing. "I wouldn't even know where to tell you to go to get really great, unbiased information," she said. "There's nothing out there for women. You want a third-party, credible source—and not to be tied to somebody who's trying to sell you on doing this—and it doesn't exist." At first, I felt pretty deflated hearing that. But her declaration also stirred in me a quiet defiance to prove her at least partially wrong; surely there was *some* helpful, scientifically sound information about egg freezing out there for women.

Pros and Cons

Late one October evening in my Brooklyn apartment, I sat cross-legged in bed, eating salad out of a Tupperware container. It was my third semester of graduate school. A string of delicate paper-lantern lights bordered shelves brimming with books. On my bedside table, a scented candle burned. My journal lay open in my lap. I needed to clarify some basics; lists are good for that. I flipped to a blank page and scribbled:

What egg freezing is:
A back-up plan
Hope and peace of mind—I think?
Promising technology; keeps getting better over time
Supported by lots of big companies
A very good option for many women

What egg freezing is not:
An insurance policy—right?
Risk-free
Inexpensive
A guaranteed way to prevent my fertility from fading
A very good option for many women

I studied the lists. I finished my salad. On my desk lay a faded, two-pocket folder labeled "Surgeries." Tucked inside were medical records, copies of doctor's notes, pamphlets on egg freezing, and a handful of Polaroid-sized pictures of my ovary. From my perch in bed, I reached for the folder and lifted a recent ultrasound image from one of the pockets. I held it up to the light. In the narrow white space beneath the fuzzy picture, I had written: *Just me and my ovary, giving this all we've got.*

I sat wrapped in a patchwork quilt I had made out of T-shirts I'd collected as a child and teenager. Running my hand across the soft cotton squares, I smiled, recalling nicknames and jersey numbers, celebrations and milestones. When it comes to having children and being a parent, I am drawn to the ineffable mystery of motherhood, the seductive veneer that nothing has been able to penetrate—at least for me, and, I believe, for many women—despite how much and how fervently motherhood and all it entails is discussed and picked apart in our culture. My mother's experiences being pregnant and giving birth have a lot to do with my romanticizing early motherhood. She talks about it in a way she doesn't talk about anything else—not her decorated career as a U.S. Army officer and government lawyer; not the few dozen countries she's visited; not even her forty-five-year-long marriage to my father. She has also made giving birth sound easy and joyful (yes, really). My mother is not a martyr, nor does she have an unusually high tolerance for pain. But she did birth three babies, all without epidurals, IVs, or pain meds—not even Tylenol. (She wasn't opposed to medical intervention had something gone wrong; she just hadn't needed it.) And when she talks of nursing my siblings and me, her normally rapid-fire voice slows and she sighs in satisfaction, in reverence, as if she's sharing a secret about some magical land she once visited. "Breastfeeding my babies is the single most satisfying and wonderful experience of my life," my mother has told me more than once. She says it triumphantly and I believe her completely.

Perhaps the in-my-heart certainty is a seed watered by my mother's stories. I am her firstborn daughter. It would not be until years later, when my friends began having kids, that I would come to realize that, for many women, pregnancy is *not* easy or joyful, epidurals are a polarizing topic, and breastfeeding is not something that all women love or even want to do. Even so, where my mother's tales of pregnancy and childbirth left off, I want mine to begin. Of course, I have no way of knowing if I will one day have the unmedicated, low-intervention birth experiences she did, but I can't help but imagine I might. And, also like her, I want to have children with a person I love and am committed to. I have always wanted this. I have always planned on it.

A few weeks before that list-making night in my apartment, I'd returned home after being out of town for my brother's wedding. I took the subway from the airport and by the time I arrived at my street it was quite late. I pulled my purple suitcase along the sidewalk and wondered how many times I'd done this exact thing, returning home alone after a trip. A fierce loneliness took hold. As I walked, I felt as if a hole in my heart was growing bigger, block by block. Inside my empty apartment, I unpacked, made a ham sandwich, stood at the kitchen island, and cried. Then I shook my head hard, as if to fling off the sobs. *Stop it,* I berated myself. *You've lived on four continents and traveled all over the world. You're close with your family. You're earning a master's degree from one of the top journalism programs in the country.* My life was full—but I felt deeply alone. I wanted to lug my suitcase next to someone else lugging theirs, then climb the stairs to my fifth-floor walk-up together. I wanted to make this ham sandwich for someone else.

My last serious relationship had ended two years earlier. I hadn't had much time or energy to devote to thinking about a new one since moving to New York, but now that I was feeling settled, I was ready to not be single anymore. I wasn't yet facing the intense time pressures I knew single women in their thirties often feel, and I wasn't old enough to worry about the expiration of my fertility. But my missing ovary was beginning to haunt me, saying otherwise. It used to remind me of painful surgeries and hospital stays; now it reminded me of too-close calls and the quiet ticking of my biological clock, of egg freezing and my forever desire to have a family.

A few months before the Apple and Facebook news broke, *Bloomberg Businessweek* reported: "Not since the birth control pill has a medical technology had such potential to change family and career planning." The questions were coming faster now: Was egg freezing really the next revolution for women's reproductive lives? Did it give women real agency, or just the illusion of it? Would I be among a generation of women buying into a grand experiment? As I sat on my bed that night, I realized I was almost certain I wanted to freeze my eggs. But I needed to do something about all these questions and figure out why egg freezing was being so readily and widely embraced and if in fact it was, or could be, as good as it sounded. To better understand the nuts and bolts of egg freezing, I decided, I needed to go back to the science, and lay out all the facts and implications as best I could.

That sounded like a lot of work. And *many* more lists.

Maybe there was a better place to start.

Maybe I could find someone who had decided to do it.

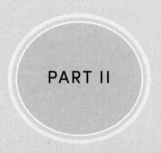

PART II

The Orientation

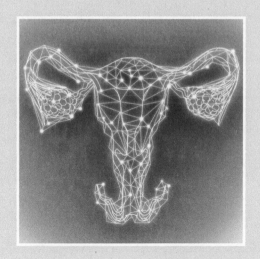

4

Hacking Our Hormones

~~~~~~

Remy: Egg Freezing Orientation

A little after eight o'clock on a cool Nashville morning, Remy opened the door to her apartment and headed straight to the bedroom. She fell face-first onto her bed, too tired to peel off her scrubs. Sophie, her cat, padded in to greet her. Remy lay on the soft white duvet for a few minutes, eyes closed, hoping to nap. But her racing mind wouldn't let her. *Get up and get it together,* she told herself. Her appointment at the fertility clinic was in a couple of hours; she needed to be alert. *Just wash your face, brush your teeth, let's go, let's go.* She took a deep breath and pushed her tall, lean frame to a seated position on the bed.

An anesthesia resident at Vanderbilt University Medical Center, Remy was used to crawling into bed when most people were beginning their days. Night shifts bled into days spent sleeping; weekends were indistinguishable from the Monday-to-Friday hustle. She didn't mind the relentless routine, really—life was busy, and good—but she found she especially looked forward to her appointments at the fertility clinic, where she would soon be freezing her eggs. The visits reminded her of the future—of *her* future, and what it held. *There's so much more to come,* she thought often.

Remy had made the decision to freeze her eggs a couple of months earlier, shortly after her birthday. Thirty-three had long felt symbolic to her. Unabashedly superstitious, Remy had always imagined having kids at this age. This year of medical residency was going to be her year for children. But things in the love department hadn't exactly gone as planned, and so now thirty-three was her year for egg freezing.

A broken engagement when she was twenty-five and in medical school. Then: a new flame, a whirlwind romance, a hasty wedding, a brief marriage, and divorce—all before she finished residency. When Remy's personal life got derailed, she couldn't help but feel she had somehow fallen behind. She hadn't thought she'd be single at thirty-three, and she definitely hadn't expected to have a broken engagement and a divorce under her belt by then—or ever. What she did have was the career of her dreams and an unshakable belief in doing whatever she could to secure the future children—future family—that felt more important to her than anything else.

And egg freezing was the way to do it.

Remy exchanged her scrubs for a long-sleeved denim shirt and faded tan jeans. She looked around for her tall leather lace-up boots, tucked in a corner next to a stuffed brown bear she'd had since childhood. She glanced at her Apple watch. Just enough time to stop for a smoked rosemary latte at her favorite coffee shop before driving south to the clinic.

It was a damp morning in February, the sky a deep gray. Nashville traffic was a pain, and Remy arrived with hardly any time to spare. The clinic's waiting room was drab. Beige walls, beige carpet, fluorescent lights. Monochrome portraits of babies hung on the wall. Two couples sat waiting to be seen. Remy walked purposefully to the receptionist's desk and offered a warm hello. The woman smiled brightly, remembering her, and presented a clipboard of forms in exchange for Remy's credit card.

Checked in, Remy settled into one of the stiff chairs. She rubbed her eyes, feeling tired but calm. She had been too busy at work to overthink today's appointment, a two-hour session about the hormone shots that were the prelude to her egg retrieval and freezing. For the past month, Remy had been treating pregnant women, her schedule a whirlwind of epidurals and C-sections. Some overnight shifts were so busy she didn't stop to eat or rest. But she was thrilled to be on OB/GYN clinical rotation this month, of all months; her workdays felt rich with meaning and connectedness. She prepped patients who were about to give birth while her brain buzzed with egg freezing plans and the babies she hoped—she knew—her frozen eggs would someday yield. She closed her eyes and concentrated on turning off her doctor brain and switching to the patient mindset. Here at the clinic, most of the staff didn't know she was an anesthesiologist, and Remy preferred it that way. She could sit back and be the one taken care of. Here, she was just another woman preserving her fertility.

At her first egg freezing appointment a few weeks earlier, Remy had met the reproductive endocrinologist who would do her egg retrieval. Dr. Ruth Lewis* had walked Remy through the process, the research, some of the risks. She wasn't particularly warm and fuzzy, but Remy trusted her no-nonsense demeanor immediately. Dr. Lewis explained that she typically didn't see women having difficulties with fertility until after age thirty-six. Remy was three years shy of that, but she already felt she was losing precious time while she waited to develop the relationship she wanted, to be able to have children with the right person. Or to decide to become a solo parent, a possibility she'd been considering. All her clocks were ticking.

In an exam room, Dr. Lewis had Remy's blood drawn to test her hormone levels and looked at Remy's ovaries via transvaginal ultrasound. When her follicles, the fluid-filled sacs containing egg cells, appeared on the monitor, Dr. Lewis counted them: eight follicles on the right ovary, thirteen on the left. Dr. Lewis told Remy she was remarkably healthy, with a good supply of eggs. She was unlikely to face issues conceiving if she tried to get pregnant in the next few years. She understood Remy's desire for the peace of mind that can come with preserving eggs at an optimal age. But having found no red flags in terms of Remy's current fertility, Dr. Lewis had told her she might want to reconsider egg freezing, save her money instead.

* Name has been changed.

Remy appreciated the doctor's straightforward way of laying it all out. But she was already committed to freezing her eggs and told Dr. Lewis she wanted to start as soon as possible.

Now she was back for her second appointment. A nurse called Remy's name and led her to a small exam room. More fluorescent lights and beige. The nurse, nodding toward a chair, instructed Remy to make herself comfortable and left. A few minutes later, there were two curt knocks and the door opened. Dr. Lewis—straightened blond hair, long white coat over a blue floral top, black ballet flats—sat down on a stool, clipboard in hand. She and Remy exchanged hellos, and then Remy introduced me as a friend who was interested in egg freezing and was also writing about it. Dr. Lewis nodded and shook my hand before turning her attention back to Remy.

"Got a lot to cover today," Dr. Lewis began. "We'll review the ovarian stimulation process, go over some risks and consent forms, then talk about the egg retrieval. Sound good?"

She launched into explaining the different types of medications that stimulate a woman's ovaries: carefully timed, self-injected hormone shots phased over about two weeks. During the first phase, the shots would kick Remy's ovaries into overdrive to produce more eggs. The second phase of shots would prevent immature ovulation, instructing her ovaries not to release the eggs too soon. The final injection, known as the "trigger shot," finishes off the eggs' maturation so that they're ready to be retrieved.

Remy leaned forward, chin in hand and elbow resting on her crossed leg. Her blond hair sat in a messy bun on the top of her head, and silver feather earrings dangled from her ears.

"Now, the trigger shot," said Dr. Lewis, resting her back against the exam table. "It's a powder, so you have to mix it. And then, don't shake it, you just—"

"Reconstitute it," Remy interjected.

"Reconstitute it *gently*," Dr. Lewis went on. "Sometimes it takes a while to clear. And then it's an IM injection."*

Dr. Lewis explained that the egg retrieval would be thirty-six

---

* Meaning "intramuscular," referring to a shot administered directly into a muscle.

hours after Remy took the trigger shot. Describing the retrieval, she said, "It's a seventeen-gauge needle, one stick per ovary. The risks are small; bleeding, infection, injury to organs is minimal. The embryologist stands next to me while I aspirate the follicle. She looks to see if there's an egg, and if she got the egg I move to the next follicle. We keep going until we get all the eggs."

Dr. Lewis shifted on her stool and continued. After the procedure, she explained, the embryologist would determine how many of Remy's retrieved eggs were mature and thus would be frozen; typically, more eggs are extracted than are frozen (more on this in chapter 8). A nurse would call Remy later in the day to let her know how many of her eggs were successfully put on ice.

When they got to discussing sedation, Remy got excited. This was the aspect of the procedure on which she had a lot of expertise.

"We usually do Versed, propofol, fentanyl," Dr. Lewis was saying, except she said it in one breath, so it sounded like "Versedpropofolfentanyl." Most patients undergoing an egg retrieval are put under moderate sedation with IV medications to keep them still and comfortable.* "You can talk to the anesthesiologist, but if people don't do all three, they tend to move around a lot and it makes it hard for me to get the eggs."

Dr. Lewis went on, explaining that the retrieval would take about twenty minutes and that the follicles holding Remy's eggs are quite fragile. As she spoke, I imagined it to be like sticking the tiniest needle into the tiniest water balloon to extract an even tinier particle. "So if I take the needle and you flinch even a little bit, it pops and I miss the egg. So I need you to just not wiggle."

Remy nodded. "Be in Zen. Got it."

Listening to Dr. Lewis and Remy discuss egg freezing specifics, I realized that Remy had a leg up thanks to working in medicine. She'd been downplaying being a doctor during her appointments at the fertility clinic but was so clearly in her element here. The two physi-

* Sedation options can vary depending on the clinic and the resources available to them. In some cases, stronger medications are used to create a deeper level of sedation, including up to general anesthesia.

cians spouted off names of drugs and protocols, abbreviations rolling off their tongues. I scribbled down acronyms and made a mental note to add them to my list of egg freezing terms to look up.

Dr. Lewis looked at the clipboard on her lap, sliding her finger down a list. "Couple more general things to go over," she said. "Avoid caffeine and alcohol when you start injections."

Remy sprang forward in her chair. "Wait. No coffee? Really?"

"I'm sorry, yes."

"A hundred percent no caffeine?" Remy looked visibly distressed. She sighed. "Oh, gosh. Okay."

"Yeah, alcohol's iffy, but caffeine's a big one. There was a study that showed even under thirty milligrams of caffeine a day affected outcomes."

"Alcohol's not a problem. Giving up this"—Remy held up her smoked rosemary latte—"is going to be the problem." She paused. "But I'll do it."

By the time another nurse came in for the final portion of the appointment, Remy's head was spinning. "So much paperwork! So many different scenarios that might happen," she said, wide-eyed, looking at me sitting rather deflated in the other chair. She sat up and arched her back against the chair, her long legs stretching out in front of her. The stack of forms in her lap was mounting. She was glad she'd remembered to move her crystals from the pocket of her scrubs, where she normally carried them, to the pocket of the shirt she'd put on that morning. She had four with her today: moonstone, helpful with transitions and new beginnings, supports all stages of pregnancy, childbirth, and fertility; elestial amethyst for empowerment; black tourmaline to feel grounded amid change; and fossil ammonite, evolution of the body and soul. A happy fertility combo pack—that's how Remy thought of them. The moonstone was roughly the size and shape of an ovary. She carried the crystals on her body most days and meditated with them most nights. Tactile and cool to the touch, they gave her something concrete to feel, to focus on.

An hour later, the nurse had walked Remy through the medications, demonstrating how to prepare and inject the hormone shots into her abdomen. Syringes, needles, vials. There was so much to remember—and she'd gone to medical school, for goodness sake! She told me she couldn't imagine a person who'd never before administered a shot going through this, and, honestly, I had to agree. We both felt drained, overloaded with information. The last part of the morning's appointment was more blood work down the hall. Remy took a deep breath and brought her hands to her head, pushing her hair back. She glanced over at me. "This is a completely overwhelming process," she announced, her tone both declarative and resigned. Then she quickly stood up from the chair before the fatigue could settle in.

The Pill's Power—and Unintended Consequences

A common question many potential egg freezers ask is, "What if I'm on birth control?" Beyond the surface-level pragmatic answer—most IUDs don't need to be removed; users of the Pill will simply stop taking it before freezing—is a more important matter: the relationship between hormonal birth control and fertility. Understanding this relationship required a working knowledge of something I knew very little about: hormones.

If there were a class called Egg Freezing 101 (there should be), hormones would be covered in the first week. That's how fundamental a role they play in a person's health, including fertility. Many women know something about hormones only in the context of their choice of birth control, which makes sense, because taking hormonal contraceptives is a common way women change up the balance of hormones in their bodies—to prevent pregnancy, to combat acne, to make painful periods more bearable. Artificially altering the mix of chemical signals in a woman's body, however, often masks the effect of those alterations, which makes it nearly impossible for her to understand how her hormones operate in a natural, non-synthetic state.

Around the end of the nineteenth century and the beginning of the twentieth, scientists began to discover the chemicals that regulate various functions in the human body, including reproduction. The word "hormone" was coined in 1905; in the 1920s, human chorionic gonadotropin, or hCG—a hormone found in high concentrations in pregnant women—was identified. Hormones are chemical messengers that travel through the bloodstream to different parts of the body. Hormones fluctuate, increasing and subsiding, and in so doing they influence the body in far-reaching and powerful ways, regulating heart rate, appetite, mood, reproduction, sleep cycle, growth and development, and more. You are your hormones. It sounds trite, but it's no exaggeration. Of the fifty or so hormones in the human body, estrogen and progesterone—the predominant sex hormones for women—are two of the most important ones connected to reproduction. To explain them, I need to go back to ovaries.

Ovaries are organs and part of the female reproductive system. An ovary is most similar in size and shape to a small walnut. At birth, you'll recall, ovaries contain around one million to two million immature egg cells, or oocytes, all held within follicles—those tiny, fluid-filled sacs—and after puberty a single follicle from the group of available follicles is "selected" as the dominant one each month and recruited for ovulation. A view inside a woman's ovaries reveals follicles, resembling a honeycomb, with their enclosed microscopic egg cells, in every stage of resting or growing. Zoom in closer and there are the granulosa cells, a halo of even smaller cells surrounding each egg that are essential to its development.* In addition to housing oocytes, ovaries also direct several key operations—most notably, menstruation. The menstrual cycle is more than just a woman's period; it is her reproductive system's rhythmic changes. This cycle is like having an additional vital sign, similar to blood pressure or pulse. All the changes that occur throughout her menstrual cycle are governed by hormones. And where are the two crucial fertility hormones, estrogen and progesterone, produced? In the ovaries.

Let's start with estrogen. There are three main naturally occurring estrogens—estradiol, estriol, and estrone—that play an important role

---

* Along with producing hormones and nurturing the developing egg, granulosa cells play a role in deciding which eggs live, which die, and which are ovulated.

in growth and reproductive development. Estradiol is the most common type of estrogen in reproductive-age women (and the one people are usually referring to when they talk about estrogen) and the one I'm going to tell you about. It's produced primarily in the ovaries, specifically within the follicles, and is involved in reproduction, menstruation, and menopause.

If estrogen is a woman's superhero sex hormone, then progesterone is its trusty sidekick, helping to regulate her monthly cycle and prepare her uterus in case of pregnancy. Estrogen is primarily secreted in the first part of a woman's cycle, peaking around ovulation. Progesterone picks up where estrogen leaves off, alerting the uterus that an incoming fertilized egg may be on its way. In a normal menstrual cycle, the hypothalamus works with the pituitary—a pea-sized gland at the base of the brain—to send a signal to the ovaries to start making estrogen and progesterone and stimulate follicle growth. Then, as I mentioned earlier, a single follicle is selected to grow a mature egg for fertilization. The anointed follicle begins to secrete estrogen. The brain waits for the estrogen level to be high enough for long enough, which is its sign that there's a dominant follicle containing a mature egg. Once the brain is alerted to the fact that there's a mature egg, it sends out another signal to the ovaries, triggering ovulation. The follicle bursts. The egg breaks free, and its journey toward the uterus begins. The other, non-dominant follicles begin to break down, and the uterus starts readying itself for the possible arrival of a fertilized egg.

It's amazing, really, how every month a woman's body readies itself for a potential pregnancy. There's a flurry of activity going on there pretty much all the time. I imagine a symphony: My reproductive system is one section of the orchestra and my brain the conductor, eliciting every note that's played by way of hormones.* The music that results from this feedback loop between my brain and ovaries (well: ovary) is determined by the cyclical changes in my hormones—especially estrogen and progesterone—which control which of my

* The orchestra's other sections: the liver, skin, immune system, kidney, heart, lungs, and muscles.

follicles are selected and develop, the release of my eggs, and my uterus primping and preparing to perform its duties as hostess in case a fertilized egg cozies up there. The orchestra could not play, would not *be,* without its conductor's ability to wave its baton.*

Human sexual reproduction is exquisitely complex. It's truly remarkable that any of us gets born. This is not part of the messaging of grade school sex ed classes, which more or less scare young people into thinking that sex equates to unwanted pregnancy every time clothes come off. The reality is, while all I've described above is happening, the story becomes even more intricate. A sperm has to make a long and difficult journey to meet a woman's ripe egg, which has made its own shorter but equally arduous trip. Millions of sperm battle to reach and penetrate the egg. After beating out its other sperm competitors, only one will break through the egg's outer layer—think of a pea going into a basketball—and this is the magic moment: fertilization.

But we're talking about what happens if there is not, in fact, a magic moment. If the star-of-the-show egg hasn't been fertilized by the sperm and there is nothing to implant in the endometrium, the egg dissolves and the uterus begins to shed the lining that it has been developing to receive a fertilized egg. A woman's period, or monthly bleeding, is the shedding of the endometrial lining. That's why the arrival of a woman's period is usually a sign she's not pregnant.

As we've just seen, virtually every part of this delicate symphony is run by hormones. And so no matter what she is using it for, hormonal birth control transforms the regulatory systems in a woman's body in a sweeping way, which can have all kinds of intended and unintended consequences.

One of those unintended consequences, it turns out, is why I'm here telling this story.

---

* For more on this remarkable feedback loop of intercellular communication involving the brain, eggs, and ovaries—and for a fascinating exploration of female anatomy in general—I highly recommend the book *Vagina Obscura* by Rachel E. Gross, in which she describes the ovary as being, beyond just a basket of eggs, "a crackling network of communication, alive with signals that pass back and forth between follicles."

. . .

After my first emergency surgery, doctors told me that while it was unusual and unfortunate that I'd needed to have an ovary and fallopian tube removed, my chances of becoming pregnant naturally weren't affected by my loss of one ovary. Once I began menstruating, about a year later, my periods were more or less regular; in a miracle of compensation, my other ovary took over, popping out an egg each month. Life resumed, and I happily went back to sports, friends, and my adolescence. Years later, though, trying to piece together my particular situation and the chain of events that caused me to almost lose my remaining ovary became an important pit stop on my journey to make a decision about egg freezing.

The summer after my sophomore year of college, a boy I adored and I broke up. We'd dated on and off for a year. There were nights staying up until dawn talking about music and sharing playlists and days spent draped on the couch together reading books like *Moby-Dick* for a favorite literature class. We enrolled in the same astronomy course only to get in the bad habit of skipping most of the early morning classes; I loved stars, but I loved staying in bed with him more. Once, after one of our "off" periods, he asked my roommate to let him into our apartment while I was out and I came home to rose petals scattered throughout my room, a love note on my pillow. He was a dreamer and I was in my Kerouac phase, enthralled by sensitive hearts and sharp minds like his. I was pretty sure we were in love, pretty sure I'd never felt so alive with anyone, and then we went home for the summer. Suddenly, all the miles between us made communicating feel like a chore; our intense connection seemed like a fire that burned too bright too fast. The relationship sputtered until, for reasons I'm not sure either of us understood at the time, it was over in the same whirlwind way it had begun.

Back on campus in the fall, I found myself thinking about him every morning when I took my birth control pill. The constant reminder that he and I were no longer having sex grew more and more frustrating until one day I chucked my pink pack of pills in the trash. No reason to continue taking the Pill if I'm not having sex and not at

risk of getting pregnant, I figured. I'd soon be leaving to spend a semester abroad in Ghana, and so, with some degree of petulance, I
decided not to bother going to the trouble of filling a prescription of
several months' worth of pills to take with me.

When I was prescribed the Pill at my college's student health center, several months before that breakup, I didn't have a conversation
with the nurse practitioner about its possible side effects—mood
swings, bloating, spotting—and I didn't know to ask. I knew the Pill
helped protect against pregnancy; that was why I wanted to go on it.
But I didn't understand how it prevented ovulation by interfering
with the natural balance of hormones in my body. And I definitely
didn't know that it suppressed the formation of ovarian cysts.

This would turn out to be something I really wish I had known.

Until I understood what it was, the word "cyst" made me think
of tumors and cancer. But "cyst" is a generic term for a fluid-filled
structure that can form almost anywhere in the body. And most
ovarian cysts, it turns out, are common by-products of ovulation;
they're actually part of the follicle that the egg comes from. These
functional cysts, as they're called, are found in nearly all women who
have a normal menstrual cycle—except those who are on hormonal
birth control. So, just to be clear, premenopausal women who *are*
ovulating and *are not* on hormonal birth control tend to develop
ovarian cysts.

Quick recap: Ovaries contain follicles. Follicles hold eggs. At any
given time, there are follicles at all stages of development in a woman's
ovaries. Ovulation occurs when a follicle releases an egg, every month
or so. After a complex series of interactions between the brain and the
hormones in the ovaries, the follicle housing the egg bursts and the
egg is released.

Once the egg has vacated the premises, the left-behind follicle seals
itself off and morphs into a yellow, fatty-looking structure known as
the corpus luteum. So this mass of cells has a new name, and it has a
new job as well. If pregnancy occurs, the corpus luteum continues
making progesterone, a hormone that stimulates the uterus to thicken
in preparation to receive the incoming fertilized egg. If pregnancy

doesn't occur, the corpus luteum stops producing progesterone, begins to break down, and, after about fourteen days, disappears. As progesterone levels drop, the uterus gets the message that there's no need for lining this month, and a woman gets her period. But sometimes, instead of shrinking away, the corpus luteum lingers and grows, filled with light yellow fluid. This buildup causes a corpus luteum cyst. This is one type of functional ovarian cyst; the other, a follicular cyst, forms when the follicle stays intact, instead of rupturing and releasing its egg. Sounds a bit aggressive, but functional ovarian cysts are usually harmless, rarely cause pain, and often go away on their own within a few months of forming.

It's when one of these normally-not-a-big-deal cysts swells up with too much fluid and becomes abnormally large, doesn't shrink away, and/or bleeds into itself that there starts to be cause for concern. That's where, in my case, things got tricky. For a long time after my second surgery, I wondered why an overgrown, blood-filled cyst had developed on my ovary and if there was any definitive explanation for the medical emergency it led to. There isn't. But as I learned more about how the Pill works, I grew suspicious. I'd been told that my abruptly going off the Pill several months before I landed in the emergency room very likely had something to do with why I almost lost my remaining ovary. I accepted this as fact when my doctors explained it to me in my post-surgery haze. I was still in a considerable amount of pain. I felt very, very grateful I still had my ovary. At the time, I didn't really want to fully understand what had transpired to land me there. Now, though, I'm able to explain.

I talked earlier about the considerable impact the Pill has had in the more than sixty years it's been around. On a more micro level, it's also had a tremendous impact on the biology of every person who has taken it. The Pill—which, in case you haven't seen one lately, is about half the size of an Altoid—doesn't just block sperm from reaching an egg; it changes the entire internal landscape of a woman's body. Tens of thousands of studies have explored how hormones influence behavior, and there's evidence that the Pill impacts several bodily systems, affecting everything from sexual behavior to appetite to emotion regulation to whom we're attracted to.* Members of my generation are among the first to be on long-term birth control for the majority of our adult lives; from the minute we're sexually active until we decide to start trying to become pregnant, many of us are "on" hormones. Birth control pills are used today by roughly 20 percent of the country's women using contraception. It took some time for reproductive biologists to figure out what the Pill was best used for, and for that reason it has a colorful history of off-label uses. Before Enovid received government approval to be sold as a birth control pill, for example, it was marketed as a cure for irregular menstrual cycles. But while doctors puzzled over the precise explanations for the Pill's effects, all that the over half a million women who started taking it "off-label" needed to know was that it prevented pregnancy.

Here's how it works. The Pill relies on synthetic hormones to prevent ovulation and thus pregnancy. "Synthetic" hormones, those produced in a lab, are modified to *imitate* natural hormones. Women's bodies, you'll recall, make estrogen and progesterone on their own. In a normal menstrual cycle, levels of these sex hormones fluctuate up and down. When you take the Pill, these fluctuations stop and levels are kept stable. Hormones, as I've said, are chemical messengers, facilitating communication between cells throughout the body. The Pill alters the normal feedback loop between the brain and the body. The ovaries don't get the message from the pituitary gland to make estrogen and progesterone, and the brain, in turn, isn't told by the ovaries to continue the cycle, so it stops directing the ovaries to select and develop a dominant follicle and release an egg. That's why women

---

* It does not, however, affect a woman's fertility long-term. That's a myth—a pervasive one, I've found. While it makes sense that many women believe that years and years of being on the Pill and suppressing their ability to conceive would, surely, have some sort of enduring impact on their fertility once they stop taking it—it doesn't. Using hormonal contraception, regardless of the type or duration, does not have a negative effect on a woman's ability to get pregnant after she stops using it. Among the many large studies on this topic, one that looked at almost nine thousand planned pregnancies found that those who had never used oral contraceptives (birth control pills) conceived at the same rates as those who had used oral contraceptives for five years or more.

who take hormonal birth control don't ovulate. (You're neither killing off nor "saving" the extra eggs; you're just not using them.)

Most birth control pills contain a synthetic estrogen, usually ethinyl estradiol, and a synthetic progesterone, called progestin. These synthetic hormones, taken in the form of the Pill, do some pretty heavy lifting to stop a woman's ovaries from releasing eggs and make the uterus inhospitable. They thicken her cervical mucus, which makes it difficult for sperm to reach the egg in the first place. They also keep the lining of the uterus thin, which discourages a fertilized egg from implanting there.* So, there's no egg in the tube, the sperm's already treacherous journey becomes nearly impossible, and the uterus becomes a far cry from a cozy, safe cocoon. When the egg and sperm can't get together, pregnancy can't happen. (And if, against all odds, they somehow still managed to connect, they wouldn't last long in such an inhospitable meeting place.)

The Pill does all this by suppressing the release of two other naturally occurring hormones: follicle-stimulating hormone (FSH) and luteinizing hormone (LH), both produced in the brain's pituitary gland. Remember how the brain sends signals to the ovaries to develop follicles and release eggs? FSH and LH are those signals. FSH stimulates follicle growth and tells the ovary to recruit and mature an egg. LH is the surge that indicates ovulation is about to occur; it sets ovulation in motion by telling the ovary to release the mature egg. So, the Pill's synthetic estrogen suppresses FSH, preventing a dominant follicle from developing, and the Pill's progestin suppresses LH, blocking ovulation. And no ovulation means not getting pregnant.

In short: When used correctly, the synthetic hormones in hormonal birth control prevent a woman's ovaries from developing follicles and releasing eggs (ovulation), which in turn prevents the growth and shedding of her uterine lining (the natural period). The Pill in essence short-circuits the brain and stops a few key aspects of the body's usual hormonal cycling, typically a delicately controlled equi-

---

* The body's natural forms of estrogen and progesterone make the uterus a hospitable place to grow a fetus; the synthetic forms of these hormones override the system, doing the opposite.

librium. The symphony has stopped, the music replaced by an entirely different composition of the powerful chemicals the Pill contains.

Bye, natural hormones. Tag, you're it, synthetic hormones.

There are hundreds of brands of birth control pills on the market, and new ones come out often. Most women take their doctor's recommendation for which kind to take and usually try a few different brands before finding one to stick with. The variety can be daunting. It's not all that easy to find the right hormone dosage, especially considering that birth control pills use different types and varying potencies of synthetic progesterone and/or estrogen. Women are encouraged to experiment with different brands of the Pill, which makes it sound fun even though it's not. The Pill's positive side effects are great ones: For many women, it eases cramps and PMS, clears up acne, and makes periods lighter and more regular. (The Pill's negative side effects, which plenty of women are familiar with, are not so great; more on that shortly.) A "period" while on the Pill, by the way, is actually called withdrawal bleeding—it's not a real period. But even though the Pill effectively puts a woman's natural hormone rhythm into sleep mode, her body still reacts when her hormone levels drop, which happens* when she takes the placebo pills at the end of the pack.* In the case of both withdrawal bleeding and a period, the decrease in hormones causes the mucus and lining of the uterus to shed and exit through the vagina. So this fake "period," while typically lighter and shorter than the real thing, can still cause PMS symptoms in some women, including headaches, nausea, mood swings, and sore breasts. These are more common in the first few months of being on the Pill and usually—but not always—go away, or a woman simply gets used to them.

No ovulation means no egg to be fertilized. It also means follicles

---

* Placebo pills—part of some but not all regimens—are placeholders; the idea is that if a woman stays in the habit of taking a pill every day, she'll be less likely to forget when she needs to take the real thing. Even though she's taking placebo pills, she's still protected against pregnancy as long as she's been taking the active pills as prescribed. Some women opt to go on a continuous-cycle birth control pill and skip placebo pills and having a light, fake period altogether.

don't grow; they're hibernating, so to speak. And no mature follicles means no corpus luteum—and no functional ovarian cysts. Ah. This very small fact—that, in addition to everything else it does, the Pill helps reduce the size of ovarian cysts and sometimes prevents them from forming at all—is, for me, a crucial piece of information that I did not have when it mattered most.

Decades ago, doctors learned that women taking birth control pills had fewer cysts, since the hormones in the Pill typically stop follicles from developing. Here's the bit I really wish I'd had some inkling about: that going *off* the Pill and waking follicles from their deep slumber can lead to a functional cyst growing too large, which in turn can cause the ovary to twist (remember that kinked garden hose?). Ovarian torsion, an uncommon but serious condition, must be treated quickly. If it's not, in rare cases it can result in the loss of an ovary—because the twisting cannot be undone.

I certainly didn't know any of this when I was in college and going on, and then suddenly off, the Pill. But I believe I should have. I prided myself on being an informed and self-aware young woman, attuned to matters of body and health. But when it came to hormones, my reproductive system, and birth control, I was mostly clueless.

It's only as an adult that I've come to understand the chain of events that led to my second surgery and how the stakes got so high. Piecing things together only happened after several long afternoons on my hands and knees, sifting through my medical records on the floor and trying to understand their contents. I'd emerge dizzy from doctor notes and jargon I could barely comprehend. One day, I called the hospital where I'd had my first surgery. I was pleasantly surprised to learn they still had my records—seventeen years after the fact—and would be happy to mail them to me. My college's health center had kept my records, too; they emailed a copy to me when I asked. Looking them over, I noticed that the nurse who prescribed the Pill to me that day had made a note about the fact that I only had one ovary, but I don't remember us talking about my girlhood surgery. It didn't occur to me at the time to ask her to describe in detail the connection between ovaries and birth control. But I wish the nurse had mentioned, even briefly, that the Pill did other things besides prevent pregnancy.

Now, of course, I'm clear: The pill I swallow each morning prevents most cysts from growing too large or even existing at all. And so for women concerned about troublesome ovarian cysts, birth control pills are extremely helpful. In my case, having only one ovary makes the Pill's risk-reduction power especially important. My doctors agree, and they've explained that I need to stay on the Pill until I am ready to become pregnant. I went back on it over a decade ago, almost immediately after my second surgery. These small pills are a daily reminder of my surgeries, my missing ovary, and my promising though uncertain fertility future.

But at the core of my complicated feelings is some degree of confusing self-blame. I realize that if I had lost my ovary—and with it, my ability to have biological children—it would have been at least partially my fault. I simply should have known better than to abruptly stop taking a prescribed medication without consulting a doctor (who hopefully would have consulted my chart or asked about any surgical history and advised me well—though there's no guarantee that would have happened). My surgeries were the result of much that was out of my control. And yet. I should have known something, anything, about how hormones work, about my ovaries—the one I'd lost and the one I'd kept. Something, anything, about the basics of birth control. It's my body, after all. As a woman, as an educated medical consumer, I should have known better. In hindsight, chucking that pack of pills in the trash was reckless. But I have sympathy for this younger me. How *could* she have known if she didn't know what to ask, and whom?

Messing with my hormones and birth control pills had consequences. If there is a moral to my story, it's that. Not every woman has such a complex saga when it comes to her ovaries. But many have a muddled relationship with birth control, a personal story about going on or off hormonal contraceptives. A gruesome IUD insertion story. Getting pregnant despite having a contraceptive implant. Being prescribed the Pill as a teenager to make painful periods more bearable. Finally getting off the Pill and feeling so much better.

My story is just one extreme example of how surprisingly little women know about birth control. Whether or not a woman uses hormonal contraception, and whether or not she wants to have children, understanding how hormones regulate her body and impact her fertility is important.

Pills and patches and rings—oh my. There are *so* many ways a woman can suppress her reproductive system. Here's a non-exhaustive list of the myriad contraceptive methods women use (some being much more common these days than others):

- Surgical sterilization procedures: tubal ligation (tying, clipping, or blocking a woman's fallopian tubes) and partial or total tubal removal (completely taking out the fallopian tubes)*
- Fertility awareness–based methods (more on these in chapter 6)
- Oral contraceptives (broadly known as the Pill)
- Intrauterine device, or IUD (two types: hormonal and non-hormonal)
- Patch: a thin beige square that looks like a bandage and is adhered to the skin; it delivers hormones and is changed once a week
- Shot: a progestin injection once every three months
- Implant: a plastic rod the size of a matchstick that contains progestin, is placed under the skin in the upper arm, is invisible, and typically lasts three years
- Vaginal ring: a small, flexible piece of latex-free plastic that delivers hormones and is inserted into the vagina once a month

---

* I was surprised to learn that female sterilization is the most popular birth control method for women—more popular than the Pill, even—both in the United States and worldwide. For most women who opt to have their fallopian tubes tied to prevent pregnancy, they've had all the children they want to have.

- Spermicide: products that work by killing sperm and are placed in the vagina just before sex; come in several forms (creams, gels, suppositories, and more)
- Diaphragm: a flexible, shallow, saucer-shaped cup (typically made of silicone) that's inserted in the vagina before sex; reusable; must be used with spermicide
- Cervical cap: a deep, bowl-shaped silicone cup (smaller than a diaphragm) that's inserted into the vagina and fits snugly over the cervix; reusable; must be used with spermicide
- Sponge: a small round piece of thick, soft plastic foam that's inserted in the vagina before sex; disposable; must be used with spermicide
- Female condom (also called internal condom): a small nitrile (synthetic rubber) pouch that's inserted in the vagina before sex

As for available birth control options for men, there are three: condom, withdrawal* ("pulling out," which works until it doesn't), and surgical sterilization (vasectomy).†

About 65 percent of reproductive-age women in the United States use contraception. Interestingly, four in ten women also use contraception for reasons other than avoiding pregnancy, such as managing a medical condition or preventing STIs. The most common birth control methods are ones that rely on hormones—the Pill and long-acting reversible contraceptives (the IUD, patch, implant, shot, and vaginal ring)—as well as male condoms and female or male sterilization. Besides surgical sterilization, the Pill is the most widely used form of birth control in the United States, but the IUD is increasingly

* There's a lot of room for error with "coitus interruptus," aka the withdrawal method, when a man withdraws his penis before ejaculating. It is not as effective at preventing pregnancy as most other forms of birth control; about one in five people who rely on the withdrawal method for birth control becomes pregnant. It also doesn't protect against STIs.

† Researchers have created a birth control pill for male mice, which proved 99 percent effective in preventing pregnancy, but experts say male birth control pills won't be available anytime soon. An injectable hydrogel that's marketed as "the IUD for men" recently completed clinical trials.

popular, as well as one of the most effective contraceptive methods on the planet. The idea of being on little to no hormones is what makes the IUD such an appealing alternative to the Pill for so many women; more than six million women in the United States have IUDs. It's a T-shaped piece of plastic, about an inch long, that's inserted into the uterus. There are two kinds. The hormonal IUD—Mirena is the most common—releases a type of progestin into the uterus; the device stays in a woman's body for about eight years. The non-hormonal IUD, called Paragard, is effective for about ten years; it's often referred to simply as "the copper IUD" because of the copper wrapped around the T-shaped flexible plastic. Sperm, as it happens, don't like copper; Paragard's copper ions change the way sperm cells move so they can't swim to an egg.

Despite their prevalence, we don't talk much about why hormonal contraceptive methods make many of the hundreds of millions of women around the world who use them feel crummy. That's partly because we don't know a whole lot about their myriad psychological and behavioral effects.* Hormonal contraception is known, however, to precipitate or perpetuate mood disorders, including depression, in some women. And, in addition to its impact on a woman's mental state, hormonal birth control—estrogen-containing oral contraceptives, in particular—is associated with a few more serious health risks, including breast cancer, blood clots, and strokes. Less serious but more common are spotting, headaches, acne, and cramps. Needless to say, these aren't inconsequential side effects. Not that women are complaining. The less serious but still unpleasant side effects are sure more manageable than an unplanned pregnancy. I once saw a meme that put it like this: "Birth control be like well do u want depression or do u want a baby" and, honestly, that just about sums it up.

When a woman freezes her eggs, she injects fertility drugs that generally work like the body's natural hormones that command ovulation. It's these pricey hormone shots that run the entire operation.

* But we do know that many women struggle to find any form of hormonal birth control that they're happy with and often stay on hormonal birth control despite the way it makes them feel.

Most reproductive technologies rely on the ability to manipulate hormones, and it's this ability that also makes it possible to have this totally new, but increasingly mainstream, conversation about egg freezing and fertility preservation. Consider, for a moment, just how incredible it is to be able to regulate your fertility. What was once a story about contraception and prevention, about Sanger and her fellow birth control revolutionaries, is now a story about intervention—and about *more*. More eggs, more control, more time.

Remy: Handle with Care

A few weeks after her egg freezing orientation, a box of fertility medications arrived on Remy's doorstep. FedEx, overnight from Florida. Red FRAGILE, HANDLE WITH CARE stickers on every side. The package happened to come just as Remy was getting home from an overnight shift—which was lucky, since a few of the medications needed to be refrigerated right away. She thanked the delivery person and, yawning, fished for her keys in her bag. Her long blond hair hung in a low messy ponytail, her moss-colored eyes smudged with mascara she'd hastily applied fourteen hours earlier.

Remy was ready to start. She'd tossed and turned the past several nights, her mind racing with possible scenarios of how the whole freezing procedure might go. Thinking through logistics usually calmed her, but there were too many unknowns right now to feel good about the process. Anticipating how she was going to manage fitting in the daily shots during her upcoming weeks of night shifts at the hospital was activating her brain's control-freak wiring. Walking into her house, though, soothed her, as it usually did. Remy had begun to nest as soon as she moved in, intent on making the small one-story house feel cozy. Now it felt like her bohemian sanctuary. Shoes stacked neatly in the cubby by the door. Peloton in the office, in front of her framed diplomas. White shag rug. Small bottles of essential oils. Several sets of blue scrubs in a chair, neatly folded. A gigantic wall calendar made of glass, covered in writing from dry-erase markers: *Injection Day* 7 scrawled in red, *Egg Retrieval Day!* marked with hearts, squares labeled *Bills* and *Budget* off to the side.

She carried the box to her kitchen and opened it, pulling out the contents item by item: vials of fertility drugs, pills in orange bottles, ice packs, syringes, alcohol swabs, needles, a red sharps container, and a receipt. For most women freezing their eggs, the sight of these medical supplies could be daunting. For Remy, though, the wow factor was zero. Still, there had been a bit of a learning curve, getting clear on the medications and how exactly she'd be injecting them into her body.

With the arrival of the fertility meds, egg freezing suddenly felt more real than ever. Remy already thought of her eggs as her future babies. Maybe it was her faith in the universe talking instead of her faith in medicine, but a few weeks earlier, when a pregnant patient asked Remy if she had kids herself, Remy had replied: "Not yet—but they're getting frozen shortly." Blond, blue-eyed babes, she hoped they'd be. She even had names picked out.

The sound of birds chirping outside the window above the kitchen sink meant it was past time for her to be in bed. She opened the fridge and pushed aside a few things to make room for the egg freezing drugs and, one by one, carefully placed the cardboard boxes of meds inside. On the counter, she arranged the non-refrigerated meds alongside the syringes, alcohol swabs, and sharps container, and surrounded the pile with four small crystals—black, light green, orange, purple. *Gotta let these meds marinate,* she thought. Her injections were here. She was nervous—but so excited.

5

Why Women Freeze

~~~~~~

Egg Freezing Appointment #2

Like many people, I've spent much of my adult life trying not to get pregnant. And like a lot of people with uteruses, I've long been nervous about it happening accidentally. But at the same time, I've been anxious about the fact that I'm not certain I *can* have biological children, since I've never been or tried to become pregnant—and the only true test of fertility is conceiving a baby. I'm aware of this continual contradiction: I want to protect my ovary, but I do not want to let it do what it was made for. Not now, anyway. These connected yet contrary worries have troubled me for more than a decade.

A memory: It's the middle of the night, the summer after college. I wake suddenly and sit up in bed, clutching my side, the cramp sharp and hot. I'm twenty-two and halfway across the world, traveling through Sri Lanka with my boyfriend of six months. We're in a house on the outskirts of Colombo. He's asleep next to me, his feet pushing against the mosquito net. I sit up, reach around for my headlamp, then slip out of bed and walk barefoot into the bathroom, where I swallow a couple of over-the-counter pain pills. In the kitchen, I put the kettle on for tea and boot up our laptop. My surgeries have left me hypersensitive and somewhat distrusting of my body; for me, pain is often indicative of a deeper problem. I've had cramps for the past two days but don't know if they are related to my cycle on the Pill or if they are the less frequent but more painful cramps caused by the scar tissue that has built up since my first surgery.

But what I'm really afraid of is that it's neither of these things. And so for what feels like the hundredth time, I type "signs you are pregnant" into Google. My periods had been irregular for years—the real periods I had before I got on the Pill, and the fake ones while on it— which made it hard to know whether I was late or it was just my cycle that was off. For a long time, I didn't understand why I still bled a bit every month or so if I wasn't ovulating, since I was on the Pill. (I hadn't yet learned about withdrawal bleeding.) And during our travels around balmy, humid Sri Lanka, it had been difficult to remember to refrigerate my birth control pills. The heat, the doctor who'd prescribed them had warned me, could make them less effective. It used to be that sharp pain in my lower abdomen only made me worry I might have another cyst threatening ovarian torsion. But since I started having sex, I worried that anything more than a mild ache near my abdomen meant either that I was about to lose my ovary or that I was pregnant. When the cramps subsided, my worries did, too—until the next time it happened and the anxiety spiral repeated itself.

One night months later, in another part of Sri Lanka, I found myself in the back of a tuk-tuk speeding to a hospital. I remember the hot, spiced air and my lower left pelvic area feeling as though it were on fire. My ovary, I'd convinced myself, was twisting, again, under the weight of another cyst. In the emergency room, I waited for hours, my thoughts spiraling. *What if I lose my remaining ovary? What if I really cannot have babies?* In a poorly lit exam room, I described the throbbing to a slightly taken-aback doctor. I explained what I needed him to do, and when he wheeled in the ultrasound machine—which looked as if it hadn't been used since the 1980s—I sighed in relief, nodding. This piece of medical technology has, on three different continents, conveyed to me what is happening within my reproductive system. It's not always good news, but this time it was: The doctor saw nothing abnormal. I left the hospital that night with one more black-and-white photograph to add to my collection. The mental seesawing—anxiously suppressing my fertility now, anxiously worrying about my ability to conceive in the future—would continue for years.

All of this was on my mind when, several months after my first appointment with Dr. Noyes, I called her office to schedule a second one. The nurse on the phone didn't remember me and asked me the usual questions. I was getting used to this—the repetitive back-and-forth, the questions about my fertility and desire to freeze eggs, my well-rehearsed answer about my one ovary. We scheduled the appointment and a few weeks later I was back in the waiting room at NYU Langone Fertility Center. More paperwork. Still single. This time, in addition to the regular questions, Dr. Noyes asked me a bunch of questions about my love life.

"You're smart, pretty, ambitious," Dr. Noyes said matter-of-factly. Then: "Why don't you have a boyfriend? You're so cute."

What are you supposed to say when a world-famous fertility doctor tells you you're cute—and asks why you're single?

"I—uh, thank you, Dr. Noyes."

"Well, I'm not worried about you, you're very young. But . . . I am surprised a little bit."

I cringed slightly at her comment (and, later, wondered why she'd made it at all). I felt some pressure to reassure this somewhat intimidating doctor that I occasionally went on dates, had a healthy sex drive, was mostly fine. I did not feel like telling her about the ham sandwich. I mumbled something about having a major crush on my brother's best friend, whom I'd known since I was nine years old and had lately been daydreaming about more than usual. About how witty and kind he was. About his meaningful work in international education. About the way he'd intently listen when we were having a conversation, the way he held my gaze and released it. About how—

"Oh, so you have a dream guy out there?" Dr. Noyes asked brightly.

"Well," I said weakly. I wanted to go back to talking about my ovary and fertility fears, which, compared to dissecting my personal life, struck me as very pleasant topics of conversation.

"Does he know?"

My face felt hot. Were my *dimples* blushing? It felt like it, even if dimples don't blush.

"He does, I think. Kind of. I—it's not easy talking about this."

Dr. Noyes waved her hand as if to sweep all the awkwardness out of her office. "Your life's on the right track," she said, closing the folder containing my medical records that had been lying open on her desk, as if the matter had been decided. I wrung my hands in my lap. At the moment, neither my life nor this appointment felt the least bit on track.

"Anyway, I remember you saying you definitely want biological children," she continued, getting back to safer ground. "And especially if you want more than one child, then we're probably gonna do two cycles. Because I want to have a really good number of eggs.

"Whether you freeze eggs or just bite the bullet and have a baby . . ." She paused, as if interrupted by nostalgia. "To go through life without kids—well, I really can't imagine my life without kids."

We got to the risks. What I was most worried about was overdoing it, hyperstimulating my ovary and causing irrevocable harm. "I'm just so nervous that if I do this and lose my one ovary . . . that's what really scares me," I said. "That's what's holding me back."

But Dr. Noyes had the confidence I was lacking. "I'm not at all worried about freezing your eggs," she announced. "Since I met you, I've done another three thousand. I'm not worried at all."

Three thousand what? I wondered, but didn't ask.

I was once again led to an exam room, where a nurse instructed me to undress and put on a thin soft gown. The strings dangled at my sides. I shivered; the gown's open front left me chilled. I lay on the table and slipped my heels into the stirrups, shifting my hips down before the nurse told me to.

"You've really done your homework," said Dr. Noyes as she squished lube onto the knob of the ultrasound wand and slid it inside me. It was cold and uncomfortable. I took a breath and tried to focus on the facts. The doctor examining me was one of the most respected in the field. She'd determined I was a good candidate for egg freezing. And while her demeanor could be a bit patronizing, I had to admit that her optimism—and clear enthusiasm for my ovary—was drawing me in. I glanced at the monitor, to where Dr. Noyes was motioning with her free hand. "Here's a picture of your ovary—whoops, sorry, it's this part that's the ovary. Okay?"

"Okay," I said, and there was something about the moment when Dr. Noyes found my ovary that allowed me to find my feelings about all this. I wanted to do it, I realized. I wanted to freeze my eggs. It felt good, such a relief, to decide. Legs spread wide, wand still inside my vagina, I told Dr. Noyes: "I'm going to do it. I'm going to freeze my eggs, here, with you, and it's gonna be great."

Mandy: "Ticking Time Bomb"

One June morning, thirty-year-old Mandy woke with a jolt. *Finally,* she thought, reaching for her phone to silence the alarm. After eleven days of hormone injections, the day of her egg retrieval was finally here. She'd been up late, hunched over her laptop checking egg freezing forums and reading blog posts with titles like "What to Expect on Retrieval Day." Had she done everything she was supposed to? With egg freezing, she'd learned, there wasn't much room for error. And yet the process seemed error prone. Just the day before, Mandy had opened the injections kit and realized the shot she was supposed to give herself that morning was missing. She then rushed to her doctor's office, where the nurse injected her with the Menopur she needed just in time.

Mandy's husband, Quincy, stirred next to her. She lay back in bed, knowing his phone would buzz soon; most mornings, they set their alarms five minutes apart. They'd both taken the day off from work. The outfit Mandy had picked out the night before lay waiting: black leggings and her favorite worn gray sweater. It was a warm early summer day in Oakland, California, where Mandy and Quincy lived, but she had been in enough chilly doctor's offices and exam rooms lately to know she'd be glad for the sweater.

Mandy was freezing her eggs at her doctors' urging. Two surgeries in her twenties had left her with half of one ovary and a quarter of the other. When Mandy was twenty, a dermoid cyst—a small, usually non-cancerous abnormal growth—on her right ovary ruptured, requiring emergency surgery. When she was twenty-eight, she had surgery to remove another dermoid cyst, on her left ovary. Unlike the more common follicular and corpus luteum cysts—the ones we talked about earlier that form in response to a woman's menstrual cycle—ovarian dermoid cysts are often present at birth, meaning they form in utero. They're not unusual but are removed if they grow too large or are at risk of rupturing, as Mandy's did.* She was lucky, doctors had told her more than once, to still have her ovaries—even if they were partial ones. A woman can still have babies with partial ovaries, but Mandy now faced an increased risk of trouble getting pregnant if and when she chose to.

It was after her second surgery that Mandy's doctor, worried about Mandy facing fertility issues, recommended she try to get pregnant sooner rather than later or consider freezing her eggs. Then, two years later, when Mandy was thirty, she learned she had a third ovarian dermoid cyst. A ticking time bomb if it was to grow like the others over the next few years—years in which Mandy's currently good eggs would start slowly diminishing. And if she needed to have yet another surgery to remove this cyst, her fertility could be further compromised. She needed to make a decision about egg freezing—now.

Mandy had first contacted me after what she referred to as "a Google-search spiral." An attempt to learn more about egg freezing after recalling the experts' advice had turned into a twisty, alarming deluge of unhelpful social media posts and aggressive ads that left her feeling overwhelmed. When she happened upon some of my articles on the subject, she got in touch right away. "The more I read, the more confused I get," Mandy said the first time we spoke on the phone. "I really can't tell if egg freezing is a good thing or a bad thing." Unable to distinguish marketing from medical advice, she was

* While ovarian dermoid cysts themselves are relatively common, it's extremely rare for one to rupture. The recurrence of bilateral dermoid cysts, a condition Mandy has, is also rare.

put off by what she found on the internet: fertility clinics with one-, two-, or five-star ratings; glamour shots of women next to their glowing egg freezing success stories; bitter writings detailing how the procedure had gone horribly wrong.

Having kids felt like a far-off possibility; Mandy and Quincy hadn't meaningfully broached the topic yet. Both Americans, the two had met in southeastern China while teaching English to high school students in a remote town in the province of Hunan. Eventually they moved back to the States, found jobs in the Bay Area, and got married. They began to save money and set goals. Things started to feel somewhat stable; Mandy and Quincy's shared life together was just beginning. They weren't ready to start a family just yet.

"It had always been, like, 'Oh, I have to go get my oil changed,'" Mandy told me when we first started talking. "'Figure out my ovary situation' was on my long-term to-do list." But it was time to make a decision. "I'm hoping that if I ignore the problem long enough, it will just go away," she said. I heard the tension in her voice, an inner conflict just beginning to bubble up. "But time is not on my side, especially with my medical history."

A few months after her thirtieth birthday, she decided to freeze her eggs.

At Mandy's initial consultation at Spring Fertility, the clinic she'd decided to go with, a doctor advised her to freeze embryos instead: combine Quincy's sperm with her eggs and put the resulting healthy embryos on ice. So that's what she'd do. Next, she attended a two-hour orientation at the clinic, where a nurse demonstrated to Mandy and several other women about to freeze eggs or embryos how to self-inject the drugs. There were boxes and vials of medications and various sizes of needles. Some meds needed refrigeration, others not. Some had to be taken at a certain time of day, others not. It was a lot of information and words Mandy had never heard before—too much for her to absorb. Later, at home, she turned to YouTube to get a grip on the process, watching hours of videos that explained, step by step, how to prepare and administer the shots. Fertility medications are usually injected either into the skin at the lower belly or upper thigh or into the muscle just above a butt cheek. Typically, ovaries are around one inch in diameter; during an egg freezing or IVF cycle, they increase to four to five inches, about the size of a clementine.* Mandy dreaded the painful shots so much that she wasn't able to do them herself; Quincy did them instead. The first injection hurt enough to make her cry, at which point she briefly considered abandoning the whole thing.† Quincy learned to go as slowly as possible with the needle so the shots hurt less.

Before long the nightly injections began to feel like a kind of ritual, and Mandy was surprised by how easily she and Quincy had fallen into such an odd routine. Each night around nine o'clock, for ten days, Mandy changed into her pajamas while Quincy surreptitiously prepared the shot in the kitchen. In the living room, Mandy lay on the couch with their dog, an Italian Greyhound Chihuahua mix named Doe, sometimes turning on Netflix to distract herself. She always looked away while Quincy iced and cleaned the bit of belly fat he'd inject the medication into.

On a warm night in late June, when Mandy's ovaries were lush with what she hoped were lots of mature eggs, Quincy injected the last injection—the trigger shot, a hormone called human chorionic gonadotropin, or hCG—just above Mandy's left butt cheek. It was exactly eleven o'clock. The timing of the trigger shot is crucial, whether the woman is preserving her eggs for later (egg freezing) or fertilizing them with sperm to become pregnant now (IVF). The follicles holding the eggs have been developing steadily throughout the days of hormone injections. The trigger shot is the final kicker, stimulating the eggs' final bit of maturation, and the carefully timed egg retrieval is thirty-six hours later.

The morning of her egg retrieval, Mandy dressed quickly and re-

---

* The degree to which a woman's ovaries enlarge during the process depends on her starting follicle count—that is, how many follicles she has when she begins fertility medications.

† Mandy learned later this wasn't a universal experience, and that many other egg freezers don't find the shots quite this painful.

read the procedure paperwork. In the kitchen, she glared at the cof-feemaker, as she had most mornings since she'd begun the egg freezing process and had to forgo caffeine and exercise.* Her phone lit up with a text message from her mother, part of it written in Chinese: *Go celebrate with Quincy after it's done,* it read. *Love you! I am with you, sweetie.* Mandy let the words and heart emojis on the screen sink in. It had been a long several days of needles. The egg retrieval seemed like the easy part after all those shots, she thought. It was also the only part of this process completely out of her hands. She would be under seda-tion and had no control over how many or how few eggs her ovaries had produced. As she puttered around the kitchen, a wave of exhaus-tion came over her. She was ready for all that had led up to today—the blood work and all the tests, the worry about success rates and probabilities, the feelings of being tired and bloated and anxious—to be over. *Tomorrow's going to be a regular day,* Mandy reminded herself, and for a moment she felt lighter. No more shots. No more stress. And all the coffee she wanted.

They piled into their reliable old Toyota Corolla, Quincy at the wheel. Mandy had gotten the car when she was in high school, a decade and a half earlier. She had driven it to take her SATs, to get married, and, now, to freeze her eggs. It was after rush hour and they had an hour to get into San Francisco to make her eleven o'clock ap-pointment. Plenty of time.

"Wait, what's going on?" said Mandy, leaning forward to better see out the windshield. Standstill traffic stretched along the San Francisco Bay Bridge—a massive traffic accident. She looked down at her phone. The maps app showed they were now due to arrive at the

---

* Ovaries enlarge during an egg freezing cycle, and the larger they become, the more vulnerable they are to ovarian torsion. Certain types of exercise heighten that risk. So, while taking the injectable egg freezing medications and for several days post egg retrieval, low-impact physical activities—walking, lifting light weights, gentle yoga—is okay. Strenuous exercise—CrossFit, running, any activity that requires jumping, twisting, or flipping the body—is not. As for caffeine, which is a stimulant that narrows the blood vessels and increases heart rate and blood pressure: The data on its effect on fertility is limited, but similar to how women trying to get pregnant are advised to stop or limit their caffeine consump-tion, women undergoing egg freezing and IVF are, too.

clinic half an hour late. She closed her eyes and tried to stay calm. No way was she going to miss her retrieval—a procedure for which she'd put several weeks of her life on hold—because of traffic.

Cars inched along. Quincy's hands were tight on the steering wheel. It was, Mandy thought, the longest hour she'd ever experienced.

Finally, Spring Fertility came into view.

In addition to aiding with age-related fertility issues, ART helps people overcome infertility problems caused by medical conditions. Some women freeze eggs and/or undergo IVF because of factors associated with female infertility such as ovulatory disorders, fallopian tube blockages, structural problems with the uterus, and low egg count. Two common diagnoses that can affect fertility are polycystic ovary syndrome, or PCOS, and endometriosis. PCOS, a disorder caused by hormonal imbalances in which a woman's ovaries develop many follicles but don't actually release an egg, can prevent ovulation. It affects about 10 percent of women in the United States, although experts estimate that more than 50 percent of women with PCOS remain undiagnosed. And endometriosis, a painful inflammatory condition in which tissue similar to uterine lining grows outside the uterus— roughly one in ten women of reproductive age in the United States have it—often interferes with ovulation and can lead to scar tissue and ovarian cysts that can impair fertility. Women who suffer from either of these conditions are more likely to have trouble conceiving and, on average, take longer to become pregnant.

The most common medical condition typically aided by ART is medically induced infertility, which is when a person experiences fertility issues or becomes infertile due to a procedure to treat another problem—most often, chemotherapy or radiation for cancer. One of the thousands of women with cancer who froze her eggs is twenty-five-year-old Olivia, a freelance music teacher from North Carolina who worked part-time at Starbucks for the health insurance. On a chilly day in March, Olivia woke up and dressed carefully for the day—makeup, hair, a determined smile, and her favorite pink purse. She was headed out to get her recent biopsy results. *If I'm about to get a cancer diagnosis, I refuse to look like crap when they tell me,* she thought. She slipped on her lucky pink sneakers. Then she drove to her doctor's office.

She was diagnosed with breast cancer later that day.

Olivia's specific cancer treatment required medication that would put her in menopause for five to ten years. Her doctors urged her to freeze her eggs right away. "It was do or die," Olivia told me. "We needed to get my ovaries turned off five days before I started chemo." She ultimately couldn't freeze her eggs but was able to freeze two embryos fertilized with her boyfriend's sperm.

While Olivia's case is a straightforward example of medical egg freezing—thousands of women like her urgently preserve eggs before undergoing fertility-compromising cancer treatments—Mandy's situation, like mine, is less clear-cut. While our medical charts don't constitute the same solid rationale to freeze eggs as Olivia's does, we are both what doctors call "cyst-formers"—as in, prone to developing problematic cysts—which, in addition to our history of gynecological surgeries and lack of two healthy ovaries, means we are at higher risk of diminished fertility in the future.

In Spring Fertility's waiting room—they'd arrived just in time—Mandy looked around at the familiar warm, calming hues. The mood lighting and modern decor gave off the vibe of a fancy spa but didn't quite mask the typical sterile feel reminiscent of a doctor's office. The place was a little over the top; *I see what you're doing,* Mandy often thought while she sat and waited before her appointments. She took a deep breath, trying not to fidget. Next to her, Quincy—her mostly serious, reliably calm Quincy—was absorbed in a Garth Greenwell novel.

A nurse called her name and led her to a small room. Mandy changed into a pink surgical gown, medical bonnet, and oversized grippy socks. In the photo Quincy took just before the procedure, her thick-rimmed glasses are slightly crooked, her spill of shiny black hair partially covered by the pink cap. Her hand is raised in a wave; her smile, nervous. Quincy kissed her and promised to save her a cereal bar from the waiting room. It was her little tradition; Mandy took one every time she visited the clinic. She didn't exactly enjoy the appointments, but at least she had the cereal bars to look forward to.

She sat alone in the procedure room, waiting. She felt anxious. Vulnerable. She couldn't stop thinking about the limitations of her body, if pushing it to the extreme with medications and hormones had been the right thing to do. Egg freezing, Mandy decided, felt like something between giving birth and being in a science experiment. And even though it was finally Retrieval Day, she still felt conflicted about the whole process. She had invested so much time, money, and emotional energy in this process that was supposed to put her in control. But all she wanted now was for the worry to cease, for relief to settle in. *Almost there,* she thought. *This will be over soon.* From the procedure room, she could see the clinicians through a large glass window. Clipboards in hand, they peered through microscopes and handled lab equipment. *Look at these men playing God,* Mandy thought. A doctor saw her staring and waved. It reminded her of the movie *Ex Machina:* technology, money, the future. She waved back at the god.

When she opened her eyes, she was in the recovery room. A doctor and Quincy stood next to her. "It went really well!" the doctor exclaimed brightly. "You got plenty of eggs—we extracted twenty." Mandy blinked, trying to clear the fog in her head. Twenty? A wave of relief washed over her. She knew that having partial ovaries meant it was unlikely she'd be able to freeze a lot of eggs; she had been careful to keep her expectations low. At one of her initial appointments, the doctor had told her that her ovaries were working very hard but her follicles weren't developing as well as he'd hoped. *We're not where we want to be yet,* he had said, choosing his words carefully, *but I'm sure we'll get there soon.* At a later appointment, he'd counted only eleven follicles. Mandy had lain on the exam table trying to read his expression, as she did at every exam, but at that appointment the doctor was more direct: *Not a great number, but we can work with it.* So twenty eggs was good—great—news.

Half an hour later, Mandy and Quincy were ready to leave. A nurse handed them a small box of Godiva chocolates on their way out of the clinic. In the elevator, Quincy showed Mandy the inside of his coat pocket, stuffed with cereal bars.

Hope and Heartbreak:
Why Most Women Freeze Their Eggs

Lots of people use ART for *non*-medical reasons as well. One's ability to be a parent is not limited by genitals; egg freezing and IVF, in particular, have made pregnancy possible for women experiencing or facing age-related fertility decline, as well as scores of people in the LGBTQ+ community. This is an important subject, which I'll discuss more in chapter 9. While the demographics are beginning to shift as more people from a variety of ethnicities and income levels pursue egg freezing, for the most part the majority of people who freeze their eggs are healthy, mostly young, cisgender women—and, more specifically, white middle- to upper-middle-class professionals. They tend to fall into one of two groups. The first group is made up of women in their twenties or early thirties; a growing number of egg freezers—roughly 35 percent now, compared to 25 percent in 2012— are women under the age of thirty-five. These women know they want to have children someday, perhaps within the next five years or so, but aren't ready yet. For them, egg freezing is a proactive measure. The second group includes women in their mid- to late thirties or early forties who know their fertility window is closing and want to give themselves the best chance of pregnancy in the near future. Many hoped to be mothers by now. They want children but aren't in a position to have them yet—usually because they aren't in a relationship with someone who feels ready.

When I began looking into the research and data behind why healthy young women freeze eggs, I expected the main motivation to be fitting fertility around ambitions and careers. But I was surprised to learn that, contrary to popular belief, egg freezing is rarely undertaken for that reason. It's actually because of what medical anthropologist and Yale University professor Marcia Inhorn calls "the mating gap"—a lack of eligible, educated, equal partners ready for marriage and parenthood. Inhorn, who embarked on a decade-long study to understand what drives healthy women to freeze their eggs, found that the majority—more than 80 percent—do so because they lack a partner. (While, obviously, one does not need a partner to have children, this cohort of women envisions rearing children with a partner.) Inhorn identified three main categories of those who froze their eggs: women freezing after a breakup or divorce, women still single despite years of dating, and women with partners who weren't ready for children. The typical egg freezer is a highly educated professional woman in her thirties, well established in her career by the time she walks into a fertility clinic. What she doesn't have is a suitable partner with whom to start a family. Freezing her eggs is "a reproductive backstop," Inhorn writes in her book *Motherhood on Ice,* "a technological attempt to bridge the gap while waiting for the right partner."

This was the case for thirty-six-year-old Valerie, who, until she froze her eggs, couldn't look at romantic relationships objectively. Valerie, who lives in Atlanta, has undergone egg freezing cycles on four different occasions, in three different states.* She's carried hormone injections on planes and more than once has excused herself from a date to self-administer a shot in the restaurant bathroom. As it happens, Valerie is a fertility doctor. The first time she froze eggs, she was twenty-eight and in medical school. Armed with the knowledge that her mother went through early menopause, Valerie initially saw egg freezing as both a means of protecting against possible fertility issues in the future and a way to pursue a demanding career without sacrificing her vision of having three kids down the road.

A few cycles in, she began to also see egg freezing as a worthwhile way to hold on to her reproductive potential while she waited for true love with the right person to come along. When Valerie went for her last retrieval, she had an epiphany. For years, she'd struggled to see her romantic relationships for what they really were, sometimes staying with an unsatisfactory partner only for the sake of the theoretical children she knew she wanted someday. Putting eggs on ice changed all that for her. She credits her frozen eggs for saving her from a miserable marriage. She says of one recent partner, whom she was living with and planned to marry: "He was wonderful on paper, but ultimately he

---

* Often, multiple cycles are needed to get "enough" eggs. We'll get into the nitty-gritty of what "enough" means, as well as egg freezing success rates, shortly.

wasn't the partner I needed for the rest of my life. And, honestly, knowing I had twenty-two eggs on ice helped me have the strength to end the relationship." What Valerie's attitude illustrates is that for many women freezing their eggs, the decision is as much about independence now as it is about family in the future. "I'm paying for peace of mind," she told me. "To be able to make decisions not based on my biological clock—which I still hear screaming in my ear."

So, egg freezing is often seen as a technology of hope for future romance. But research has shown it can also be described as what some call a technology of despair. Most women who freeze their eggs are hopeful, heartsick, or a mix of both. Inhorn's work is based on the largest egg freezing ethnographic study to date. What she and her team of researchers learned was that for many women, relationship dissolution, as Inhorn refers to it—divorce, separation, a broken engagement—is one of the primary pathways to egg freezing. A woman pursuing egg freezing at the end of a failing relationship has left or been left by someone she has loved. She's at a critical reproductive juncture, depending on her age, but even if she's in her twenties, she's old enough to internalize the breakup as an assault on her sense of self and her hopes for the future. She freezes her eggs in the midst of heartache, perhaps even a sense of hopelessness. "For women whose anticipated life course trajectories had been disrupted or broken, egg freezing provided them with a temporary biological reprieve, allowing women to heal their relationship wounds [and] recalibrate their sense of identity," writes Inhorn in *Motherhood on Ice*. "Egg freezing also fueled some women's visions for different futures, in which partnership no longer became an end goal."

A few days after Remy's injections appointment, she went for a long walk after work in her favorite park. She was still processing everything the doctor and nurses had gone over. Her egg freezing to-do list was growing longer. *Submit pharmacy paperwork. Ask Sarah in San Diego for her extra hCG shot to save some cash. Apply for a new credit card to help pay for meds.* She was all but certain she was going to break the "no caffeine for a month" rule—she simply could not wrap her head around *that* scenario—and figured if it was the one thing she did off protocol, it wouldn't be the end of the world.

It was a brilliantly sunny day, a welcome reprieve from the recent dreary ones. As Remy walked and prepared to jog for a bit along her usual loop, she noticed women about her age, one after another, pushing babies in strollers. Normally, the sight of so many stay-at-home moms (she presumed; at least some probably were) would have given her pangs, a stinging reminder that she was single and nowhere close to having children of her own. But today it affirmed for her that her experience of having a baby would likely be quite different from theirs, and that was liberating. She felt run-down and ragged—sleep deprivation was a fact of life these days—but she also felt calm and in control. Yes, she was single, again. But she was taking advantage of the fact that that meant she could live a little selfishly. She had only herself to take care of, to consider; no one depended on her, except, in some ways, her patients. Life consisted of going to work and coming home. She might not have this kind of selfish period in life ever again. That had been on her mind ever since she made the decision to freeze her eggs; it was an optimal time to do it. She was totally on top of the fertility thing now. She was being proactive about motherhood. Her stroller-pushing days were hopefully not too far away, but if they were, that'd be okay.

Everything in medicine was constantly telling her she was late. Late, late, late. At least Remy was two years shy of that dreaded "advanced maternal age" classification. She knew more than she'd like to, maybe, about high-risk pregnancies and how common infertility diagnoses were.* She was determined not to have a high-risk pregnancy and wanted to avoid, at all costs, the heartache that often came with undergoing fertility treatment at an older age. Remy was freezing her

---

* An estimated one in six adults globally—17.5 percent of the population—are affected by infertility. Being diagnosed as infertile doesn't mean a woman can't get pregnant; it just means something is preventing her body from getting pregnant on its own. Another fact worth noting—and this is important, so let it sink in for a moment—is that infertility affects women and men equally. About a third of infertility cases are the result of issues in the woman, a third can be attributed to men, and the remaining 33 percent or so either are a combination of both or can't be explained.

eggs to buy herself time to date, pursue relationships, and look for the husband she ultimately hoped to have. He was out there somewhere, putting in the time to develop himself and ready himself to be a committed partner. This was Remy's way of doing that, too, controlling the unknown as best she could.

Remy loved lists. Even more, she loved checking off items on lists. Life's big moments and decisions had neat square boxes next to them, and as Remy progressed through her twenties, she checked those things off her list. Go to medical school, get engaged, get married: check, check, check. But life wasn't always sunshine and checked boxes, Remy learned. Going through a broken engagement with one man and then a divorce with a different man convinced her that choosing the right person—to share life with, start a family with— was one of the most important life decisions she'd make, if not the most important.

She began to jog at an easy pace, her thoughts swirling as they propelled her back to her last egg freezing appointment. She remembered when a woman who identified herself as the clinical business coordinator had poked her head in the door. "Finished reading through everything? There's one form I have to notarize when you're done." Remy held up one of the forms from the pile in her lap. "This is more about, like, couples doing it—IVF, I mean. But I'm just freezing eggs. And the top of this page says it needs to be completed by a significant other."

"Yeah, you still need to fill it out, though," the woman said.

Remy read from the paper. " 'In the event of my separation or divorce' . . . 'transfer ownership to' . . . 'donate reproductive . . .' " She looked up. "Is that, like, in the event that I die?"

"Huh," the woman said. "I don't know that you would need to fill that out." She left the room and returned a few moments later. "Dr. Lewis said to write, 'Not applicable.' "

"Not applicable," Remy repeated slowly.

"Just put 'n/a,' " the woman said, as if that was that.

Remy ran hard, wanting to wear herself out. She could still feel the heaviness of that moment; it was sad to think about dying before using her eggs. Ultimately she had written her mother's name on the form, later adding both her parents' phone numbers, which felt a bit strange. Her mom, Remy knew, would have a strong opinion about where her eggs should go in the event of Remy's death. But would anyone else? If signing the blizzard of forms and making rushed decisions about what would happen to her frozen eggs and who would care were supposed to make her, as an egg freezing patient, feel better, she didn't.

That night, Remy felt uneasy. When she sat down to meditate, she couldn't find her moonstone ovary crystal anywhere. She rummaged through her apartment, checking the same spots over and over. She found it, finally, tucked deep inside the plastic rim of the door of the washing machine. She had forgotten to remove the stone from the pocket of the denim shirt she'd worn to the appointment the other day. The moonstone lay soaked in water, glistening. It reminded Remy of what an ovary looks like under a laparoscopic view.

Later, after getting into bed, she texted her father to let him know that he and Remy's mom would be in charge of her eggs if something happened to her before she could use them. He texted back that he'd take care of her "twins," joking about raising them in Arizona, where they'd live in a trailer and fish off the dock. Remy read the text and giggled. She texted back: *Just as long as you raise them humble.* As in, with a sense of humility—a virtue she couldn't imagine her children not having, no matter who raised them.

Since emphatically deciding *Yes!* at my last appointment with Dr. Noyes, I was beginning to see how egg freezing might be the long-lost key to the Have-It-All Castle. Like Remy, I feared waiting until too late. I was wary of being part of an older couple, or being a single woman, who wanted a family. Like Mandy, I worried about my ovaries, or lack thereof, and felt pressure to protect against possible future regret by grabbing whatever my ovary could yield now. The facts were adding up: I wanted biological children in the future. I was single, and in a demanding graduate school program that consumed most of my time and energy. My eggs were not getting any younger. Egg freezing technology had vastly improved since its early days. Underlying the facts was a bit of subliminal messaging that resonated with me: *Smart women think ahead. Smart women are uncompromising about what they want—and have a backup option in case life does not go according to plan. Smart women are proactive and in control.* There was that idea again: *control.* There was a part of me that found it incredibly appealing.

Twelve days after my second egg freezing appointment, I met Ben.

We "met" on a dating app. After a bit of flirtatious banter over the app's messaging platform, we arranged to meet in person at Brooklyn Public House, a bar a few minutes' walk from my apartment. He was late and I was cranky—great start!—but what I thought would be a casual drink turned into four hours of conversation. A few of the coincidences were striking. We each had a parent who was a retired U.S. Army colonel (his father, my mother). His sister and my sister-in-law shared a name. He and my brother had the same name, too.

Ben spoke passionately about his work in the renewable energy industry. He wore glasses and a red Patagonia pullover over a wrinkled button-down. He was the first person I'd ever met from Wisconsin. Sometime after midnight, we stepped out onto the sidewalk and kissed under the bright moon. He pulled me into his chest and I felt a quick shiver of pleasure as his hands moved down my jeans and gripped my hips. "Where have you been all this time?" he said softly, his arms wrapped around my waist.

Our next date found us ducking inside a pizza shop for 99-cent slices and two bottles of Snapple after a concert at Madison Square Garden. We ate on a dirty street corner outside the entrance to the subway. I was exhausted, anxious to get home. Ben had pizza crust crumbs all over his collar. "You still haven't told me what you write about," he said.

For the most part, the men I dated never wanted to hear about any of this. They'd ask me what kind of journalist I was, what sorts of subjects I covered. "Lately, fertility and egg freezing," I'd reply, and they'd cock their heads or reach for their beers. "Like, chicken eggs?" a guy once asked me. I took a big bite of pizza, stalling. *Here we go,* I thought. *When I was twelve* . . . I always began. I was used to telling friends, or anyone who knew me well enough to ask, the story of my surgeries for years. I had never felt reluctant to talk about why I only had one ovary. Until now. I didn't know how to begin explaining my possibly uncertain fertility future—especially since that future suddenly seemed close to the present. Two weeks had passed since my last appointment at the clinic, where I'd excitedly announced I was going to freeze my eggs. The man standing in front of me with crumbs in his beard could someday have a vested interest in my fertility, my ability to have children. It was only our second date—in fact, he was the first guy from the dating apps I'd gone on a second date with. But I had that knowing feeling, deep in my gut.

I looked at Ben, my mouth suddenly dry. The thought was so clear in my mind: *I cannot fall in love with you and freeze my eggs at the same time.* It wasn't a logical thought—women freeze their eggs while dating and starting relationships all the time—but I felt a creeping sense of overwhelm. I took a swig of iced tea and shook my shoulders, as if to clear away the dramatics looping in my mind. A taxi blared its horn. "Well," I began. I couldn't think of another way to answer the question. "When I was twelve . . ."

I could almost hear my ovary mutter in exasperation.

I don't remember all of what I said. I do remember his rambling reply. "Yeah, fertility, yeah," he said eagerly. "I read this article the other week, about free IUDs in Colorado? Some sort of program for low-income teens and women, have you heard about it?" he continued, explaining the program. While he'd been talking, we had walked down the stairs leading to the train platform. "So, are you still considering egg freezing?" he asked. His tone, unlike my brain at the moment, was very matter-of-fact. I searched for what to say. "I think so, yeah."

Ben opened his arms to hug me. "It sounds like what you're doing and writing about is important," he said. My face pressed into his chest and he kissed the top of my head. I felt exposed, vulnerable. He looked behind me and squinted at a Metro-North sign. I wanted to keep talking, but he had a train to catch.

"Can we do this all the time?" he asked.

I stared. He wanted to talk about my missing ovary all the time?

"Can we hang out all the time?" he clarified, smiling.

"Well, no," I replied, smiling back.

That weekend, Ben slept over for the first time. Before he arrived, I removed the four-by-six ultrasound image of my ovary from its prominent spot on the fridge.

As a reporter, I had a lot of questions about egg freezing technology and the money and medicine behind it. But on the personal side, things were looking up. The optimism I had felt leaving Dr. Noyes's office lingered. And: I had a plan. When the clinic called me with the results of my blood work, I'd get a clearer picture of the current state of my fertility and learn whatever the tests—what did the tests actually test, again?—said about my ovary and my eggs. Then I would move forward with the next steps of egg freezing. I wasn't actually sure what the next steps were, but I'd figure it out.

And in the meantime, I would keep seeing charming, easygoing Ben.

6

Optimizing Fertility

~~~~~~

Cerviva or Bust

It didn't start out as a quest to give cervical fluid a more palatable name. It started, as so many things do, because of love. And sex.

"'Cerviva,'" said Will Sacks, seated in a coffee shop near his home in Boulder, Colorado. He wore a blue T-shirt that matched his eyes; behind his trim beard was a warm smile. "We wanted to start calling cervical fluid 'cerviva.' Cer-VEE-va. Pretty good, right?"

It was a brisk fall morning, and Will, an entrepreneur in his late thirties, was telling me about the connection between cervical fluid—also called cervical mucus—and Kindara, a company he co-founded that develops apps and products for fertility tracking. And cervical mucus, a fluid secreted by the cervix, changes in texture, color, and amount during a woman's menstrual cycle, especially around ovulation. Until recently, most of what I knew about cervical mucus involved words like "sticky" and "egg-white." But I'd done my homework before meeting with Will, because I realized that in order to grasp what Kindara did for its hundreds of thousands of users, I would need to understand cervical mucus and ovulation. And to talk about ovulation, I quickly learned, requires a working knowledge of the cervix.

A woman's cervix acts as the gatekeeper to her uterus. The

cervix—the "neck" of the uterus, about one inch long, positioned at the top of the vaginal canal—decides what and when things go in and come out. Tampons, sex toys, fingers, and penises can all get to the cervix, but they don't get past it. And things like menstrual blood and perhaps a baby need to get out. The cervix's job is to safeguard the uterus—like a bouncer poised outside a fancy, VIP-only hotel—and keep this crucial part of a woman's reproductive system happy and healthy. Outside the cervix, sperm are lining up and competing to get in. Cervical mucus, acting as a protective barrier to the uterus, has two jobs depending on where a woman is in her cycle. Either it prevents sperm from entering the cervix or it nourishes and protects the sperm as they move through the cervix and reproductive tract to fertilize an egg. So at this particular party, if a woman is nearing ovulation, cervical mucus keeps the sperm alive, sweaty and dancing, while inside the uterus an egg makes its way down to the lobby. Once the cervix determines which lucky sperm are worthy enough to enter, the fun really begins.

I had asked Will to coffee to learn more about Kindara, and about fertility- and period-tracking apps in general. Most women I know—whether trying to conceive, actively avoiding pregnancy, or falling somewhere in between—use an app to track their menstrual cycle. And each swears by the one she uses. Kindara, in particular, intrigued me because of what it's based on: fertility awareness-based methods of birth control, also called FAMs or FABMs. "Fertility awareness" is a general term for the set of practices used to determine the fertile and infertile phases of a woman's menstrual cycle. A woman is fertile only a handful of days each month—around ovulation, when the egg is released. Fertility awareness-based methods are essentially about answering one question: *Am I fertile today?* People using FAMs identify and track fertile days and draw upon that information to avoid or achieve pregnancy. A woman does this by tracking the hormonal fluctuations that occur during her menstrual cycle, paying close attention to signs of ovulation in particular. Two primary ones are her basal body temperature and the consistency of her cervical mucus. Taken together, these physiological indicators can help her monitor her ovulation patterns and reliably identify the days when pregnancy is possible.

One August, more than a decade ago, Will was twenty-nine and in need of a change. Originally from Quebec, he was living in Toronto and had recently quit his job as an energy efficiency consultant. He dreamed of being an entrepreneur, using his engineering background to create companies that would have a net-positive impact on society and the environment. Companies that did things that mattered. He decided to attend his first Burning Man festival, which he was pretty sure was a thing people his age did when they were having a quasi-existential crisis. He booked a plane ticket to the desert and, upon arriving at the Reno airport, posted a message on Craigslist saying he was headed to Burning Man, had a rental car, did anyone need a ride? Kati Bicknell, a young woman from Brooklyn, answered. Petite and fair-skinned, with wavy brown hair and dark blue eyes, Kati worked for TED Conferences. They talked the entire drive into the desert.

After Burning Man, they started dating. "We got along like a house on fire," Kati told me. It was a long-distance relationship from the start, maintained with overnight buses between New York and Toronto. One weekend night in November, a few months later, the couple had a conversation about birth control. For Kati, fertility was a familiar topic. Her mother was one of the two million women who had been fitted with the Dalkon Shield, the defective IUD. Kati's mother struggled to conceive her. And Kati had had an IUD earlier that year, but it was so painful she'd had it removed. That, along with a bad experience on the Pill—she'd reluctantly taken it in her late teens and early twenties to "correct" her irregular periods—led her to swear off hormonal birth control.

It's commonly assumed that women, especially those in long-term relationships, will bear the responsibility of preventing pregnancy by using a contraceptive method like the Pill or an IUD. The ubiquity of hormonal birth control makes this even more commonplace. As an adult, Kati developed strong feelings about how the division of labor in birth control plays out in women's lives. She also found it deeply unfair that women are saddled with dealing with hormonal birth control's side effects. She was done with the Pill and IUDs, but after settling into their relationship, neither she nor Will wanted to continue using condoms. Kati, a trained FAM instructor, had been charting her fertility for the past year. She mentioned this to Will one day. When Kati began telling him about fertility tracking, Will told me, he laughed at her. "There's no way that can be real," he recalls saying. "I've heard of the 'rhythm method.' It doesn't work." That was the end of the conversation. The next day, Kati handed Will her worn copy of *Taking Charge of Your Fertility,* the formative book about reproductive health and natural birth control by Toni Weschler, and told him to read it. Will was more than skeptical. But as he paged through the book and learned more about FAMs, his skepticism splintered into questions. "I said to Kati, 'Wait a minute. You're telling me there's a method of birth control that's nearly as effective as the Pill, has no side effects, is hormone-free, and costs nothing—and that nobody knows about it?" He found it hard to believe, yet was deeply intrigued. "I was like, 'How is this possible? There's no way this is possible.'"

Will is polite, measured, always paying attention. He avoids caffeine, which maybe has something to do with his calm demeanor. He locks eyes when he's speaking. He says things like "There's, like, four forces that are coming to me as you're talking" and "I just really think it's the patriarchy." He had crumbs in his beard for most of our conversation. "I thought I was a progressive man," he mused, sipping from a mug of herbal tea. "I'd have conversations about hormonal birth control. I understood the different methods. And then I read this book and I was like, 'Oh my God. I don't know anything about how women's bodies actually work.'"

Will recounted all this to me matter-of-factly, with an air of confidence that indicated his ignorance hadn't lasted for long. It sounded like the ripe beginnings of a good origin story: An enlightened woman meets a self-assured man who is woefully misinformed about the female body. Then, a plot twist. It turned out that Will reading a thick book about fertility would change both his and Kati's lives for the better.

A national bestseller, *Taking Charge of Your Fertility* is the FAM bible. The book was originally published in 1995 and has become one of the most universally lauded health books on the market. In it, Weschler describes FAMs and explains the concept of charting menstrual cycles as a way for women to practice effective natural contraception, maximize their odds of getting pregnant, and command their gynecological and sexual health. "Your menstrual cycle is not something that should be shrouded in mystery," Weschler writes in the book's twentieth-anniversary edition. "The best thing to come out of my years using the fertility awareness method was the privilege I felt in being so knowledgeable about a fundamental part of being a woman."

Will was intrigued by *Taking Charge of Your Fertility.* He learned that there are a few different FAMs that help a woman track her ovulation and fertility patterns, and that FAMs are used by women all over the world who are drawn to them simply because they don't involve the kind of chemicals associated with hormonal methods of birth control like the Pill—and because they minimize the frequency with which they'd choose to use condoms, a diaphragm, or other barrier methods of birth control. He learned that many couples use FAMs to avoid getting pregnant, but that they can also be an aid when trying to conceive. And he learned that charting fertility is a good way for a woman to be on top of her gynecological health in general; it's easier to tell what's normal and what isn't when you're tracking what's going on down there.

Will's initial quick leap to misassociate FAMs with the rhythm method is, unfortunately, a common one—and it's a major reason there remains some stigma and confusion surrounding it. The rhythm method involves simply counting the days starting when a woman's period ends and then abstaining from sex around day fourteen, the assumed midpoint of her cycle and when she is supposedly most fertile. Will had been mostly right in his comment to Kati, as the rhythm method is one of the least effective methods of contraception. What he didn't know was why: because it falsely assumes that all women have twenty-eight-day cycles and that cycles are reliably consistent over time. The length of a woman's menstrual cycle is the number of days between periods, counting the first day of your period until the day before your next period starts. The notion that a normal menstrual cycle is twenty-eight days is a routinely accepted myth, perpetuated by a slew of medical sources, from diagrams in sex ed classes to birth control pill packaging. In fact, cycle lengths vary among women, ranging anywhere between twenty-one and thirty-five days, and often vary for an individual woman as well. A woman might ovulate on the twelfth or the twentieth day of her cycle. The idea that ovulation happens on day fourteen, then, is arbitrary—and getting it wrong can have serious implications for contraception science.

Having learned the basics about women's fertility, Will found the bit about cervical mucus particularly fascinating. Composed of nutrient-rich electrolytes, proteins, and water, cervical mucus shares a purpose with semen: to help sperm reach and fertilize an egg. Ovulation triggers the cervix to produce various kinds of secretions; the wetness a woman might notice on the crotch of her underwear at different times of the month differs depending on where she is in her menstrual cycle and usually follows a predictable pattern. She can check her cervical mucus every day, looking for changes in quality and quantity—dry, sticky, creamy, egg-white—and have a pretty good sense of where she is in her cycle and if ovulation has occurred.* She can also take her temperature in the morning every day before getting out of bed. This is basal body temperature, or BBT, your body's temperature when it's completely at rest.† BBT measures ovulation; pro-

---

* A few days before ovulation, cervical mucus is clear, heavy, and slippery—think raw egg whites. This consistency helps sperm swim up to meet an egg at ovulation.

† Technically speaking, you can take your temperature vaginally, orally, or rectally to chart your BBT. The books classically say to use an oral glass mercury thermometer immediately upon waking to get the most accurate reading. Digital oral thermometers work well, too, as long as they have the appropriate accuracy and precision.

gesterone, the hormone that prepares the uterus for a fertilized egg, causes BBT to rise, signaling that ovulation has occurred.

Somewhere around page 164 of the book, Will told me, he had an epiphany. He'd read that conception is only possible from about five days before ovulation through to the day of ovulation. Sperm can live for up to five days in a woman's body, so if a woman has sex up to five days before the egg is released, she can get pregnant. After ovulation, the egg can live for up to twenty-four hours, which means that once it's released from an ovary, the egg can be fertilized as it travels through the fallopian tube toward the uterus. Fertilization happens when a sperm cell successfully meets an egg in the fallopian tube. Known as the fertile window in a woman's cycle, these six or so days are the only time each month when having sex can lead to pregnancy.* So, the length of a woman's fertile window takes into account the combined life span of an egg (about twenty-four hours) and sperm (roughly five days). The trick is figuring out exactly when that window is—and, like menstrual cycles, fertile windows vary from person to person. All this is why determining the few days around ovulation is the crucial component of fertility tracking.

So then Will got it. By observing and tracking signs of ovulation like cervical mucus and basal body temperature, as well as using a calendar to chart her menstrual cycle, a woman could estimate her fertile days. And *that,* Will realized excitedly, was information he and Kati could use. They could choose not to have sex on the days that made up Kati's fertile window, or if they did, they'd use a condom or another barrier method of birth control. That was it; he was sold. FAMs would be their natural birth control. It would require careful, daily monitoring, but the nerd in him was more than up for that. Will finished the book—and told Kati he was in.

Using FAMs and tracking fertility patterns helped Will better understand Kati and helped Kati better understand herself. And gone were the days of "I'm wearing a condom, so I'm responsible" or

---

* If you're trying to get pregnant, the more often you have sex during this window, the better. Especially one or two days before you ovulate, because the egg starts to deteriorate quickly after it's released from the ovary. Think of it like a sperm cell waiting in the wings, ready to greet the egg cell as soon as she emerges.

"She's on the Pill, so she's responsible"; by practicing FAM, Will and Kati shared the responsibility of protecting against pregnancy. But amid the newfound intimacy in their relationship, Will couldn't stop thinking how mistaken he'd been about how women's bodies work. He knew this kind of ignorance was pervasive. And he was fairly certain there were many, many more people out there who, once they realized they didn't know what they didn't know, would feel forever changed by discovering a form of natural birth control that, if practiced correctly—and this is key, practiced correctly—was very effective at preventing pregnancy.* And those people, Will predicted, would likely need some help figuring out the best tools with which to reliably use FAMs. *This will change the world,* he thought. Kati agreed.

Their vision was to use technology to empower women through body literacy, while simultaneously helping to improve how men and women relate to each other. Will, an engineer, and Kati, a product designer, set out to find the best tech with which to track Kati's cycle—and quickly realized it didn't exist. So they decided to create it themselves. That winter, they ditched their jobs and moved to Panama to save money. In a rented house near the ocean, they secured freelance gigs to cover their living expenses but spent most of their time devouring studies and the latest scientific research. They returned north a few months later and, with pitch in hand, started filing patents for an app and a digital BBT thermometer that would make it easier for couples to chart ovulation and fertility patterns.

I tried to imagine this bearded, herbal-tea-drinking man in a boardroom, pitching a bunch of all-male venture capitalists while clicking through PowerPoint slides about periods, fertile windows, and carefully timed sex. I could picture a few men loosening their power ties; someone coughing, clearly embarrassed; and maybe some of them wondering why they'd never heard about any of this before. "We got pooh-poohed by a lot of people," Will said, gripping his

---

* They're most effective when multiple FAMs are used together. Using FAMs perfectly correctly and consistently throughout the menstrual cycle, though, can be difficult to do. With typical use—using FAMs the way the average person does, which is sometimes incorrectly or inconsistently—pregnancy rates increase.

mug. I asked why; he gave me an *isn't-it-obvious* look. "Because I was talking about cervical fluid and starting a business. People were like, 'What is that? I don't want to hear about that. It makes me uncomfortable and, also, what the hell are you talking about?'" But he wasn't deterred.

The couple moved to Boulder, a town that had recently been named as having the most tech start-ups per capita of any city in the United States, and set to work translating their ideas into a company. Two years later, in the summer of 2012, they launched the fertility-tracking app that they had designed themselves. In between, they got married at Burning Man, on the first anniversary of the day they met. Will and Kati started with limited cash and skills, but the venture capitalists stopped scoffing—Kindara raised around $10 million in funding—and the couple built Kindara into one of the first venture-capital-funded digital women's health companies in the world.

The app's main features—an ovulation calculator, BBT chart, and period calendar—can be used not only to help a woman get pregnant or avoid pregnancy but also to help chart her menstrual cycle simply for her overall health. Users can input days they have sex and days they menstruate, get ovulation predictions, and record changes in cervical mucus and BBT. For Erin, twenty-eight, a loyal Kindara user, the best part about the app is the self-knowledge factor. "Fertility tracking has helped me to understand so much more about my body, my mood, and overall health," she told me. "Really getting to know their own unmedicated cycle should be something all women are encouraged to do."

I've met my fair share of entrepreneurs and start-up founders who talk about being a force for good, but Will and Kati struck me as the real thing. They have moved on to other ventures since starting Kindara—the company has been acquired by another Boulder-based women's health company—but remain visibly stoked about normalizing the conversation around FAMs and helping people feel empowered when it comes to sexual well-being and fertility. "We get all kinds of letters and emails from people saying, 'Oh my God, I understand my body for the first time now. Thank you,'" Will told me. "That's been the best part of the whole ride." From the beginning,

Will's relationship with Kati inspired how he thought about Kindara. "I think we're fucked up about sex and intimacy from an early age," he said. "I was like, 'I want every couple to have the experience we were having—feeling that connection, learning about each other's bodies, having that level of intimacy.'" The steep learning curve was worth it. Will summed it up to me like this: "I don't think there are a hundred people in America who know more about fertility awareness than Kati and me."

I was struck by the realization that the man sitting across from me knew a great deal more about the female reproductive system than I did. Which absolutely delighted me. Maybe I shouldn't have been surprised by Will's openness. Still, it was so refreshing to talk about sex, birth control, and the role technology plays in the future of fertility education—and with a man not too much older than me that I hardly knew. To talk about these things with a man at all! I had reached out to Will to learn the ins and outs of starting a women's-health-focused technology company. But as we talked in the coffee shop that day, I realized I was just as interested in the why behind Kindara, the ways in which he and his partner—in business and in life—navigated the potentially awkward, messier parts of their relationship, the ones having to do with sex and contraception and romantic things like cervical mucus. I listened to him describe his journey from stunned ignorance to cool-as-a-cucumber "wokeness" with some envy. When was the last time I'd had a frank, science-based discussion about vaginas and penises with a man? Had I ever?

His comments about the burden of birth control nagged at me, too. Will and Kati's head-on conversations around contraception struck me as progressive, and that didn't sit well with me. I would like to believe that safe sex—protecting against pregnancy and STIs—was a shared responsibility between two people sleeping together. But in my experience it seldom played out this way. In fact, on the potential pregnancy front, I could not recall a man ever initiating a conversation about protection before we had sex. In most of my relationships and sexual encounters throughout my twenties, I'd offer up the fact that I was on the Pill early on in conversation and that was that. What bothered me—and, based on the experiences of many other women I've discussed this with, them too—was the *assuming,* how men frequently wait until the woman asks him to put on a condom before doing so and doesn't ask before sex if she's on some form of birth control or not.

My frustration in this regard was relatively new; for years, I thought nothing of taking primary responsibility for pregnancy prevention. But my tune had changed. It wasn't just that I found the double standard irritating. An unplanned pregnancy is a consequence for both parties, so leaving women to shoulder the burden of preventing pregnancy struck me as just plain dumb and irresponsible. Now this thought is never far from my mind when I'm deciding whether or not to have sex. Do men really just not think about this? Or if they do, is it merely a passing thought, dismissed with the assumption that the woman's got the protection handled? The most troubling bit underlying that assumption, I realized, was that it actually *wouldn't* be on both my partner and me. Because it's my body, my decision—at least ultimately. Right?

I haven't worked out the answer to this question yet. Yes, it's my body, my business—not his. But men *should* be asking their sexual partners about birth control; both men and women should initiate the conversation about protection. Just like both men and women—all people—should know the basics about both female and male fertility. The burden of birth control, I had come to realize, extended to the management of women's fertility. Men do not experience the same pressures to manage their fertility, and in the same way that pregnancy prevention is often left to the woman, so too are the expenses and decisions related to preserving fertility, particularly for young women freezing their eggs.

"Fitbit for Your Period": The Rise of Fertility Trackers

While Will and Kati were hustling to get Kindara off the ground, the fertility-tracking space was heating up. In 2013, a year after Kindara's app launch, Max Levchin, co-founder of PayPal, helped launch a period-tracking app called Glow, which raised $23 million in venture funding in its first year. The race to hack women's menstrual cycles was on.

If learning about hormones and menstruation led me to Kindara, then Kindara led me to the world of femtech. Depending on whom you ask or what you read, femtech is a concept, a movement, or some Silicon Valley lingo. Actually, it's kind of all three. Ida Tin, the Danish entrepreneur and co-founder of Clue, a popular period-tracking app, is widely credited with coining the term, which refers to products, software, and services that use technology to improve women's health. Femtech, powered mostly by female entrepreneurs, is geared toward improving healthcare for women across a number of conditions specific to people with ovaries, including maternal health, pelvic and sexual health, menstrual health, fertility, and menopause.

"The Fitbit for your period" is a good sales pitch, and Will used it when talking with investors about Kindara. On the heels of Kindara came a boom of other female-focused apps and technologies to support women of reproductive and post-reproductive age. The market for digital women's health and femtech products is big: women from puberty to menopause. Personalized testing products and do-it-yourself healthcare have never been so popular, and a slew of pioneering developments—from period-tracking apps to at-home hormone tests to wearable fertility-monitoring devices—have burst onto the scene. Meanwhile, mobile technology has rushed in to fill the reproductive health knowledge void in the same way it's rushed into virtually every other part of our lives. The trendy companies behind these new digital applications focus on a range of issues, from charting ovulation via AI-based apps to supporting women experiencing low libido to marketing period care goods to financing fertility procedures like egg freezing. Part of broad shifts in digital medicine, they also illustrate femtech's potential to revolutionize women's health. There are Bluetooth-connected breast pumps, pelvic floor exercisers, digital bracelets that track ovulation, subscription-based services that deliver organic tampons to a woman's front door, and a lot more. Wearable and digital fertility monitors, period-tracking apps, and at-home fertility hormone tests are the major ones I'll go into here.

Can Silicon Valley get you pregnant? Many femtech companies are screaming yes. Do women want to manage their reproductive health with their smartphones? Oh, absolutely. The global femtech market is projected to be worth more than $100 billion by 2030, and investors—primarily the world's mostly male venture capitalists, who customarily all but ignore women's health—are now paying attention.

Smart wearables have been booming for some time, since biosensors in mobile devices make it easy to record, store, and analyze data about the user's body and behaviors. The most popular ones in the femtech world are external and internal electronic devices and digital fertility monitors—a catch-all term for any device that helps a woman track her fertility, especially regarding ovulation and potentially getting pregnant. Fertility monitors do this in a few different ways—such as measuring hormone levels and BBT in order to predict fertile windows—and work in much the same way as FAMs. Some analyze urine samples (the user pees on a wand, then sticks the wand into the device); others measure BBT or cervical fluid via a vaginal sensor while a woman sleeps (she inserts a discreet, tampon-esque device at night and, after removing it in the morning, holds it near the back of her phone while her data downloads to the device's corresponding app).

One of the most popular digital wearables is the Ava Fertility Tracker, a cycle-monitoring sensor worn like a bracelet overnight. It's the first—and, as of this writing, the only—FDA-cleared stand-alone fertility-tracking wearable. The device detects the user's menstrual cycle phase—and fertile window, with 90 percent accuracy, according to a recent study—by tracking physiological signs such as skin temperature, heart rate, and respiratory rate, which act as markers for fluctuating hormone levels. Fans of Ava say it's easy to use and is more convenient than ovulation test kits. Some users credit their pregnancies to their Ava bracelet—$279 a pop, as of this writing—and for those who pay more for premium packages, the company offers a full refund if the user isn't pregnant within six months or a year.

Other popular fertility-monitoring products on the market include digital ovulation kits, insertable cervical mucus monitors, and BBT thermometers. Some people use fertility monitors to help them avoid pregnancy without taking birth control, but more commonly women use these products when they're trying to become pregnant; tracking ovulation helps couples conceive, but manually charting cycle symptoms can be arduous, and these tools streamline the process and make fertility monitoring much easier. They're not omnipotent, though—none of the devices are approved to prevent pregnancy— and aren't a replacement for seeing a doctor, which is sometimes necessary; even the most high-tech digital fertility monitor can't diagnose problems that could explain why a couple is struggling to conceive, such as low sperm count or endometriosis.

So many women wake up to their fertility only after struggling to become pregnant. Others go through early adulthood at least aware of their monthly bleeding and PMS symptoms, even if that awareness never quite shifts to a true understanding of what's going on. As they tell a woman about the whens and hows of her cycle—in addition to cluing her in to her overall health—digital fertility wearables and devices are powerful tools that help bridge this gap. So are period-tracking apps, which are among the most frequently downloaded kind of health app in the App Store. Also called ovulation trackers, cycle trackers, or just fertility apps, they're used by people wanting to prevent pregnancy, people trying to have a baby, and people looking for an easier way to monitor menstrual-cycle-related health issues. A user is invited to input intimate details every day— the length and heaviness of her menstrual flow, types of period-related pain such as cramps and headaches, whether she had protected or unprotected sex, fluctuations in libido—which the app uses, along with dozens of other optional data points the user chooses to input, to make its predictions. As with digital fertility monitors, fertility apps rely on the same physical fundamentals that FAMs do, those externally observable physiological signs that indicate where a woman is in her menstrual cycle (the two major ones being BBT and the color and consistency of cervical mucus). Each app has its own algorithm, but all draw upon user-inputted data to generate predictions around ovulation, fertile windows, and estimated period start dates.

I use Clue, an early pioneer in the femtech world whose app has over eleven million users in 190 different countries.* Clue's co-founder, Ida Tin, suffered side effects from hormonal birth control for years; like so many femtech founders, she set out to build something after personal experience left her frustrated and declaring, *There's gotta be a better way.* I use "Clue Period Tracking" mode, but it also has a "Clue Pregnancy" mode, which I could transition to in the future. The app makes it easy to review my cycle history and symptoms, and gives me predictions based on my tracking. In other words, it does a lot more than simply tell me when I should expect to bleed each month.† Clue helps me calculate the average length of my cycle and uses that information to help me predict my next "period" (not a real period, remember, but rather withdrawal bleeding, since I'm on the Pill). It offers a multitude of options for what I can track. I can toggle on all sorts of reminders related to my period starting, fertile window coming up, birth control pills, time to check BBT, and more. I don't need most of these toggled on, since I don't closely observe my fertility signs, but I like that Clue is designed to support FAMs. I like that it was easy to set up and is intuitive to use. I like that it teaches me about my body and personal biology. I like that it's transparent about citing the research and data it draws from. I like its clean, modern interface and inclusive tone. And I really like that it's not pink.

Because I tell Clue every day that I've taken my birth control pill, it doesn't show me predicted fertile days (the feature that shows a user her high- versus low-risk days in terms of possible pregnancy isn't displayed if she's told the app she uses hormonal birth control). But the app takes into account how my specific birth control method may be affecting my cycle and fertility. Nearly every day, I open the app and chronicle period-related symptoms I may be experiencing—

---

* I use Clue Plus, the paid version of Clue's app, which gives access to many features and modes. As of this writing, it costs $10 per month or $40 per year; the price varies depending on the user's region.

† These apps can also be quite useful for alerting the user to trouble with their cycle. Clue has a whole section, for example, for when one has recurring cramps and what that might represent. Or whether it's normal to have a nine- or eleven-day period (which, again, helps close the information gap from our childhood).

cramps, fatigue, stress—as well as make notes, if I want to, about sleep, exercise, eating, and a whole host of other factors, all of which impact my cycle. I also tell Clue when I've had sex. This admittedly felt a bit weird at first, my iPhone usually knowing more about my sex life than any human in my life does. But it's helpful: On days I am "intimate" I make a quick note as to whether it was protected or unprotected sex. Since I'm on the Pill and take it exactly as I'm supposed to, this feature doesn't matter so much—except for the very infrequent mishap, like when I went on a last-minute reporting trip out of town and left my pack of birth control pills at home. I logged "missed pill" in the Clue app, at which point it shouted at me (nicely) to use a condom if I had sex that weekend.

"The sex ed you never got," Clue's website touts. Clue's customer service team receives thousands of health-related inquiries from users about sex, menstruation, fertility, and more. The most common questions: *Why is my period late? Why is my cycle irregular? Do I need to seek medical care?* Because being on the Pill stops me from ovulating, I'm honestly not always sure whether changes in my body from month to month are a result of the synthetic hormones or if they have nothing to do with my non-cycle at all. But over the years I've switched up the brand and type of birth control pills I take, and every time I do, my body takes a while to adjust. Keeping track of symptoms helps me identify patterns and better understand hormonally influenced changes to my body—a small but very real comfort. When I open the app and input a piece of information—that I took my pill that morning, say, or that I broke out with a bout of acne—a little wheel at the top spins and it tells me "Clue is getting smarter . . . ," and that makes me feel a bit more tuned in to my body and all that's going on in places I cannot see.*

Fertility tracker apps aren't perfect. When researchers at the University of Washington collected data from two thousand reviews of

---

* For women who are trying to conceive, fertility tracker apps can be a helpful tool, particularly when using the app to transition from preventing pregnancy. Also neat: Several fertility-tracking apps have a feature that lets users share their ovulation info and cycle monitoring with a partner or a friend.

popular fertility-tracking apps and surveyed nearly seven hundred people about them, they found that users were dissatisfied with the apps' lack of accuracy and their assumptions about their sexual identity. Most are geared toward heterosexual and cisgender women, many responded, and they disliked the emphasis on pink, flowery interfaces at the expense of customization.

And it's true. A major drawback of period-tracking apps is their propensity for inaccuracy. Many of the apps assume that a user's most fertile days are her ovulation date and the five preceding days. But, again, this so-called regular cycle—meaning she always gets her period every twenty-eight days—is not the norm for most women. Also, ovulation tends to shift from month to month. And so the fertile window the app tells her could very well be wrong. The more carefully and consistently the user tracks her cycle, the more accurate the app will be. The app's estimations improve over time because the longer a user tracks and the more information about her cycle she supplies, the more data the app's algorithm has to work with. Most of the apps let you program them to send you input reminders, as I've done with Clue. Still, it can be easy to forget to be diligent about updating and engaging with the app every day. If a woman is using the app as a reliable digital record of her menstrual cycle, the stakes are low if she misses a day here or there, especially if she uses hormonal birth control. But if she's relying on the app to avoid getting pregnant and doesn't use any form of birth control, being just one day off can result in an unintended pregnancy.

Another drawback is privacy concerns. Millions of women around the world use apps to track their cycles, and that treasure trove of data is often passed on to third-party companies such as Google and Facebook. Apps in general offer very little in the way of data privacy rights when it comes to the information that's shared with them, and fertility apps are no exception. Some of the apps allow users to remove their identity from the data it has stored on them, but many don't, meaning that a user's information isn't anonymous. A 2022 *Consumer Reports* study that evaluated privacy practices and data security for several fertility apps concluded that while some make it easy for users to understand what information is collected, *all* the apps "share some user data with external partners for purposes such as targeted advertising. And then those partners may share or resell a user's personal information to third parties, who of course make no promises to the user about how they handle it."

No woman who tells an app whether she had unprotected sex or an abortion wants such deeply private information shared in a way that could identify her. This became a major issue in the summer of 2022, when data privacy issues and fertility-tracking apps took on a new, scarier meaning after *Roe v. Wade*'s reversal. This sparked action in some states with regard to safeguards for consumer health data collected by companies, but new federal regulatory frameworks are needed. While the United States has strict privacy laws that govern how entities such as hospitals and health insurers share information about patients, these laws don't apply to mobile health apps, which fall under consumer privacy laws—and offer much lower standards of protection. In other words, the personal health data people enter into consumer apps isn't protected by federal safeguards for patient privacy—including, notably, HIPAA, the federal health information privacy law.

There is a plus side, though, to anonymously sharing information of this nature, and that's the data it provides for scientific and medical research about menstrual and reproductive health. Modern medicine was developed with male physiology as the default, and women have historically been underrepresented in medical research, clinical trials, and biology textbooks; it wasn't until 1993 that including women in federally funded clinical research was required by law. A 2022 McKinsey report found that just 1 percent of biopharmaceutical and medical technology investment goes toward female-specific conditions beyond oncology. *One percent.* Considering that people with ovaries constitute nearly half of the world's population, it's both nonsensical and infuriating that female health remains so overlooked and underfunded.

Several fertility apps say that medical researchers use anonymized information from their apps to study female-focused health concerns. Sharing sensitive health data after telling users their information would be kept private isn't okay.* But the benefits of personal data being put to good use shouldn't be ignored, either. *The New York Times* pretty much nailed it in an article about the troubling data-sharing practices of Flo, a popular period tracker: "And here lies the crux of the problem with women's consumer health technology, or 'femtech' as it is known in investor speak: The sheer volume of data collected in apps like Flo is ripe for privacy violations, but that same data may also open the door to unraveling some of the biggest, understudied riddles of female health."

Private Little Revolutions:
The Truth About Hormone Testing

At her home in New York, twenty-six-year-old Margaret Crane sat at her desk, assembling a plastic paper-clip holder, a test tube, a dropper, and a small angled mirror. It was 1967, and Crane, a freelance graphic designer, had recently been hired by the pharmaceutical company Organon. While touring the company's lab in West Orange, New Jersey, she noticed multiple lines of test tubes suspended over a mirrored surface. She was told they were pregnancy tests, and that when combined with a pregnant woman's urine, the test tube would display a red ring at its base. "I thought how simple that was," Crane recalled of seeing the tests for the first time. "A woman should be able to do that herself."

Margaret Crane wasn't a scientist, nor did she have a chemistry background; the company had brought her on to work on a new cosmetics line. But she went home inspired, and set to work developing a simplified version of the test. Her first attempts to design the device were unsuccessful, and she was frustrated. Then one day she sat at her desk looking absentmindedly at a stylish plastic box she used to hold paper clips. She realized the container was the perfect size to hold the components needed for the test. A few months later, she

---

* Explicitly asking users if they want to share their anonymized information is, obviously, the best practice here; Clue, for example, invites users to opt-in to doing so and "be part of closing the diagnosis gap for some of the most common yet most under-diagnosed and under-researched health conditions."

presented her kit—it resembled a toy chemical set—to Organon, and in 1969 the company applied for a patent in her name. Two years later, her home pregnancy test, named Predictor, went on the market in Canada, and then, after gaining FDA approval in 1976, in the United States. When it hit the shelves, the Predictor cost $10, the equivalent of about $50 today.

The home pregnancy test was one of the most revolutionary products of the twentieth century. Before Crane invented it, women had to go to their doctor's office and wait two weeks or more to get their results. With the Predictor, women could find out if they were pregnant in as little as two hours, in the privacy of their own bathrooms. Today's at-home pregnancy tests are the size of Popsicle sticks and deliver results within minutes, but they work on the same principle of detecting hCG, a hormone found in high concentrations in a pregnant woman's urine.*

"Unlike medical tests that reveal something otherwise unknowable about a body, a pregnancy test can only speed the delivery of information," writes Cari Romm in an article about early home pregnancy tests in *The Atlantic.* "Regardless of who pees on what, a pregnancy has other, more obvious ways of making itself known with time. The home pregnancy test, then, wasn't just about knowing; it was about taking charge, a sentiment that fit in nicely with the ethos of the time." When the Predictor and a handful of other similar tests came to market, *Our Bodies, Ourselves,* the seminal book about women's health and sexuality, was six years old and abortion had been legal in the United States for three. Early advertisements for home pregnancy tests emphasized what they offered beyond a yes/no pregnancy result: privacy, autonomy, knowledge of one's body. A 1978 print ad for an at-home test called it "a private little revolution that any woman can easily buy at her drugstore."

But, as Romm notes, not all of the doctors, who saw their authority being overthrown, were happy about a changing status quo. In an

---

* While hCG was identified in the 1920s, it wasn't until the 1960s that scientists turned to immunoassays—tests that combined hCG, hCG antibodies, and urine—and discovered that if a woman was pregnant, the mixture would clump together in certain distinctive ways.

editorial published in *The American Journal of Public Health* in 1976, one physician argued against the use of home tests: "I feel that the reputations of both the commercial concerns and the profession of medical laboratory technology will suffer unless legislation is introduced to limit the use of such potentially dangerous kits." In a note following the piece, the journal's editors were firmly on the side of the tests: "Not everyone," they wrote, "needs carpenters to hammer in their nails."

At-home pregnancy tests are now ubiquitous, and other private little revolutions have joined their ranks. In addition to testing their pregnancy status, women can now also test their fertility from the comfort of their couch. Understanding your fertility hormones now, the thinking goes, gives you more options later. Several online companies and fertility clinics now offer ways to do diagnostic fertility testing at home. The tests, taken via a blood sample, work by checking the levels of hormones associated with egg production and ovulation. I mentioned FSH and LH earlier, two of the hormones that concern fertility. Let's recap those and get into a few more:

- Anti-Müllerian hormone, or AMH, is secreted by the small follicles found in a woman's ovaries. The level of AMH in the blood helps to approximate her egg supply.
- Follicle-stimulating hormone, or FSH, is responsible for stimulating egg growth and starting ovulation.
- Estradiol, or E2, a form of estrogen, is one of the primary hormones tied to ovulation and regular function of reproductive organs. Along with FSH, it offers clues on the state of a woman's ovarian reserve, which is a fancy word for egg count.
- Luteinizing hormone, or LH, is another key hormone responsible for ovulation. It also regulates the length of a woman's cycle.
- Thyroid-stimulating hormone, or TSH, regulates thyroid health. The thyroid plays a role in metabolism, heart function,

the nervous system, and more, and affects things like
ovulation, mood, weight, and energy.

- Free thyroxine, or fT4, plays a role in thyroid health and is
  often tested alongside TSH.
- Testosterone, or T, is, in women, secreted in small amounts by
  cells in the ovaries and contributes to ovarian health, bone
  health, mood, and libido. Recent research suggests it also
  plays a key role in which follicles develop, and are ultimately
  recruited, each month.
- Prolactin, or PRL, stimulates milk production and pauses
  ovulation after a woman gives birth.

Having hormones tested by a reproductive endocrinologist at a
fertility clinic can cost anywhere from $800 to $1,500. Products such
as Modern Fertility's kit—the company calls it "the most comprehensive fertility hormone test you can take at home to be proactive about
your fertility"—retails at $179, as of this writing. The average Mod-
ern Fertility kit user is thirty-one, and after she does the at-home
finger prick test and has up to eight hormones analyzed, she receives
her clinician-reviewed customized report, which is based on her hormones, age, birth control, health survey, and latest research by physicians. She can then opt to have a one-on-one consultation with a
fertility nurse (at no extra cost) to discuss her results.

It's remarkable, really, that a few drops of blood can tell a person so
much. Testing a woman's hormones can help identify if there's an
imbalance that could get in the way of the ovaries releasing an egg, or
that could be affecting more than just fertility; hormone imbalances
can impact weight, sleep, and even generally how a person feels. The
tests also shed light on what a woman's timeline might look like—for
example, if she could hit menopause earlier or later than average.*
And they offer clues with regard to egg freezing or IVF outcomes,
such as if the user can expect to collect more or fewer eggs than average in these procedures.

I first spoke with Modern Fertility's Afton Vechery in 2019. She

---

* The average age of menopause in the United States is fifty-one.

and her co-founder, Carly Leahy, had started the company in Vechery's apartment two years earlier. No one was talking about "proactive fertility." But, Vechery said, "we were hell-bent on bringing this thing in the world because we believed with every ounce of our bodies that it was our right as women to have power over our reproductive future." Modern society is much more focused on preventing pregnancy than on planning for it, and this was at the heart of what Modern Fertility hoped to change. They built Modern Fertility with a specific demographic in mind: people with ovaries who were not yet actively trying to conceive. A major part of the company's message became: *We don't accept "wait and see" as an answer in any other part of our lives— and we won't accept it with fertility.* Like many other female femtech founders, Vechery and Leahy saw reproductive health as a mainstream wellness issue, something that can be tracked and monitored, much like how much sleep you get or how many steps you take.

How difficult it was to access and afford fertility hormone testing was another thing Vechery wanted to change. Most women don't think to ask their primary care doctors or gynecologists about their ovarian health. When Vechery first tested her fertility hormones, she was billed $1,500 out of pocket and had to have multiple discussions with doctors to understand the results—a major one being that she had undiagnosed PCOS. Hearing Vechery's frustrating tale about trying to get a full hormone assessment, I thought about a friend of mine who, when she was twenty-eight, was able to get a basic diagnostic fertility workup only after she lied to her gynecologist, saying she'd been trying to get pregnant for a year. Most insurance plans do not cover proactive fertility testing. Initial diagnostic testing sometimes is, depending on where you live and your health insurance plan, but qualifying for coverage often requires an infertility diagnosis. And to obtain that, couples generally have to prove to their doctor and insurance company that they've been trying to conceive for at least one year (more on this in chapter 9). Single women who are not currently trying to conceive but are trying to gain valuable insight into their fertility are usually out of luck.

Kindbody, a health and technology company that provides fertility, gynecology, and family-building care, is also in the business of DIY fertility. I'll talk more about Kindbody in the following chapter, but in addition to its brick-and-mortar locations, the company has mobile clinics in several cities, where it invites potential clients to hop aboard a cushy, bright yellow van to have an exam and fertility testing done, sometimes for free.* "Reproductive health is the only vertical of healthcare where you wait until something bad happens before taking any steps to correct it," said Gina Bartasi, Kindbody's founder and former CEO, in an interview. "It's backwards. We're here to change that." In the same way a person doesn't wait to have a heart attack to eat well or exercise, Bartasi wants to help consumers take more initiative in learning about their fertility. In 2022, the company began selling at-home fertility hormone tests for both women and men, in addition to other pre-conception, pregnancy, and postpartum products. The launch of Kind at Home, as the company's consumer products division is called, is part of the company's goal to be the single door for all fertility healthcare.

At-home or in-van fertility tests have their drawbacks. They can't detect every type of hormone that plays a role in fertility, nor can they diagnose other health conditions that could be affecting a woman's fertility. The tests often don't account for women with irregular cycles. And for women on hormonal birth control—who are preventing pregnancy by manipulating their hormone levels, thus influencing their body's usual levels—the tests can typically assess only two of the eight hormones I listed above: AMH and TSH. In any case, testing fertility hormones in isolation isn't as helpful as actually *looking* at the ovaries and the number of follicles they contain, which renders the results of a fertility hormone test, particularly AMH and FSH levels, more useful and provides a fuller picture.† During a transvaginal ultra-

---

* Initially, the vans typically parked on high-traffic corners and were a marketing tool. Now they're used in various communities to serve self-pay and privately insured patients, as well as employees of companies that Kindbody has contracted with; employees interested in using their Kindbody employee benefit can pop into the mobile clinic parked at their work campus during their workday to learn more and do initial testing.

† Though not the full picture; there is currently no reliable biomarker that tells a woman how many eggs she has left.

sound, a fertility doctor counts the small resting follicles to see how many eggs a woman has waiting in the wings. The antral follicle count, or AFC, is a good predictor of a woman's egg supply that month—known as ovarian reserve.* Taken together, the ultrasound and the blood work are what's known as ovarian reserve testing. It refers to the number of follicles in a woman's ovaries and gives an indication of how her ovaries might respond when stimulated with hormone medications used in ART procedures.

Ovarian reserve is *part* of the overall picture of your fertility health; understanding it in context is important. Your age, lifestyle, and medical history are also important factors in determining how likely you are to get pregnant. Ovarian reserve testing is a standard component of an initial assessment at any fertility clinic because it provides a helpful baseline for anyone considering egg freezing or IVF; every egg freezer has her AMH and other fertility hormones tested and her ovaries examined in order to assess how she might respond to fertility medications. But for a woman who hasn't yet tried to get pregnant and who is wondering about her current natural fertility, an AMH value isn't all that helpful in that context. While a woman's AMH level can help estimate the number of follicles she has inside her ovaries, it cannot determine exactly how many eggs she has or, crucially, what condition those eggs are in. It's also not necessarily a good indication of when a woman ought to freeze her eggs. This is the biggest misconception concerning ovarian reserve and especially AMH testing: that it is a "female fertility test." While ovarian reserve testing offers some valuable insight into a woman's fertility and a sense of potential outcomes if she undergoes egg freezing or IVF—how many eggs her ovaries might yield when stimulated with fertility drugs—it is not an accurate predictor of a woman's ability to conceive through

---

* A woman's AFC can vary month to month, and both AMH and FSH levels can fluctuate not just within but also between menstrual cycles. Also, women on hormonal birth control, take note: Hormonal birth control suppresses the ovaries and ovulation, which, according to some studies, can impact AMH and suppress follicle count (not permanently; just while on birth control). For a more accurate AMH result, it's best to test while not on hormonal birth control.

sex now or at a specific point in the future. This crucial fact is missing from virtually all the hype around fertility testing.

A major 2017 study in *The Journal of the American Medical Association* (*JAMA*), the results of which were replicated in 2022, showed that AMH does not reveal a woman's reproductive potential and that ovarian reserve tests are often useless for many of the women to whom they're marketed, for the reason I've just given. The study, the largest to examine the impact of AMH and FSH levels on ability to conceive naturally, tracked 750 women ages thirty to forty-four with no history of infertility. The women, who were followed for a year, were tested for three common ovarian reserve biomarkers—AMH, FSH, and inhibin B*—found in blood and urine. To their surprise, the researchers found that AMH levels were not significantly correlated with later pregnancy and birth. Women with a low AMH value or a high FSH reading—markers of diminished ovarian reserve (DOR), a condition in which the ovary loses its normal reproductive potential, compromising fertility—didn't differ from women with normal levels in their ability to conceive. In other words, women who didn't have normal levels of the two primary hormones associated with fertility were not any less likely to get pregnant from intercourse and give birth than women with normal levels.

Lead author Dr. Anne Z. Steiner, the reproductive medicine specialist and OB/GYN professor mentioned earlier, told *Vox* in an article about the study: "These tests are great measures of ovarian reserve, how many eggs you have. But they don't work to predict a woman's reproductive potential." Steiner and many in the medical community thought the tests *would* be a good predictor of a woman's natural fertility, because in people using ART to conceive, hormone values like AMH and FSH, as I've said, often correlate with how well a woman will respond to fertility medications—how many eggs she'll yield—and her likelihood of getting pregnant with IVF. But the *JAMA* study, and other similar trials in which researchers looked at

* A peptide hormone that's associated with the maturation of follicles in the ovaries.

AMH and FSH levels as a marker for predicting natural fertility, showed that's not the case.

A low AMH and a high FSH do mean that it's harder for a woman to conceive via ART. That's because the chances of egg freezing or IVF leading to a baby are directly tied to the number of eggs a doctor retrieves, and a woman with a higher ovarian reserve is more likely to respond robustly to the hormone meds she takes during a fertility treatment cycle, producing more eggs than a woman with a lower ovarian reserve.* But these tests are not all that useful for a woman who has yet to try to conceive naturally, because regardless of her AMH and FSH levels and AFC, if she's having menstrual cycles she'll naturally ovulate one egg per month. So, the chance of natural pregnancy depends directly and exclusively on the chance that that month's egg is a healthy one—not on how many are left in the reserves for the future. In this case, quality trumps quantity. So for women wanting to get pregnant through sex, the only real way to test fertility is to try to conceive.

That's rather unhelpful to women who have no interest in becoming pregnant now. And while one could argue that at-home fertility hormone tests are a waste of time and money for a woman not planning on using ART to get pregnant, these tests have proved worthwhile for plenty of women. Case in point: When she was twenty-nine, Caroline Lunny, a former contestant on *The Bachelor* and a former Miss Massachusetts USA, took the Modern Fertility hormone test, expecting to find she was, as she put it in a blog post, "fertile as hell." Instead, she experienced a rude awakening when she discovered she had the AMH levels of someone who was about to go through menopause. She discussed the results with her doctor, as well as the fact that her mother had gone through menopause relatively young. Lunny went through nine rounds of egg freezing and ultimately put eleven

---

* Since lower AMH levels can indicate diminished ovarian reserve, a fertility patient with low AMH might need to undergo multiple cycles of IVF to get pregnant or multiple cycles of egg freezing to get a sufficient number of eggs on ice.

eggs on ice.* Requiring this many rounds was very likely a result of her low AMH, as the above study lays out, but Lunny is glad she pursued egg freezing and wishes she had taken the Modern Fertility test even sooner.

So while the tests aren't a good predictor of a woman's fertility or egg quality and are not intended to replace the more in-depth diagnostic testing conducted by a physician, some of the information they provide could be well worth knowing. Hormone levels can, for example, detect—though not diagnose—underlying conditions such as PCOS. And hormone imbalances in general, as I said earlier, can impact a lot more than fertility. If the at-home test returns an unexpected or abnormal test result, the user might be alerted to a problem they otherwise wouldn't have known existed and then have a sense of urgency to see a doctor for a comprehensive fertility evaluation. A reproductive endocrinologist can investigate potential issues related to infertility, from ovulatory disorders to fallopian tube blockages, and look for structural problems with the uterus that could affect pregnancy, such as fibroids and polyps.

On the other hand, uncertain results without adequate interpretation can cause increased anxiety, and acting on the results—for example, rushing to freeze eggs after receiving a dreaded finding of diminished ovarian reserve—may be misguided. Too often, women get their "numbers" without a true analysis of what those numbers mean for them personally, or their fertility and family goals. It's common, for example, for a woman to learn she has a low AMH level and be devastated, assuming this means she's infertile. Low AMH likely *does* mean doctors would have a harder time retrieving a lot of eggs in an egg freezing cycle but, at least based on the information in the *JAMA* study, it seems those women should have no reason to assume they'll have a harder-than-average time conceiving naturally.

As testing fertility hormones outside a physician's office becomes more common, some doctors are becoming increasingly worried that

---

* If the eggs Lunny froze don't result in a viable embryo, she'll use some of her sister's frozen eggs; Lunny's sister also froze her eggs and donated half—ten frozen eggs—to Lunny in case she needs an egg donor down the road.

women might be falsely alarmed by results outside the norm, particularly low AMH—when the reality is, as I've just explained, that they are very likely to go on to get pregnant naturally. It's not hard to imagine a woman with slightly abnormal hormone levels being pressed into egg freezing out of concern that her fertility is falling off a cliff when, in fact, that might not be true. Companies like Modern Fertility are quick to acknowledge their kits as one tool in the fertility assessment toolbox as well as to encourage women who use their product to follow up with a doctor. Kindbody similarly acknowledges that AMH testing is only one tool used to help gauge fertility. But I find the free AMH testing offered at Kindbody's pop-ups troubling because of its debatable usefulness and the fact that the company targets women in their twenties and early thirties.* It's also concerning because of motive. Kindbody's end-to-end brand is built around the consumer, and the company has every incentive to play up AMH testing as a valid measure of fertility. A woman stops by a Kindbody van on her lunch break, gets her hormones tested, and learns a thing or two about ovaries and eggs she didn't know before, and when Kindbody emails her her test results—whether they're in the normal range or not—the company reminds her that a Kindbody clinic is just down the road in case she might now want to consider egg freezing.

So, using an at-home fertility test or having hormones analyzed in a van is fine, but not truly valuable on its own. Testing fertility hormone levels in a vacuum can be misleading, especially if the user is a healthy woman who merely wants insight into her current reproductive potential. It's great that she wants to learn more, but it's imperative that she also knows that the data points the tests provide, particularly AMH, are not markers of whether she can or cannot become pregnant and that ovarian reserve testing alone can't estimate a woman's chances of conception in a given month. What's important

---

* In addition to AMH tests, Kindbody's mobile clinics also have the ability to do full initial consultations, pelvic ultrasounds, lab panels, genetic carrier screening, and well-woman exams.

is understanding what the tests are and are not measuring, as well as their limitations, and knowing if and when to see a doctor to follow up on the results.

Hormone levels are one important piece of the quite intricate fertility puzzle. An adequate supply of good eggs, healthy fallopian tubes, and receptivity of the uterus are other ones. At the end of the day, though, the most important factor in determining a woman's fertility is—you guessed it—her age. As much as we may want at-home magic answers and a crystal ball telling us everything we want to know about our fertility, they don't exist. On the bright side, though, is the fact that all this increased testing and knowledge means that more is being learned about the true complexity of human fertility—by women themselves.

The bottom line is that these at-home hormone tests can be a helpful starting point. When a nurse from Dr. Noyes's office called me to tell me my AMH level, I'd written the number down in my notebook and circled it. When she didn't offer any context, I scribbled a question mark next to it so I'd remember later to find out if the number was good or concerning—which going down this AMH and fertility hormone test rabbit hole helped me to do. It's good for women to know that ovarian reserve screenings are available, but there's a fine line between educating women about their reproductive life span and exploiting their fears about it, although many in the fertility industry won't say as much. But now you know. If you're well informed as to what the tests mean and their limitations, checking your hormones can add to your understanding of your fertility trajectory. Because both AMH levels and egg count gradually decrease, keeping tabs on hormone levels over time can offer some insight into how steep the decline of your fertility "hill" may be. Having inaccurate or incomplete information, however, can be more damaging than having no information at all.

Remy: Shots, Shots, and More Shots

Remy couldn't remember ever being this eager for her period to start. It was late March, and the fertility medications sat in her fridge, just waiting to be opened. Most women freezing their eggs begin the hormone injections on the second or third day after menstrual bleeding starts. Any day now, she'd get her period and be able to start the regimen of fertility drugs. She'd also be able to stop taking the Pill. Some women are put on an oral contraceptive pill before undergoing egg freezing, which can help follicles grow at a more similar size and rate and give a woman and her doctor more control over the timing of her egg freezing cycle.* Inclined toward most things that help a ship run tighter, Remy hadn't minded taking the Pill to temporarily control her ovulation. She was just glad she hadn't needed to change up her regular birth control method, a copper IUD, during the egg freezing process; it could stay right where it was for the retrieval.

Remy is the kind of person who always has a five-year plan of one kind or another, like the one that said this was the year she was going to start trying to get pregnant. That mindset—healthy habits, healthy pregnancy, healthy eggs, healthy baby—kept her motivated. She had been drinking green juice every day for three weeks, wanting to be in peak condition before beginning the shots. Breakfast as usual, every day: oatmeal with almond butter, blueberries, and dried cranberries. Weaning herself off coffee in anticipation of starting the injections had been rough. She'd gone from having several shots of espresso a day to three cups of coffee to a single cup. Baby steps. It was making her feel cranky, and she got a little depressed every time she thought about the toll the fertility medications might take on her body. She'd heard somewhere that by the end of all the days of shots, it would feel like she was carrying around a sack of potatoes.

But at least the process felt less daunting once she realized how structured it was. Remy took pride in putting on autopilot all the components of her life that could be managed that way. It was the giving up control of outcomes she wasn't so good at; she didn't like

---

* Fertility clinics tend to have their own preferences and policies on this, but know that there are potential suppressive side effects to using oral contraceptive pills directly prior to an egg freezing cycle. The available data is somewhat conflicting, but several studies have concluded that doing so can result in a longer stimulation cycle that requires more medication—and can actually negatively affect the number of eggs that are retrieved.

that it was hard to picture what her body was about to go through. As a second-year anesthesia resident, she had put IVs and epidurals in patients hundreds of times, but she didn't particularly like sticking needles in herself. At the fertility clinic, when the nurses demonstrated how to prepare and administer the hormone shots, she'd become overwhelmed. The way the nurses did it wasn't the way she would have done the injections—but she was the patient this time, not the doctor.

A few nights later, it was finally time to start. Remy went through her normal evening routine, doing more or less the same things she usually did. Since she had been on call at the hospital the night before, she slept all afternoon. When she woke up, she drove to her favorite trail and ran six miles listening to a podcast episode for company. It was sunny and cool, perfect weather for her last run for a while. Post-run smoothie back at home and then another walk, catching up with an out-of-state friend on the phone. Finally, a long shower with candles and donning her staple comfy clothes: Lululemon leggings and a tee. She sat at her kitchen table, damp hair wrapped in a towel atop her head, and opened the packaging.

The two cocktails on the hormone injections menu that night: Gonal-F—it came in a fancy pen, to be dialed up to the right amount—and Menopur. She reconstituted the medications, her anesthesiologist brain in full-focus mode. Her nerves were shaky; the anticipation had her feeling all jazzed up. She had resolved to do the hormone shots herself—it felt symbolically important somehow—but all of a sudden she wanted some company. At the last minute, she picked up her phone and FaceTimed Christina,* her best friend. She needed a distraction and asked Christina to tell her a silly story. While Christina rambled on about a time her mother had all the shoes stolen out of her car, Remy pinched the skin around her lower stomach, let out a deep exhale, and plunged the needle in. It hurt a lot more than she expected. But she was psyched. *Bring it on.*

---

* Name has been changed.

7

Not Our Bodies, Not Ourselves

~~~~~~

Shame and Stigma

In 1940, when she was eighteen, the poet and activist Grace Paley tiptoed into her doctor's office and lied about being married so she could get a diaphragm. "We all knew that birth control existed, but we also knew it was impossible to get," begins her essay "The Illegal Days," part of Paley's collection *Just As I Thought*. "You had to be older and married. You couldn't get anything in drugstores, unless you were terribly sick and had to buy a diaphragm because your womb was falling out. The general embarrassment and misery around getting birth control were real."

When we talk about controlling women's bodies, abortion typically bookends the conversation. A woman's right to choose has dominated the reproductive rights discourse for decades. Paley, who died of breast cancer in 2007, spoke openly and famously about the illegal abortion she had in Manhattan at age thirty. Her remarks on how difficult it was to obtain birth control are less well known but, I find, are similarly disturbing. While less drastic than Paley's, hurdles have persisted for generations of women since. In 1975, my mother waited until she was away at college to visit Planned Parenthood for the first time so as to avoid running into someone she knew at her small town's clinic. In 2006, a girl I went to high school with exaggerated her period cramps so she'd be put on the Pill without her parents knowing she was sleeping with her boyfriend. As of 2023, twenty-four states restrict minors' ability to obtain contraception without parental consent—a stark difference from 2006, when no state or federal laws required minors to get parental consent in order to get contraception.

I recalled a conversation I'd had with a woman named Cynthia, a young mother of three who grew up in rural southwest Virginia. Cynthia was raised in a Pentecostal family; James, her husband, is a strict Catholic who doesn't believe in birth control. When we first spoke, Cynthia had just turned twenty-six. She told me she'd had four miscarriages, and while she and her husband wanted to have more children, she felt overwhelmed by the prospect of trying again. Mostly she was scared about gaining weight again so quickly. Normally she weighs just one hundred pounds, and each of her pregnancies had been difficult and severely stressed her body. Her second baby had been too big to deliver naturally; her doctors said a vaginal birth would have caused her hips to break. And complications with C-section scar tissue after her last pregnancy resulted in her needing surgery to have her bladder repaired. "So I'm not really in a rush to have more kids, like, right now," she told me.

Cynthia doesn't remember having sex ed in school. She had no idea what a period was when she first got hers. When she was sixteen, the doctor in her small town of two thousand people prescribed the Pill because of her painful periods—but didn't bother to tell her its primary purpose was to help prevent pregnancy. She didn't take it regularly. Then, the first time she had sex, on the night of her high school graduation, she became pregnant, though they used a condom. "No one told me you could get pregnant even if you used condoms!" she exclaimed. "I didn't know they came in different sizes. In my town, they don't tell you about birth control. They just give you a little bit of knowledge and send you on your way." I asked Cynthia if she would have made different choices if she had known more. "I think about that a lot," she said. "My kids are my entire life." She paused. "But if I could go back, if I had the knowledge I have now, I would've waited."

Only a couple of incidents come to mind when I look back at my major milestones of learning about my body and what goes on inside it. They were all unpleasant. While I had more choices and knowledge than Cynthia did, it still wasn't smooth sailing.

Periods. I got mine after school one day in eighth grade and taught myself how to insert a tampon. The brownish, sticky blood alarmed me. It was a year after 9/11 and my mother, a colonel in the Army, had recently been deployed overseas. I can't recall if I bought the tampons myself at the pharmacy a few blocks from my middle school or if I had surreptitiously added them to my father's grocery store list. But I remember the complicated instructions inside the box, how having to decipher them alone made me feel small and scared—like a young girl who needed her mom. *But Mom's not here,* I told myself, *so you're going to have to figure this out on your own.*

Going to the gynecologist. The first time I had a pelvic exam, I was so nervous I apologized to the doctor for how much I was sweating. It is a specific kind of unnerving, spreading your legs in a harshly lit room while a stranger peers into your vagina. The speculum and probing fingers are even worse. Most of the OB/GYNs I have seen as a patient have been polite but brisk. I'd usually leave their offices with a few unanswered questions I was too intimidated to ask, but with a vague sense of having been invaded. The OB/GYN I saw when I was twenty-two was a different story. He was in his fifties and from Romania, with a rough accent and rougher hands. In the exam room, I gave my *I-only-have-one-ovary* spiel and summarized my surgeries. He asked if I was sexually active. My boyfriend and I had been sleeping together for a while, I replied, but I was frustrated: My irregular "periods" were causing regular what-if-I'm-pregnant scares, despite being on the Pill. "So that's why we use two forms of birth control," I explained. I felt self-conscious; talking about my sex life with a stranger—even if he was a doctor—was awkward. The OB/GYN raised his eyebrows. "Oh, my dear," he said, shaking his head. "That's very unnecessary. Stop using condoms and live your life!" He closed my chart with a flip. "Your boyfriend will thank me," he chuckled. We didn't stop using condoms, but fuming about this interaction to my boyfriend did make it a bit easier for the two of us to talk about sex and sex-related things.*

And then there was a more recent kind of milestone that happened as I was listening to the doctors at the EggBanxx event. They were lecturing a roomful of mature, well-educated women about their reproductive systems rather than assuming the women in attendance were well informed already. As I sat there, memories came flooding back of my sex ed days: teachers showing pictures of genitalia on overhead projectors, older high school girls whispering about hand jobs and how boys liked "shaved" girls better. I remembered the swirl of nervous-excited feelings in my stomach as I sat on the classroom floor with other girls, the boys down the hall. I remembered learning about a lot of things but never really talking about any of them. At best, sex ed explains some of what young adolescents have started to experience as they come into their bodies. But for most of us, it also sows seeds of confusion and stigma that grow as we get older. That evening at the EggBanxx party, it was those seeds I saw being watered.

Entire books have been written about the brutal cycles of women's health through the centuries. In a *New York Times* book review of Elinor Cleghorn's *Unwell Women,* Janice P. Nimura writes, "Taught that their anatomy was a source of shame, women remained in ignorance of their own bodies, unable to identify or articulate their symptoms and therefore powerless to contradict a male medical establishment that wasn't listening anyway." Most women find it difficult to get a sense of what's normal and what isn't when it comes to their bodies. We swap stories about contraception methods and bemoan uncomfortable visits to the gynecologist. At some point we realize we've never quite recovered from the grisly pictures imposed on us in health class all those years ago. Superficial, often poorly

---

* Later, I learned that about one in ten women uses two methods of contraception, such as condoms and the Pill, simultaneously. So maybe also using condoms with my boyfriend was overkill, but the doctor really could've reacted better.

taught sex ed and a pervasive cultural *shh* leave many people in the dark, missing out on or avoiding candid conversations about sex and all it entails.

Cynthia's story is a powerful illustration of the direct connection between women's lack of knowledge about fertility and lack of agency regarding reproductive choices. Beyond being poorly educated about their bodies, women continue to face challenges in their efforts to access comprehensive sexual healthcare and resources. Paley's account about procuring a diaphragm, along with Cynthia's story and other conversations I'd had with women about sex and fertility, got me thinking: How does a person gain access to the knowledge and resources they're entitled to?

Not so much in schools, as we've established. Not so much from medical providers either, it turns out. A study by Yale researchers found that about 50 percent of reproductive-age women had never discussed their reproductive health with a physician.* OB/GYNs routinely cover contraception but rarely assess their patients' quantity and quality of eggs; a survey of five thousand U.S. OB/GYNs found that less than one-third of clinicians counsel patients under age thirty-five on reproductive aging and fertility preservation. So why do these discussions rarely take place? Not enough doctors and not enough time is one reason. Nearly half of U.S. counties do not have a single OB/GYN. For patients who do see a gynecologist regularly, appointments are typically brief, with barely enough time for a woman to refill her birth control prescription and ask if she's up to date with her HPV vaccine shots, much less inquire about the quality of her eggs or check her hormone levels.†

---

* Dr. Lubna Pal, a professor of obstetrics and gynecology at Yale School of Medicine who co-authored the study, noted: "We found that 40 percent of women in the survey believed that their ovaries continue to produce new eggs during reproductive years. This misperception is of particular concern, especially so in a society where women are increasingly delaying pregnancy."

† The lack of communication is, in part, because health insurance doesn't reimburse doctors for spending more time talking to their patients. Also, some OB/GYNs don't discuss fertility with younger patients because they don't want to unintentionally add to the pressure to have children that many young women already face.

To be sure, teens learn about sex from a range of sources beyond school. But what kids learn in health class doesn't align with what the internet and popular culture tells them—not that TV, music, and movies are all that illuminating on the subject. It's also out of sync with what they hear from Mom and Dad. Most American parents, sex educators repeatedly point out, either ignore the subject completely or teach their children myths about where babies come from when they are very young, and leave it at that. In light of the horrid shame of Paley's generation, my mother giving me the American Girl body book was quite progressive.

And then there's easy-to-access online porn, which reporter Maggie Jones, in a *New York Times Magazine* feature, described as the de facto sex educator for American youth, filling the vacuum left by the country's deficient sex education. "There's nowhere else to learn about sex," one boy told Jones. "And porn stars know what they are doing." The media we consume and watch undoubtedly influences how we act in real life, and the most popular porn sites are among the one hundred most-frequented websites in the world. Jones notes that it's not easy to discern what's fake and what's real in porn; the line between fantasy and exaggeration can be blurry. It's not a huge deal for an informed adult watching porn for fun, but it's another matter entirely when we consider that hardcore porn is where a great many teenagers learn what to do to each other, and that porn is a primary influencer in young people's lives, shaping their early ideas about sex and their sexual behaviors, too.

So. Sex ed teaches girls to be ashamed. Our doctors are very busy and we don't know what questions to ask them anyway. Porn and pop culture distort our thinking, providing a script for sex that leaves many young people feeling insecure and alienated. It's not all that surprising, then, that many young women grow up having an aversion to their periods and feeling pressure to shave their pubic hair, entering adulthood all too often having never uttered the word "labia" and without knowing what a clitoris is, where it is, and/or what to do with it. And so I couldn't blame the doctors at the EggBanxx event for assuming we needed their Fertility 101 talk, nor could I fault the women for not knowing more. It was clear to me now that filling in our knowledge gaps at any age is neither straightforward nor easy, and that young women's lack of crucial knowledge about their bodies inhibits their ability to make informed choices, as adolescents *and* when they're older—especially with regard to their fertility.

It was around this time that I talked with a group of ten or so young women gathered at the home of one of them in a suburb of Washington, D.C. We sat around a dining room table, eating chips and hummus. The young women* were between the ages of twenty-two and twenty-nine, represented various ethnicities, belonged to middle- to upper-middle-class families, and had all grown up in northern Virginia, a mostly prosperous and progressive part of the country. When I had invited them, I'd explained I wanted to ask the group a few open-ended questions related to sex and fertility: what they knew and how they'd learned it. Before I turned on my audio recorder and started asking questions, I looked around the table and paused. I told the group about some of the articles I had written, hoping to break the ice before launching into intimate territory.

Then I kicked things off by asking them what they remembered from sex ed classes. They all laughed at once, exchanging knowing smirks. Beyond learning about STIs and the structure of the vagina and the penis, they all agreed they did not recall learning much. "It's kind of the same as when they were teaching us about drugs in elementary school," said twenty-three-year-old Taylor. "We were like, 'What are drugs?'" she went on, describing the pattern of young people being told about the inherent danger of something at the same time they were taught what the thing actually was. "So now it was like, 'Huh? What's oral sex?'"

The conversation turned to another taboo topic: female pleasure. "I didn't even know that women were supposed to enjoy sex," said Alexis, a college senior with a slender frame and fiery opinions. None of the women recalled talking about female masturbation in sex ed. "It wasn't mentioned that girls would touch themselves, or ever do

* Names have been changed to protect their privacy.

anything like that," Alexis continued, her tone bristly. "It was like, 'This is your uterus and that's all you need to know.'"

"This is where you carry babies when you're thirty," chimed in Madison, twenty-four.

"I totally masturbated in high school and I lied to my boyfriend about it," said another girl, in jeans and a black top. "I was like, 'No, only you. You're the best.'" Around the table, eyes rolled.

On the topic of reproductive angst, several of the young women shared that they hadn't ever had a pap smear, and a few had never been to the gynecologist—a fact that caused me to blurt out, "Wait, seriously?" even though I was trying to sit and mostly listen without interjecting.

Almost everyone at the table had a specific reason for believing her fertility had somehow been compromised—because of an eating disorder, or years running track and field, or Accutane (a strong drug used to treat acne), or PCOS, or fragile X syndrome (a genetic condition), or months in a row of missed periods. "I don't even know if I'm fertile," said Alexis, looking down at her hands. "Like, because I'm so reckless. I make bad decisions in terms of sex. I stopped taking birth control because I'm not good at taking medication. And I don't remember the last time I used a condom with someone that I was seeing on the regular. So, I don't know. I'm on a non-plan plan, I guess."

"I'm going to put this out there," a girl named Michelle said suddenly. She wore a pink blouse and nervously played with her dark hair. "I've had an abortion."

At first, the table fell silent. And then:

"I have, too."

"Me, too."

"Yeah. Same."

A few others murmured affirmatively, their eyes cast downward at the table.

Michelle shared her story of having an abortion at fifteen weeks. When she described walking into Planned Parenthood wearing a sweatshirt with the hood pulled up over her head, she began to cry. The girls looked at Michelle, then among one another. "There were old ladies literally throwing paper balls at me," she said, referring to protesters who often stand outside abortion clinics and harass women entering them. I looked around and saw expressions of sad recognition on almost every face. It turned out that more than half of the group had had an abortion, and while their experiences were not all as harrowing as Michelle's, they shared worries that the procedure had somehow impacted their ability to give birth in the future. When I asked why, no one could articulate why their concern felt as real as it did.*

Even a couple of the women in the group who had already given birth to healthy babies were concerned about their fertility. For years, twenty-five-year-old Stefanie and her partner did not use protection while having sex. After a while, Stefanie assumed she was infertile. "It got to a point where I was like, 'Oh, I can't get pregnant,'" she said, leaning back in her chair. "It would have happened by now." But it did; her son had just turned one. Still, she says, "I know I obviously *can* have a baby. But we didn't happen to get pregnant until after three years of having unprotected sex. So I don't know how long it's going to take when I actually want to *try* to have a kid." Kayla, another mother in the group, said that her first doctor's appointment after getting pregnant at age twenty-six felt like a sit-down interview. The way the doctor phrased her questions made Kayla feel the need to defend her decision to keep the baby. At the same time, the doctor's gentle probing gave Kayla pause. "I thought to myself, 'Am I worthy of having a child right now?'" she said. Like Stefanie, Kayla and her partner did not use contraception. "I knew better, but I just got comfortable. We'd been together for eight years by the time I got pregnant."

Am I worthy of having a child right now? Later, I'd consider Kayla's choice of words, reflecting on the value judgments often wrapped up in young women's perception of motherhood, as if having a baby is something one must earn and deserve. At the same time, not using birth control suggested a flippant attitude toward the possibility of

---

* Having an abortion very rarely affects a person's fertility or ability to become pregnant in the future. But many women have been socialized to think that it does.

pregnancy, a shrug at what could happen. It was a confusing juxtapo-sition, and normally I would have asked a challenging follow-up question or two. But at the time, *Roe v. Wade* was still in effect, and as our discussion came to an end, a certain tenderness hung in the air, so I chose not to press the point any further. I felt a kind of quiet kinship with these women, I realized, and wondered if that made me a less-than reporter, if it compromised my purported objectivity in some way. It was becoming more difficult to compartmentalize my work as a journalist from my work being a woman.

To me, the most striking aspect of our informal discussion was the young women's shared frustration about the lack of open dialogue around so many topics related to sex, fertility, and reproductive choices. And not just with family members or sexual partners, but among their peers and friends. The conversation that evening wasn't the first time those women had been confronted with this deficiency, but collectively airing their frustrations cracked something open. When the talk shifted to abortion and the women who'd had one shared their experiences, I saw a real catharsis happening. Shame was replaced with solidarity, and the feeling of acknowledgment and *you're not alone* that played out at the dining room table was heartening to witness.

The Knowledge Gap

One winter night a few months into our relationship, Ben and I shared ravioli and a basket of bread at an Italian restaurant in Brook-lyn. I picked at the red-and-white checkered tablecloth as I relayed details of my second surgery: the familiar pain I'd felt in my side, the doctors plunging their hands between my legs, the deep fear. I tried to keep my tone even and unemotional; after all, I was fine now, wasn't I? But I felt compelled to explain how important this all felt to me. Still.

Ben listened, eyes wide. I couldn't quite tell how much he was grasping; most men I explained my surgeries to—women, too, for that matter—began squirming at "transvaginal ultrasound" and "ovar-ian torsion," which I'd take as my cue to wrap up quickly. As I talked,

Ben sat very still, a look of concerned compassion on his face. "Do you think about these things when we're having sex?" he asked when I'd finished, his voice quiet but not shy. I looked down at my hands, twisting my thumb ring, not sure how to answer.

My adolescence, that tender time of puberty and growing into one's body, had been bookended by medical emergencies starring my ovaries. Ben's question spurred flashes of memories from the years between and after those traumas: painful recollections of when my body felt as if it didn't belong to me; moments that left me feeling exposed, alone, gone away. My list is long, my stories not particularly unique. Operations. Instances of sexual violence. Being the subject of medical studies, when I was just out of college and in need of cash, for which I received paltry amounts of money. A physician prying me open like a clamshell; a stranger forcing himself on me; a boyfriend's hands on the back of my head while I was going down on him, pushing deeper without asking me first until I gagged. The truth was, from adolescence to my mid-twenties, my understanding of my body was marked by a sense of things being done to me. Those experiences no longer defined my relationship with my body, but they did—do—inform it.

But I wasn't ready to tell Ben any of this. "No, not really," I finally answered, my heart still in my throat. Ben hesitated before he spoke. "Because I don't want to mess anything up," he said. "I don't want to hurt you."

The sit-down conversation with the young women and my attempts to talk with Ben more vulnerably about my past medical traumas stirred familiar frustrated feelings about young women's collective ignorance. Knowledge is power, and in the particular situations described by the women with whom I'd spoken, they had had little of either. The same had been true for me at various points in my teens and twenties. But it went deeper. At first I thought the knowledge problem centered around the troubling fact I'd learned about how college-age women are only cursorily informed about their cycles. But then I had to add the realities of age-related fertility decline to the

list, as well as the basics about hormones, once I'd learned that most
young women know very little about the birth control pills they swallow, the IUDs they have inserted, the reproductive parts they may rely
on one day to have a child.

The issue was not merely what we weren't taught or told but what
came to exist in the vacuum. The implications of all this not knowing
extended to an entire new chapter of obliviousness or misguidance
when women reached their thirties. Sex ed was long gone, dusty and
mostly unhelpful as it faded in the rearview mirror. Now the vast
bubble of ignorance and silence centered around fertility—around
two troubling facts in particular. One, too many women have unreal-
istic expectations about how long their bodies can biologically bear
children. And two, too many women don't understand fertility until
they learn they no longer have it.

Like Will before he met Kati, I didn't learn about fertile windows
until well into adulthood. A woman can only get pregnant on the day
she ovulates: false. A woman can get pregnant all the time: also false.
The more I learned about ovulation and hormones, the more I realized that my newly gained knowledge about a woman's ability to get
pregnant meant untangling myths and misconceptions I'd long believed to be true.

Also like Will, I woke up to how little I knew when I first thumbed
through *Taking Charge of Your Fertility.* The book is clear and comprehensive, but also warm and approachable. I've dog-eared the pages
and scribbled question marks and exclamation points in the margins.
There are pictures and helpful diagrams and straightforward, easy-to-
understand explanations for incredibly complex things. My copy was
a gift from my mother after I began writing this book, many years
after the American Girl book. She inscribed this one, too. *Dear Natalie,* her familiar, comforting cursive reads. *I've had this book a few days
now, and yesterday, I set it out to write a note before giving it to you. Last
night I dreamed I was breastfeeding my baby girl! I certainly must have "fertility" on my mind. Use this book to enhance your knowledge. Use the knowledge you gain to be a better informed, and more relaxed, mother-to-be. I have*

not a doubt in the world that you will be a mother . . . and a great mother.
I'm so happy to be <u>your</u> mother.

It was becoming clearer to me now that my relationship to my body was not separate from my decision about egg freezing. The broader truth was this: How women learn or do not learn about the basics informs if and when they learn about fertility and circumstances impacting their reproductive futures. One of the common frustrations voiced by women over the years, doctors told me, is that they wish they had known how much egg quantity and egg quality matter—and they wish they'd learned this earlier, *before* they found themselves seeking fertility treatment in their late thirties and early forties. Doctors I spoke with also confirmed what I had heard anecdotally to be true: that many women undergoing egg freezing wish they'd realized earlier how big a role age plays in the ability to conceive, instead of looking to celebrities having babies in their mid- to late forties—often through donor eggs, surrogates, or gestational carriers, though their ART interventions usually go unmentioned—to guide their sense of what's possible.

It's not just younger women who are in the dark. It's common for women in their forties to blithely assume they can get pregnant, merely because they *feel* young and healthy. It's an easy trap to fall into. Women think that because we are looking younger and living longer, the expiration of our eggs should be extended, too. But as I discussed in chapter 3, the realities of a woman's fertility have mostly remained unchanged; in this area of life, thirty is definitely not the new twenty.

Okay, so by this point I'd come to terms with the social and personal reasons women are procreating later in life. I'd learned about the sex ed we never got and begun to grapple with the long-term implications of Not Knowing. But what to do about the pesky problem of biology? Try as we might to ignore or discount it, this biological truth is not easily swept under the rug. ASRM's Ethics Committee reminds us: "Older female age increases the risk of inability to conceive due to reduced oocyte quantity and quality, with increased chromosomal abnormalities leading to more fetal abnormalities and pregnancy losses." Translated: As the years accrue, fertility diminishes. Healthy eggs are hard to come by. Miscarriages and babies born with developmental issues become more common.

"Fertility meant nothing to us in our twenties; it was something to be secured in the dungeon and left there to molder," writes Ariel Levy in *The Rules Do Not Apply,* her memoir about the loss of her pregnancy, partner, and home. "In our early thirties, we remembered it existed and wondered if we should check on it, and then—abruptly, horrifyingly—it became urgent: Somebody find that dragon! It was time to rouse it, get it ready for action. But the beast had not grown stronger during the decades of hibernation. By the time we tried to wake it, the dragon was weakened, wizened. Old."

Her words were a warning. Coupled with the words of NYU bioethicist Arthur Caplan that I quoted before—*there is this notion that you can get pregnant whenever you want, the technology is here, we've got the answers, it's in your control*—they haunted me. For educated, middle-class women, the list of things in life we can control and succeed at is long and growing. We live in an aspirational age; very little today ever slows down or de-escalates. It should come as no surprise that the message as we get older is that fertility is something we ought to be controlling—preserving, protecting, investing in. And infertility, then, is in many ways the ultimate loss of control.

"We lived in a world where we had control of so much," Levy continues. "Anything seemed possible if you had ingenuity, money, and tenacity. But the body doesn't play by those rules." And so we intervene before our bodies can betray us. Deploy technology to not only command but enhance our reproductive systems, what and when they will produce. Capitalize on the scientific advancements that have made it possible to exponentially expand our ovaries' capacity to generate eggs, thereby improving our chances of having a biological baby only when we are ready, completely or at least mostly on our own terms. Take action now to mitigate against loss of control down the road. These are the solutions women are encouraged to embrace. The nature of the game has changed, and the savvy among us will realize we no longer have to shrug and accept our bodies skirting the rules.

At least that's what our can-do society is promising us.

Egg Freezing Up Close

I had gotten some clarity on the basics, and why I hadn't known what I didn't know until now. The next step, it seemed to me, was to learn more about the mysterious technology that my fertility doctor and the physicians at the EggBanxx event all spoke of as being the solution to the hard-to-get-around biology problem. And to better understand the whole process, I needed to see egg freezing in action.

I paid a visit to a lab belonging to Extend Fertility, a boutique egg freezing clinic in midtown Manhattan. On a snowy winter day, I hurried along West 57th Street to watch an embryologist demonstrate the actual technique of freezing a woman's eggs. It was my first time visiting a fertility clinic as a reporter rather than a patient, but the potential egg freezing customer in me took note of Extend Fertility's warm and inviting vibe, the orchids at the reception counter, the sunny, window-filled consultation rooms. Privacy rules prevented me from watching a patient have her eggs retrieved, but Leslie Ramirez, an embryologist and the company's assistant director of its embryology laboratory at that time, offered to walk me through a sped-up demonstration of the process.

Most of the conversation around egg freezing centers around the several days of hormone injections and the day of the egg retrieval. But while the day a woman's eggs are retrieved is in many ways the end of her experience, the journey for her eggs is just beginning. The actual "egg freezing" part of egg freezing begins immediately after a woman's eggs are no longer inside her body. Amid the hype surrounding the whole procedure, the all-important step of vitrification— the ultra-rapid cooling technique that significantly improves egg survival and pregnancy rates—tends to be overlooked.

A crucial component of egg freezing, the delicate process of vitrification occurs shortly after the retrieval. While the woman is waking up from anesthesia, her eggs are hand-delivered to the lab and placed in an incubator for a couple of hours. Then, an embryologist inspects the eggs under a microscope to determine which ones are mature before exposing the mature eggs to cryoprotectants, the chemicals that shield the eggs from the stresses of freezing and thawing. Next, the embryologist attaches a few eggs at a time to labeled plastic strips (each about the diameter of a piece of spaghetti), called straws, and dips them in liquid nitrogen, where they freeze almost instantly; all biological activity in the eggs, including aging, stops. Once the eggs are flash-frozen, the straws are attached to a longer piece of plastic, called a cane, and placed in a sealed tank that looks like a propane canister used for a barbecue grill. The storage tank, which has been filled with liquid nitrogen and maintains a temperature of −196 degrees Celsius (−320 degrees Fahrenheit), keeps the submerged eggs cold—and preserved indefinitely.

Decorative snowflakes on the embryology lab's door matched the cobalt blue scrubs I had been instructed to change into. Ramirez gestured for me to come in. I pressed "record" on my phone and shoved it inside my waistband, hoping it wouldn't slide down my pants leg and clank onto the white-tiled floor, then stepped inside, pulling the heavy metal door closed behind me. The brightly lit lab had the faintly metallic smell of hospital-grade disinfectant. High-powered microscopes sat beside micromanipulators that resembled videogame consoles and white machines with pink or blue labels that said things like TransferMan 4m and incubator c16. There were also custom air filters, designed specifically for an embryology lab like this one. Because eggs and embryos are exposed to open air when being transferred in and out of petri dishes, keeping the air as sterile and contaminant-free as possible is important; even a lab worker's perfume can impact the quality and development of an embryo.

Ramirez, a thirtyish, petite, Mexican-born Harvard-trained scientist with a PhD in biotechnology, was looking down at a petri dish that sat on the counter. Inside the pool of clear liquid, she told me, lay two human eggs. I moved closer to get a better look, careful not to bump against any of the expensive-looking equipment. Most cells are too small to be seen without a microscope, but a human egg—0.1 millimeters in diameter, about as wide as a strand of hair and right at the level of visibility—*can* be seen with the naked eye, though it's a lot easier to see a group of eggs than just one. I could just barely make out the minuscule eggs in the petri dish, each about the size of the period at the end of this sentence. "Ooh," I exclaimed softly, looking up at Ramirez. She smiled back at me, then briskly returned to explaining. The liquid solution, or culture media, mimics the nutrient-rich environment the egg has in the female body while the embryologist inspects them to determine maturity. Usually, only mature, viable eggs—typically 75 percent of retrieved eggs—are frozen because they're the ones that can be fertilized, hopefully, later on.* The petri dish in front of me, labeled DISCARD in handwritten black capitals, held oocytes that had been extracted from a woman whose retrieval had yielded several mature eggs that had been successfully frozen. The patient had given permission for her leftover, unviable eggs to be used for training purposes.

Ramirez placed the dish on the stage of a microscope and, using a pipette, moved the eggs from their nutrient-rich bath into a different petri dish. The liquid solution in this dish is where the vitrification magic happens: In a series of chemical processes, the cryoprotectants in the solution draw out water from the eggs. On the monitor attached to the microscope—the image of one of the eggs blown up, making the action look more dramatic—I could see how it immediately shrank. In its dehydrated state, the egg, projected on the screen, resembled a small, shriveled pea. Then, the egg expanded again, as the cryoprotectant filled the cell. Almost instantly, the egg regained its normal, perfectly round shape. Ramirez stepped aside and motioned for me to look through the microscope's eyepiece myself. A tank of liquid nitrogen hissed; a machine whirred and beeped. I squinted my eyes and peered into the petri dish at the tiny scraps of life it contained.

I once heard it explained that preserving eggs is akin to preserving the crystals of a snowflake—except the eggs are far more delicate and even more vulnerable. In the laboratory environment, as they are transferred from a woman's ovaries to a plastic straw to inside a tank of liquid nitrogen, these smaller-than-small cells are incredibly sensi-

---

* Only mature eggs can be fertilized. But some clinics freeze immature eggs as well, because there's a small chance some might mature after the thawing process. Also, since egg freezing is intended for the long term, there's the hope that new technology or techniques will be developed in the future that would make it possible to use these oocytes.

tive to any variation in temperature. Fluctuations of a few degrees can destroy them. As I watched Ramirez demonstrate transporting and submerging eggs in their liquid nitrogen bath, the decorative snow-flakes on the lab's door caught my eye and I found myself smiling. A coincidence, a small irony, maybe, or both. I wasn't sure I was firmly grasping what I was seeing—literally, a woman's fertility put on ice—and what it meant. My last biology class was in eleventh grade, which was also the last time I fumbled around with a microscope. Back then, more or less pretending I knew what I was looking at and why it mattered amounted to a teenage shrug and an A-minus. But standing in the lab that day, wearing borrowed scrubs and scribbling unfamiliar words into my notebook, I couldn't even pretend I possessed the robust scientific background required to understand the most intricate parts of egg freezing.

But I hadn't come this far to stop asking questions. I reminded myself that I'd already begun to go beyond the technology's surface-level explanations. And so, burgeoning science journalist that I apparently now was, I would keep going, keep delving deeper to confront egg freezing's implications beyond its sheen of complex science and oh-so-shiny promises.

Seesawing and Second Thoughts

Early spring. The end of a long day, back-to-back classes, and hours writing at the NYU library. Ben and I met friends for dinner on the Lower East Side. On the drive home, I rolled down the passenger-seat window in Ben's rattly Civic and watched the twinkling Manhattan skyline recede in the side mirror. Cars bound for Brooklyn were backed up, their headlights piercing and brilliant. It was a velvety mid-March evening and the air had a pulse to it: the promise of see-sawing seasons, of bloom. We climbed the five flights of stairs to my apartment and fell into bed, exhausted. Ben was, predictably, sound asleep within minutes. I lay awake, my mind racing, for no particular reason, just a lot of reasons. I felt completely overwhelmed by all I was juggling: my thesis and graduate school work, my fascinating internship at a magazine, my new relationship with Ben. And on top of my overcommitted day-to-day was this business of trying to figure out my fertility and make a decision about egg freezing, all of which was proving to be more complicated than I had bargained for.

Outside, bodega doors banged shut and an occasional siren wailed. My head rested on Ben's bare chest, his arm wrapped around me and his hand cupping my breast. I blinked at the darkness. I wanted to be comforted by our tangle, our intertwined parts that at times fit perfectly, but his arm became heavier, our skin sweatier, the street noise louder, until all I could hear and feel was my galloping heart.

Something had shifted in how I'd come to think about egg freezing—and my fertility in general—since meeting Ben. While I know I can be a parent on my own, having children has, for me, always been tied to the idea of a committed relationship. I have always imagined having kids with all the basics in place: a fulfilling career, a savings account, health insurance. And a partner.

I broached the subject of kids with Ben sometime after our first weekend away together and before he met my parents. He told me he had no doubts that he would make a great father someday.

"Oh, yeah?" I chuckled. "And how do you know?" I tried to keep my tone casual—could I have asked for a better reply?—but I could feel my dimples giving me away.

"I'll just do everything my dad did, because he was the best dad ever," Ben answered.

My heart fluttered. He had said it so simply, so sincerely that I immediately trusted the pure place it came from. I murmured something in response, then sat back to savor the moment. I took a long look at Ben. He was nursing his beer, his tan, floppy loafers hanging off the barstool's bottom rung. I had come to recognize the affable smile he wore, confident and a little coy. I imagined him approaching fatherhood with this same self-assuredness. I could easily picture him as a dad, running around a grassy backyard with a toddler on his shoulders and another at his feet. But imagining him accompanying me to egg freezing appointments and plunging hormone injections into my butt cheek? Couldn't see it. And not just because Ben had a paralyzing fear of needles. I couldn't imagine it because the scene did not fit in the nice narrative that had formed in my head about the story of my life.

I initially saw egg freezing as an independent, solo thing, a way for me to claim ownership of something that had never felt as if it was in my control. Now that I was in a relationship—getting serious quickly, in a good way—why did it make sense for me to freeze my eggs? I didn't know how or whether Ben fit into my egg freezing decision. He'd been supportive since day one and showed genuine curiosity about all I'd been learning. I wondered if he had an opinion about if and when I might do it, although I wasn't sure I wanted to hear it. Maybe, I thought, I should forgo freezing and start trying to get pregnant earlier than I had planned.

But still, lying in bed most nights with Ben's arm wrapped around me, I'd find myself seized with anxiety about the possibility I might never be pregnant with my own eggs. That perhaps my missing parts wouldn't amount to anything. Thoughts swirling, I would remember similar disquieting nights, like the ones in Sri Lanka years ago when I'd jerk awake, gripping my right side, in some kind of phantom pain summoned by memories of my long-ago surgeries.

Middle-of-the-night thoughts and nagging worries that come and go over years, as these do for me, tend to have connective tissue that is as strong as it is stubborn. When would the thought of accidentally becoming pregnant stop seeming like such a catastrophe? When would the possibility of never being pregnant stop haunting me? How much information and empowerment would it take to banish this angst from my—from every woman's—head?

It had been several months since my last appointment with Dr. Noyes. She had sold me on the powerful potential of egg freezing; her ringing endorsement lingered in my mind. I had been surprised and pleased by the strength I heard in my voice when I told her I was going to freeze my eggs. But since that feet-in-stirrups declaration, I felt less sure. When I asked for help understanding the basic mechanics of egg freezing, I had secretly hoped that if I could understand at least at a rudimentary level how the process worked, I would have an aha moment that would make it easier for me to feel good about the decision I'd made. Because I *had* made a decision, lying there in my floppy gown, a goofy grin on my face because my ovary was doing great. *You know too much,* Dr. Noyes had said to me at my second appointment. *That's the problem.* She'd said it facetiously, but I was beginning to think she was right. Observing egg freezing in action had helped demystify the science some, but it had left me with more questions, not fewer. It was almost as if, the more time I spent piecing together what I was learning about egg freezing, trying to get it all straight, the more of a Pandora's box it all seemed to be.

I slipped out of bed and walked to the kitchen in my underwear, the wood floor cool beneath my bare feet. My phone screen read 1:11 A.M. I filled a glass with water and untwisted a half-empty bag of candy. In the living room, I curled up in my favorite wicker chair, which I'd had since college. Round and deep, a worn-in nest. The velvety air and laughing with friends that had punctuated the evening earlier felt so distant now. I closed my eyes and dozed fitfully, waking with candy stains on my fingers. It was still dark out. I opened my copy of *Taking Charge of Your Fertility* and, with a pink headlamp strapped to my forehead, read about cervical mucus and G-spots until it began to grow light.

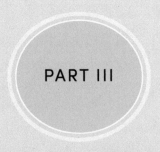

PART III

The Stimulation

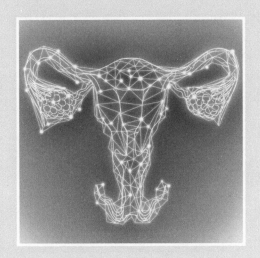

Ready, Set, Trigger Shot

~~~~~~

Remy: Bring On the Eggs

By the end of the several days of hormone injections, Remy felt like she was about to pop. *Legitimately feel like I am a goose waddling around with a gut full of (very expensive, like 14-karat) eggs,* she texted me on the last day of her shots. We'd kept in touch since she'd started the egg freezing medications. She felt more or less okay, save for the intense bloating that was unlike anything she had ever experienced before. As her egg retrieval day neared, anxiety began to creep in, laced with humor in her texts: *I'm so scared of something happening to them hahaa I'm hyper-conscious of my every move. MUST PROTECT THE EGGS AT ALL COSTS.*

I flew to Nashville for Remy's trigger shot and egg retrieval. This would be the first time I saw these parts of the egg freezing process up close. The night of that crucial last injection, I drove from my hotel to an apartment on the other side of town. Remy's good friend Leah,★ also an anesthesia resident, lived there. When I arrived, Remy and Leah were draped on an overstuffed couch, watching *Crazy Rich Asians* on Netflix. A typical millennial Saturday night, save for the various vials of drugs and needles scattered on the kitchen counter.

★ Name has been changed.

The two women howled at the movie, heads thrown back in laughter. Remy had been up for twenty-two hours by this point, having come off one of her long hospital shifts. She was wearing black leggings and a roomy gray sweatshirt, her hair in a high ponytail. Her feet were bare—pink toenails, from a recent pedicure—and her face fresh, makeup-free. She looked twenty-three, not thirty-three.

Outside, the skyline was gray and darkening. Leah turned off the TV. After ten days of injecting the hormone shots herself, Remy had decided to ask Leah to do this final one. This shot would go just above Remy's right butt cheek. Remy's biggest takeaway from the injection demonstration appointment at the fertility clinic had been learning what not to stress about throughout the egg freezing process and what to *definitely* stress about. In reassuring words, the nurse had told Remy not to worry too much about always injecting the shots at the exact same time each night. But Dr. Lewis, Remy remembered, had been explicit about the timing of the trigger shot. "If you take it too early," she'd warned, "you'll ovulate too soon and release all your eggs and I'll have nothing. If you inject it too late, the eggs will be immature and I'll have nothing." At the time, Remy had half-groaned, already worried that she'd make a mistake and mess up the timing. The clinic had provided Remy with a video tutorial to review before taking the trigger shot, which she watched, but she still felt somewhat confused and nervous because it had different directions than the other meds she'd been injecting.

When it was nearly time, Remy and Leah stood at the kitchen counter and took stock of the vials and syringes spread out in front of them. Remy got to work reconstituting. The trigger shot is a powder that needs to be dissolved in saline. Mixed, but not shaken.

"Does that look ready?" Remy asked Leah.

Leah peered at the vial. "Maybe swirl it one more time."

Remy reached for a long needle. "Are you sure the twenty-seven gauge is the one you inject with?" Leah asked.

"Hundred percent sure," Remy replied. "I mean, I think so. It's really long but it's not supposed to go all the way in. They told me if I hit the bone it wouldn't hurt, not to worry. The periosteum is so sensitive, are you kidding me? That would fucking hurt."

"It would definitely fucking hurt," Leah echoed.

"I still don't understand how women who aren't in medicine do this," said Remy, glancing at her watch to check the time. "I mean, reconstituting meds is our life. But this isn't easy stuff."*

A few minutes later, the trigger shot was ready. Remy pulled down her leggings partway. She looked at Leah. "I trust you, I love you, let's do this." She closed her eyes, turned around so her backside faced Leah, and braced against the kitchen sink. Leah stuck the needle into the skin just above Remy's butt cheek and pushed the syringe, then pulled it back out. Remy exhaled loudly. "Okayyyy," she said. "Wait. That was the least painful of all of them. Why was that so easy?"

"Well, your butt's not as sensitive as you'd think," Leah said, at which Remy gave a sarcastic laugh.

"Man, I made a big deal of this," said Remy, adjusting her leggings. "Wasn't that shot supposed to be a big deal?" She leaned over to hug Leah. "Oh my God, I'm so happy you did it. Thank you so much."

Leah grinned, hugging Remy back. "I just gave you a baby!"

"Like, thirty babies," Remy said, giggling with relief.

They started cleaning up the counter, disposing of the needles and plastic wrappers. Over the next thirty-five hours, Remy's follicles would finish maturing all the eggs that had been developing since she started the hormone shots.

"Now what?" said Leah.

Remy, already on her way back to the sofa, tightening her ponytail, replied: "Now we finish watching *Crazy Rich Asians.*"

So far, egg freezing had been straightforward for Remy. Yes, injecting herself with fertility hormones was complicated, but watching her going through the process up to this point showed me that the experience itself didn't have to be. She made it look doable. That she was a doctor and so comfortable with the shots, the blood work, and all the

---

* In most areas of medicine, nurses and pharmacists administer medications, but in anesthesia, doctors directly dilute and administer meds. Remy and Leah were pros.

acronyms certainly helped—and it made our situations less comparable. But it was also her attitude, how confident and self-assured she'd
been since the moment she decided to freeze. She'd advocated for
herself and been proactive every step of the way. Her optimism was a
welcome breath of fresh air. I envied her certainty—and her two
healthy ovaries. When I met Remy, I'd already decided to freeze my
eggs. I hadn't changed my mind, but I was stalling. As much as I wanted
my egg freezing experience to look like Remy's and that of other
women I'd met who had done it, I knew it probably wouldn't. The
stakes were different for me. Higher. I had one ovary; if anything went
wrong, I had much more to lose. On the other hand, what if some
other bizarre thing happened—another ruptured cyst, another emergency surgery—and my ovary had to be taken out? If that happened, I
would forever regret not freezing my eggs when I'd had the chance.

Checked Boxes and Longings

At five feet tall and just under 115 pounds, my mother doesn't look
like your typical U.S. Army colonel. She was commissioned into the
Army in 1978; hers was the third class of ROTC college graduates to
include women. My mother has been many things: high school vale-
dictorian, state supreme court legal clerk, Girl Scout troop leader,
battalion commander, mother of three, an ethics attorney for the Department of Justice. She has jumped out of airplanes; she's prepared
soldiers for immediate deployment after 9/11. She gardens and bakes
cookies. Some mothers teach their daughters how to ski, or cook, or
work a sewing machine. Mine taught me the military phonetic alpha-
bet, how to hold a rifle, and the most efficient way to lick cookie
batter off the beaters of a mixer. My mother was a trailblazer who also
liked to mow the lawn on hot summer days and tuck her daughters
into bed, reading us library books out loud. She maxed out on the
military physical training test every year—push-ups, pull-ups, running a fast mile—and loved a good manicure. She didn't change her
last name when she married, not because it was post-1960s and she
felt like being radical but because her parents had always told her:
Don't do something just because everyone else is doing it.

The world my mother became pregnant in is nothing like the world I live in. But I was raised to do what I wanted to do, and I grew up believing I had permission to live as fully as my mother did. Women of my generation were promised by a liberated society that we could do and be anything we wanted. It's a promise we are not apt to forget. We are taught to never give up, to always be striving, to pursue happy endings—whether by holding out for them or by manifesting them. This mindset is true in love and in the pursuit of motherhood, where discussions are rife with talk of miracles and perseverance. On the surface, anything seems possible. But when we dig deeper, we find we are following the same myths I've been focusing on: the illusion that any woman who tries hard enough can have whatever she dreams of, whenever she wants it, as long as she takes matters into her own hands.

It was starting to make more sense to me now why young women like me are quick to buy into the notion that when it comes to fertility, taking action is required if a woman is to maintain a sense of agency in her life. If the 1960s saw the rise of birth control and sexual liberation for women, the 2010s were the decade that freed women from thinking they have to settle, ushering in the second phase of trying to have it all. This was, after all, the time of *Lean In* and #girlboss and the possibility of the United States' first female president. When I was a girl, the message was: *It doesn't matter that you're female! Go be whatever you want to be.* Now there's a backlash of sorts, with biology and culture telling us otherwise, that being a mother is a not-to-be-missed experience, that being a wife is a status upgrade because we live in a world that regards romantic partnership as the sine qua non of content adulthood.

And so it's not difficult to see how women being given the potential to pause their biological clocks—or at least muffle the ticking—is as potent a possibility as it is. In the context of social pressures and expectations, egg freezing is an easy sell. At first glance, it seems like an ideal technological solution to a long-standing human conundrum: How can women postpone having children until the exact time in their lives that makes the most sense for them?

I recalled Remy telling me about how, in her twenties, she had approached certain aspects of life as if they were boxes to check off.

Namely, becoming a doctor, but also dating. She had approached romantic relationships with the same checklist mentality with which she approached her career, and she expected return on investment in both. But as she entered her thirties, she realized that despite her best efforts—sincere, time- and energy-consuming efforts—the neat and tidy boxes of some of the most important parts of her life were, well, not so neat and tidy after all. "Turns out that's not really how life works," Remy told me. "A lot of the life components that I viewed as checked boxes ended up being the least stable. I obviously didn't pick the right partner, either time. What ended up being the most stable was my career."

I remember when the checked boxes I envisioned for myself began to shift. It was the day I moved back to the United States from Sri Lanka and was given a warning. "Your passport is full," the officious customs agent had said. It was a Friday afternoon in July; the immigration lines at Washington Dulles International airport were hours long. The agent glanced at my short hair and thin cheeks, then back down at a picture of me taken dozens of countries and a lifetime ago. "You are not permitted to leave the U.S. again until you get a new passport."

"That's fine," I replied, adjusting my heavy pack. I had been back in the States for seventeen minutes. "I'm not going anywhere for a while." Every page in my passport was covered with stamps and visas. I had lived on four continents, sometimes for years at a time, and had just returned from a yearlong Fulbright scholarship. I loved traveling and was confident it would remain a major fixture in my life. But I was beginning to yearn for roots, the kind that would make staying in one place for a while the adventure rather than the default. I was still young, but I was also making plans—the kind I wanted my boyfriend at the time, whom I'd been living halfway around the world from for the past year, to be a part of. My worn passport was ready for a rest, and so was I.

Several years later, I can still feel the sweat underneath the straps of my backpack, the buzz of activity in the airport terminal. I was in my early twenties then, and the concept of marriage and babies seemed abstract, even though certain events had caused me to consider the baby part. But I was very much in love, and I remember how arriving back in the States coincided with a strong feeling of self-imposed pressure to put my relationship and romantic future ahead of my nascent career ambitions for a while. Then, less than a week after I returned home, my boyfriend broke up with me—later I'd come to understand his reasons, but at the time it felt so out-of-nowhere that it almost didn't seem real—and the aftershocks of our painful breakup pushed all thoughts of roots and future children out of my mind.

Now life was different, especially in the relationship department: I was falling more in love with Ben. We'd experienced a lot together since we started dating. Christmas with my family, Thanksgiving with his. We'd been each other's date at our best friends' weddings, we'd shown each other our college campuses. His comments about fatherhood had moved me, and the more time I spent with him, the more clearly I could picture him as a father—putting together the crib, doing dozens of Target runs, him getting out of bed at 2 A.M. instead of me when the baby cried. Every now and then I'd feel a pang, a sort of longing ache, at the thought of being pregnant with our daughter or son.

I had been rethinking my exuberant *Yes, let's freeze my eggs!* declaration I'd made at the fertility clinic. I'd had the preliminary assessment, done the blood work. Next up was deciding when to attend the mandatory egg freezing orientation session at the clinic, where I'd learn about injecting the medications. Yes, I'd been putting off scheduling this next appointment, but I still had a lot to look into. Among the rabbit holes I had yet to fully immerse myself in was the efficacy. It was time to find out how successful egg freezing actually was.

Does Egg Freezing Work?

I took a deep dive into what's known about the number of women freezing their eggs and egg freezing's success rates. And what I found was conflicting statistics, cherry-picked figures, and just straight-up impossible numbers. I noticed that articles and studies discussing egg freezing's popularity relied exclusively on data from the Society for Assisted Reproductive Technology (SART), so I reached out to them, hoping someone could help me whittle down my growing list of questions. SART's president at the time sent me spreadsheets of raw data and explained several figures to me over a few phone calls and emails. Later, other folks at SART provided me with updated statistics and helped me arrive at clearer numbers. I mentioned them in chapter 1, but I'll unpack them here.

Between 2009 and 2022, nearly 115,000 healthy women in the United States underwent egg freezing. In 2009, the number of healthy women choosing to freeze their eggs in the United States was 482; in 2022—the latest year for which official data is available, as of this writing—it was 22,967.* That same year also saw a 73 percent increase in the number of egg freezing cycles from two years prior. And in terms of fertility preservation as a whole, I was surprised to learn that in 2021, 40 percent of all ART cycles performed in the United States were cycles in which all resulting eggs or embryos were frozen for future use. This is significant, considering that for nearly the whole time ART has been around, the main type of ART has overwhelmingly been IVF—that is, women attempting to get pregnant *now*, not at some unknown future date. This marked rise in fertility preservation is a growth trend that is all but certain to continue, and likely increase, in coming years.

Okay, so, egg freezing has grown sharply and is continuing to soar. But what's been happening with all those thousands of frozen eggs? And more importantly, what happens when they're thawed? Turns out that it's difficult to determine, with any real certainty, how well egg freezing works. When we talk about its success rates, the conversation gets convoluted fast. It took me weeks of focused research to figure out exactly what we do know and what we don't, and why. To get to the bottom of the efficacy of the process, I needed to understand what data the procedure's success rates are based on. After more digging, I learned the bad news: Reliable data is paltry, mostly be-

---

* In this statistic, "healthy" means patients freezing eggs to preserve fertility, versus patients undergoing egg freezing for medical reasons. The data do differentiate, and today, the vast majority of women who freeze their eggs do so to preserve their fertility.

cause it's proved difficult to compile the kind of information from which helpful conclusions can be extrapolated.

There are a few reasons for this. The first has to do with the technology. The bit of good news I found reaffirmed that the science behind egg freezing has come a long way since it was developed roughly thirty years ago, particularly in terms of more dependable thawing methods and more effective ovary-stimulating medications. Vitrification—the science involved in the actual freezing of eggs—was, as I've mentioned, a game changer for the procedure. The downside of this otherwise optimistic news is that a lot of the egg freezing data available today was compiled from non-vitrified eggs, when clinics were using the less effective slow-freezing technique, which means it's not reflective of the advances in egg freezing technology used today. This has muddied the waters and makes comparing "what was" to "what may be" in terms of frozen eggs' pregnancy potential difficult to predict. What's more, many of the studies done early on focused on younger women who froze their eggs due to cancer diagnoses. That's a very different demographic compared to older women without medical conditions who are pursuing fertility preservation, which characterizes most egg freezers today.

A second, significant issue is that we simply don't have reliable data—and won't for some time. One obvious way to measure whether or not egg freezing works, I figured, would be to look at how many healthy babies were born from those eggs that *were* used. Problem is, it's just not known how many babies worldwide have been delivered from a woman's own frozen eggs. By most estimates, it's in the low thousands—a number sure to increase over time. I had assumed egg freezing's popularity could be attributed to the fact that it worked—and that there were firm numbers to prove it. But there aren't, simply because most women who have frozen their eggs haven't gone back to use them.

A small but important study published in the scientific journal *Human Reproduction* in March 2017 found that only 6 percent of those who froze their eggs between 1999 and 2014 had used them to try to become pregnant. A 2023 *Journal of Clinical Medicine* study—the first to review the worldwide literature on outcomes of egg thaw cycles following social egg freezing—showed that "the average return rate is low, around 12 percent." Other sources have concluded similarly, finding that fewer than 15 percent of American women who have frozen their eggs have thawed them. The reasons vary. Some women never find a suitable partner, or else they end up conceiving through sex; others are postponing returning to their frozen eggs in case of a divorce or in hopes of having a second or third child down the line. In these cases, the eggs represent a contingency plan that these women—so far—haven't chosen to use. This illuminates a few crucial facts often left out of conversations about egg freezing. One, how few women have tried to get pregnant using their frozen eggs. Two, that many women don't attempt to use their eggs for several years after freezing them. And three, that many women won't end up using them at all—but it will be years until we can say that with any degree of certainty.

A common mistake when talking about egg freezing's live-birth rates is to point to a single statistic and call it a day. I know this to be true because it's what I did before I got into the weeds with the numbers. A few years ago, there was an oft-discussed scary statistic from ASRM referenced by many journalists and media outlets writing about egg freezing. I latched on to this stat myself in one of the first articles I published on the topic—and learned just how easy it is to misinterpret egg freezing data. At the time, ASRM's stat put egg freezing success rates at between 2 and 12 percent—disastrous! But that statistic refers to live-birth rates per egg retrieved, using the older freezing methods. Live-birth rates from eggs frozen using vitrification, as I'll get into in a moment, are more promising. But the main reason that statistic is misleading is that it's the live-birth rate *per egg*—and virtually no one freezes just one egg.

Once I understood why there is so little data on vitrified eggs from women freezing for non-medical reasons and why studies reporting outcomes in women returning to use their frozen eggs are scarce, I turned to evidence from other contexts. Much of what we *do* currently know about egg freezing, I found out, relies on egg freezing cycles for egg donation or for medical reasons (more on egg donors in chapter 10) as well as statistics extrapolated from IVF data. When doctors talk about egg freezing success rates, they tend to compare the procedure to IVF or egg donation. Both of these ART procedures involve ovarian stimulation, as egg freezing does, but they are not the same, and chiefly are used by different subsets of patients. IVF is often done with fresh—that is, recently retrieved—eggs; egg donation often uses frozen eggs from women in their early twenties. And, as a *Time* article noted, "While anecdotal evidence suggests egg freezing is comparable to IVF because frozen eggs behave like fresh ones, IVF itself is hardly foolproof—even in women under thirty-five, the majority of cycles don't result in a live birth. But because IVF is such a common procedure, women are often reassured when they hear the comparison." The good news is that the smattering of existing findings indicates similar pregnancy rates whether using fresh or frozen eggs for IVF and that freezing eggs and thawing them for use later has no detrimental effect on a woman's pregnancy potential. So, while these are extrapolated conclusions, this is encouraging information for women hoping to become pregnant with frozen eggs down the line.

In an effort to help fill the void, some fertility clinics have taken it upon themselves to compile and publicize their own statistics. NYU Langone Fertility Center, one of the longest-standing clinics in the field, has completed more than three thousand egg freezing cycles since their egg freezing program began in 2004. In 2022, a study published in the journal *Fertility and Sterility* analyzed fifteen years of data from 543 patients who froze their eggs at NYU Langone between 2002 and 2020.* The study showed that 74 percent of eggs survived the thawing process and nearly 70 percent of those surviving eggs were successfully fertilized. It also found that the overall chance of a live birth from frozen eggs was 39 percent. The average age when

* For all patients who underwent the procedure after 2011, their eggs were cryopreserved using vitrification, making this study relatively robust in terms of data on eggs frozen with the more modern, non-slow-freezing method.

women froze eggs was thirty-eight, and on average they waited four years to return to the clinic to use them. Among women who were younger than thirty-eight when they froze their eggs, the live-birth rate was 51 percent. It rose to 70 percent if women younger than thirty-eight also thawed twenty or more eggs. So the study's conclusion is no surprise: The younger a woman was when she froze her eggs, the greater a chance she had of a live birth.

At first glance, these live-birth rates from frozen eggs may not seem very encouraging. The pregnancy rate is not as good as a lot of women think it will be. But it's crucial to understand that the current data on live-birth rates using frozen eggs doesn't offer a clear picture on how well egg freezing works because *the numbers aren't there*. As frustrating as that may be, it's the reality. We simply do not have robust data yet on unused frozen eggs. Unthawed eggs, then, do not represent any kind of failure; they can only be characterized as such if they prove unviable when they are unfrozen.

Another takeaway from the NYU Langone study and others like it is that their data reaffirms what fertility doctors have talked about anecdotally for years now: that many women who freeze their eggs do not get pregnant because of the age at which they preserved them and/or because they did not preserve enough eggs. It's the same quantity-and-quality idea from our egg discussion in chapter 2. Getting many high-quality oocytes is key with egg freezing, and younger women have a distinct advantage both because they produce more eggs and because a higher proportion of their eggs turn out to be good. Egg quality: Younger women's oocytes are more likely to create chromosomally normal embryos. Egg quantity: Younger women are more likely to respond better to the hormone injections and thus have more oocytes extracted in a single cycle.

And the more eggs a woman successfully retrieves, the better. Why? Because not all eggs will become viable embryos. First of all, remember that usually not all extracted eggs are mature, and only mature eggs can be fertilized. Then, some eggs won't survive the thawing process. And not all eggs that make it to the fertilization stage will merge properly with sperm to form early-stage embryos. Finally, not all fully developed embryos will be genetically normal. Using frozen eggs to have a successful pregnancy is a multistep process, with many eggs or embryos lost along the way; one egg frozen does not necessarily equal one child. Which brings us to attrition rates.

When a woman is ready to use her frozen eggs, IVF picks up where egg freezing left off. Here's how it works. First the eggs are thawed. Then they are injected with sperm. The next day, an embryologist will assess which eggs were fertilized, and the fertilized eggs are left in a petri dish for five to seven days, with some developing from early-stage embryos into what are known as blastocysts.[*] Some of the blastocysts will grow into viable, chromosomally normal embryos.[†] One of these embryos is then transferred into the uterus, where the hope is that it attaches to the uterine wall and implants successfully.[‡] Fertility specialists sometimes describe the success rates of thawing eggs, fertilizing them into blastocysts, and transferring a resulting viable embryo to the uterus as resembling an inverted pyramid: You start with a certain number of eggs and lose some at every step.

Let's say Alex freezes twenty-four mature, good eggs. Eighty to 90 percent will survive the thaw, meaning about twenty of the eggs will make it to the fertilization stage, which is when the eggs are injected with sperm. It's about a 75 percent fertilization rate, so that's fifteen fertilized eggs. These fertilized eggs are left to grow for a few days, becoming early-stage embryos that are graded on certain characteristics. Most will reach day three of growth—in Alex's case, that leaves twelve early-stage embryos—and some will make it to day five of growth, at which point they become blastocysts. An embryo that

---

[*] After fertilization, the embryos are grown in a nourishing liquid nutrient solution—the kind I mentioned in chapter 7 when I visited Extend Fertility's lab—that mimics the internal environment of the reproductive tract.

[†] It's only possible to assess whether a woman's thawed eggs are chromosomally normal after they are fertilized and the resulting embryos are tested; more on this when we get into the pros and cons of freezing embryos versus freezing eggs in chapter 11.

[‡] Increasingly, patients across all age groups choose to transfer a single embryo. Transferring more than one embryo increases the likelihood of multiple-fetus pregnancies, like twins or triplets, which in turn increases the probability of premature births and related health problems (lower average birth weight for the offspring, higher risk of gestational diabetes for the mother, and more).

reaches the blastocyst stage of development consists of two types of cells, those that will develop into fetal tissues and those that will develop into the placenta. Finally, with an approximately 40 percent blastocyst conversion rate—50 percent is considered excellent—Alex will end up with four to six chromosomally normal embryos. Each has a 55 to 65 percent chance of resulting in a live birth. If Alex is twenty-eight years old when her eggs are frozen, about three-fourths of her embryos will be normal. If she's thirty-eight, half will. And if she's forty-two, one-fourth of the embryos will be normal.*

While there is no magic number for how many eggs a woman should freeze to feel confident about the procedure "working," a 2021 *Journal of Assisted Reproduction and Genetics* article that summarized the existing evidence around social egg freezing found that, on average, twenty eggs are recommended to achieve a pregnancy, with the minimum number being eight to ten. And the 2023 *Journal of Clinical Medicine* study I mentioned emphasized quantity being a crucial factor, determining that "irrespective of age at freezing, a significantly high live birth rate was achieved when the number of eggs frozen per patient was 15 or more."†

Two researchers at Brigham and Women's Hospital and Harvard Medical School were among the first to try to assign probabilities to egg freezing based on a woman's age and the number of eggs retrieved. Their analysis, published in April 2017 in *Human Reproduction,* uses a mathematical model based on data from more than five hundred healthy women in their twenties or thirties who underwent IVF (because of their male partners' fertility issues) without freezing their eggs to extrapolate to women who elect to undergo IVF with frozen eggs. The study predicts that patients under thirty-five who

---

* The figures in this example are general averages; a lot of attrition data is clinic-dependent, so the numbers vary.

† The researchers involved in the 2021 study, on the other hand, plainly stated that the available data "clearly suggest that age is the main factor that dictates success rates, and even with the most optimistic predictions, a live birth cannot be guaranteed." The point is, both a woman's age at the time of freezing and the number of eggs she has retrieved significantly impact her chances of having a baby with her frozen eggs.

froze ten to twenty eggs have between a 70 and 90 percent chance of at least one live birth later on. The most oft-cited favorable stat from their predictive model—note the word "predictive"; the study wasn't based on actual births from egg freezers—indicated that a thirty-six-year-old woman who freezes ten eggs has a 60 percent chance of producing a live birth with one of those eggs. That's pretty good. What's really exciting, though, is that their study offers one of the best new tools for predicting egg freezing success rates, which, as we've seen, are difficult to parse. A calculator based on their work can be found online; SART, CDC, and a few fertility clinics also have publicly available calculators that women can use when trying to assess their individual chances of having a child using their frozen eggs.

You can see how the varying percentages and patient-specific factors make it challenging for fertility doctors to thoroughly inform their patients. But the good ones try to, because they know how important it is for women to take into account the many steps involved in attempting to use their frozen eggs. Dr. Temeka Zore, a reproductive endocrinologist at Spring Fertility in San Francisco, is explicit about what is and is not known about egg freezing's success rates when she counsels patients considering the procedure. At the initial consult appointment, she shows a slide describing the attrition rates associated with frozen eggs. She walks the patient through the embryo development stages and explains that of all the eggs a woman freezes, only one-quarter will become chromosomally normal embryos that are suitable to be implanted in her uterus.

"Egg freezing is not a guarantee," Dr. Zore told me. "It provides you with greater options for the future, but no one can guarantee that egg freezing will lead to live births." Other fertility doctors I spoke with echoed one of Dr. Zore's major concerns: that most women undergoing egg freezing don't end up with enough eggs on ice. "Many patients think that, as an example, freezing eight eggs means eight chances at a baby," she said. "It doesn't. Because not all of those eggs will make it to embryos. I think that needs to be well stated by physicians. We have to be very clear as a field about the data—about what happens after you freeze and thaw eggs."

To the common question of "How many frozen eggs do I need?" responsible fertility clinics and doctors offer a range. The more eggs a woman has frozen, of course, the better the chances of selecting the best eggs that will then be used to make chromosomally normal embryos and lead to a successful pregnancy. This is why many women do more than one cycle to retrieve more eggs. Those aware of the importance of getting enough eggs—who've really sat with what "enough" means in this context—often undergo multiple cycles to retrieve more eggs. For these patients in particular, the total number of eggs frozen is the end point, their awareness of what happens if they try to use their frozen eggs a good deal less clear. Not their fault—clinics aren't always forthcoming on that part of the process. And while most fertility doctors understand that age-specific success rates are highly dependent on the number of frozen eggs a woman banks, many don't explain to patients the possible need for additional cycles. Hence why hearing about Dr. Zore's straight talk with egg freezing patients was so refreshing. As her explanation made clearer than most fertility clinics ever do, the reality is, most frozen eggs will not result in a baby.

So: Until more women who froze their eggs return to use them, we won't have reliable numbers to predict more accurate and, hopefully, higher success rates. In the meantime, we glean what we can from the small studies that have been conducted—particularly the more recent and relatively more robust ones, like the NYU Langone study, acknowledging the caveat that the varied factors make it difficult to apply the extrapolated data to the general population—as well as from patient-specific egg freezing predictive calculators.

All in all, I found that the data surrounding egg freezing success rates is both encouraging—and not very. Here are my takeaways after analyzing the numbers and research:

- Egg freezing is, by and large, a numbers game.
- One of the few indisputable certainties is that the younger you are when you freeze eggs and the more eggs you retrieve

when you do, the better your shot at producing a chromosomally normal embryo(s) and having a healthy baby.

- Egg freezing success rates are described as general rules and broad averages. New useful tools like online egg freezing calculators help on an individual level, but to more accurately predict personal fertility health, you need to get the facts about your egg quality and quantity.
- While many thousands of women have had their eggs frozen, the vast majority have not had their eggs thawed.

As for what I'd learned about the lack of reliable data—honestly, all that left me feeling pretty disheartened. Remy, Mandy, and thousands of other millennial and Gen Z women are intent on securing their reproductive futures. But considering how tricky it is to get a handle on egg freezing success rates, it's easy to see how they pin their hopes on limited data. How tempting it is to fall prey to a false sense of security. This really frustrated me. The more I learned about egg freezing, the more I understood that it was an expensive and intense process. Now I was learning that it was riddled with uncertainty. One doctor puts egg freezing this way: "I always tell patients, 'There's not a baby in the freezer. There's a chance to get pregnant.'"

Except that's not how we think about egg freezing. Its popularity is predicated almost entirely on providing a kind of insurance—saving viable eggs now in hopes of using them later. But egg freezing carries no guarantees. "If you buy insurance, you're guaranteed a benefit if you need it," said Dr. Julie Lamb, director of fertility preservation at Pacific Northwest Fertility in Seattle. "Egg freezing isn't an insurance policy, because it doesn't pay out all the time." This was so counter to how I was used to hearing it talked about that I wrote the doctor's words on a Post-it note and taped it to my bathroom mirror. *Egg freezing is not an insurance policy.* Brushing my teeth, I'd read the note and shake my head. How many articles had I read, how many doctors had I heard say the exact opposite? But I got it now, especially after all the time I'd spent sifting through the success rates (or lack thereof): Egg freezing isn't a dependable safeguard against age-related infertility.

"The message about egg freezing's benefits is much stronger than the message about its uncertainties," said Dr. Karin Hammarberg, the lead author of the first *Human Reproduction* study I mentioned, when I called her up to ask about all those women not coming back to use their frozen eggs. And then she reminded me of something else that really threw a wrench into my thinking about all this: that while women who bank their eggs at younger ages are more likely to have those eggs work, they're also far less likely to have to rely on them. Dr. Lamb had said something similar during one of our conversations: "The fear-based advertising is a huge ethical dilemma because a lot of those patients are never going to need those eggs."

Egg freezing, then, is a possibility, not a promise. And therein lies the enormous question mark when we talk about its role in the reproductive medicine revolution. The Catch-22 of egg freezing is that its effectiveness will remain unknown until more women return to *use* their frozen eggs. But even though its efficacy remains somewhat shrouded in mystery, that's not stopping the growing numbers of women who are doing it.

FertilityIQ

Somewhere between trying to analyze egg freezing's success rates and getting bogged down by acronyms, I heard about a fertility education start-up that reviewed fertility clinics and doctors. It had a name that particularly appealed to me: FertilityIQ. On a warm weekday morning back in Brooklyn, I opened my notebook and dialed the company's founders, Jake and Deborah Anderson-Bialis, a married couple living in San Francisco. Their company was relatively new, but from what I'd learned up to this point about the lack of data surrounding assisted reproductive technologies, it was clear that what they were doing was unique—and desperately needed.

FertilityIQ's mission is to provide the latest research on every kind of fertility treatment, including outcomes and costs. It does this through a robust online platform, a website chock-full of educational courses and guides on every ART subject. This, along with FertilityIQ's verified assessments of reproductive endocrinologists and clinics, make it one of the only in-depth resources for a person pursuing fertility treatment in the United States. It offers the comprehensiveness of Google business reviews paired with the intelligence sorting of Amazon and the old-school veracity of *Consumer Reports.*

When I talked with them for the first time over video, I was struck by their genuine and down-to-earth demeanor. Our follow-up conversations were just as invigorating. Jake and Deborah's enthusiasm—for the company they'd created, for speaking with someone also personally invested in the fertility field—was apparent in every sentence. After one of our conversations, I read through some of the witty and irreverent "Founder's Notes" blog posts on FertilityIQ's website. One read: "Maybe we're all masochists, but according to a Gallup poll, 90% of us want to have a child. . . . Normally, conceiving a child involves a steamy shower, a bottle of rosé, and Enya's greatest hits. But when you are infertile, or sub-fertile, the majesty of conception is supplanted by teeth-gnashing anxiety (on-par with developing cancer, according to a Harvard study), skyrocketing expenses (one round of IVF depletes two years of household savings) and mating acts so unnatural even Seaworld would boycott in protest."

I soon realized that what FertilityIQ did was totally novel in the ART world—offering dispassionate facts, extensive assessments of fertility specialists, and straightforward explanations about treatment plans and protocols. I often saw their data cited in *The New York Times* and other major news outlets. In our initial phone and video calls, Deborah and Jake explained their goal to me: get patients the best information during the most trying process of their lives. Now, FertilityIQ has a far reach—the company, which is growing and profitable, helps 85 percent of all fertility patients in the United States—but the founders started out just trying to solve their own needs. They met when they were both pursuing advanced degrees: Jake at Harvard Business School and Deborah at Georgetown Law. The couple married in 2012 and planned to start a family. They wanted biological children but faced a potential complication: Deborah had a history of ruptured ovarian cysts, and she risked losing an ovary if it happened again. Even so, there was no reason at the beginning to think this wasn't an issue they couldn't overcome. But they didn't want to waste time finding out. "I don't know if we made an appointment from our 'Just Married' car, but if not, it was by the time we got to the hotel," Jake told me, smiling.

They were in their late twenties and could count on one hand the number of people they knew who had ever been to a fertility clinic. Of those, only a few had positive things to say about the experience. Like so many other couples, they knew they wanted a family—even if they didn't know exactly how or when that family might take shape. But they had no idea what fertility treatment entailed and, try as they might, couldn't find helpful information, online or off. With the sense of urgency and spunk she was born with, Deborah led the charge, doing her best to balance their foray into the fertility world with their demanding schedules. Jake was a partner at Sequoia Capital, a Silicon Valley venture capital firm. Deborah worked as an attorney for a start-up called Rise, a mobile nutrition app. Over the next two years, the couple traveled coast-to-coast and spent $75,000 pursuing IVF—to no avail. The timeline and costs are typical, although most people undergoing fertility treatment don't travel to multiple states. Deborah and Jake grew increasingly frustrated and exhausted in their efforts to have a baby. After miscarriages and three unsuccessful rounds of IVF, they gave up.

The silver lining of their arduous journey was that it inspired them to start FertilityIQ. Not in a hurry to monetize it, Deborah and Jake turned away potential investors when they were launching their company. At first, FertilityIQ was self-financed, and it was entirely free until it added pay-to-access courses. Unlike other companies that act as an intermediary between patients and fertility clinics, FertilityIQ doesn't get any referral fees; it has no affiliations or partnerships with doctors or clinics.

There are a number of ways patients can use and interact with the site. Prospective patients use FertilityIQ's assessment data when they are trying to find a fertility specialist who would be a good fit (the site's find-a-doctor database is free to use). This is a huge benefit, since one of the most important things a woman considering fertility treatment can do is to find the best doctor for her particular situation, as quickly and as accurately as possible. But finding one who matches your needs and won't abscond with your time, money, or hope is easier said than done. "For most of us, picking a fertility doctor looks a lot like how a first-time entrepreneur chooses a venture capitalist," said Jake, the former venture capitalist. "Decisions are made on a short fuse, fraught with emotion, swayed by unsubstantiated claims of success, insensitive to economic implication, and clinched on brand cachet alone. Ninety percent of patients we talk to don't bother to interview a second doctor—and yet most run out of patience with their first doctor well before they run out of hope or money." The anecdotal doctor recommendation from a friend or colleague is usually unhelpful, since it represents a tiny percentage of all the patients that a fertility specialist or clinic sees at any given time. "You simply don't know what you're getting," said Deborah. "That may suffice for picking a sandwich shop. Not when lives, budgets, and relationships are on the line."

Click "Find a Doctor" on FertilityIQ's home page and a quick guide about their doctor rankings pops up, followed by an easy-to-navigate list of physicians, including their specialty, proximity, and photo. Most of the physicians have at least a dozen detailed assessments—provided by unsolicited fertility patients—and several have more than one hundred. I've looked up my own fertility doctors on the site—their reviews felt accurate to me—and have directed friends to FertilityIQ's database to compare clinics and specialists before booking appointments. Unlike sites like Yelp or Zocdoc, FertilityIQ is ad-free and has protections in place to ensure that assessments are vetted and written by real patients. The fertility industry is plagued by paid referrals, which makes FertilityIQ's efforts to connect women with patient-reviewed physicians and reliable data on procedures such as egg freezing all the more valuable.

I was most impressed, though, with FertilityIQ's nearly three hundred courses.* They're taught by reputable doctors and leading fertility experts—names I recognized and individuals I'd come across in my reporting, even—and are geared toward current or prospective fertility patients wanting to learn more about specific treatments and pre-

---

* In fifty-five countries, taught by regional experts in the native tongue.

paring them for decisions that they'll be making along the way. "Once you're in treatment with a doctor, there are myriad hard decisions you still need to make," Deborah explained. "Each has trade-offs." With IVF, it's things like how the eggs are fertilized, whether to do preimplantation genetic testing (PGT), and how many embryos to transfer. If you're an egg freezer, it's how many rounds to do, whether to freeze eggs or embryos, if you want to store all your frozen eggs at the same place, and more. "Most doctors don't have time to give patients the balanced details each of these life-changing decisions warrants," she said. In lieu of that, she continued, FertilityIQ offers full courses on a wide variety of fertility-related subjects, "so that the degree to which patients are educated is not a function of how busy a doctor might be that morning." A few examples of course titles: Fertility for Lesbian Women Becoming Moms. IVF with Donor Eggs. Fertility 101. Endometriosis. Mental Health and Fertility.

Zeynep Gurtin, a sociologist of women's health at University College London, told *MIT Technology Review* that "when it comes to making a decision on egg freezing, it's vital that people be fully informed on four issues: the success rates, the risks, the side effects, and the costs." FertilityIQ is a solid resource in this regard, and a great place to start. Now that I was mulling over the incongruities between the realities of egg freezing and its promises, there was still a lot I didn't understand. What does having this option actually afford women? Who are the doctors putting all these millions of eggs and embryos on ice? Who owns the clinics? And what accounts for the many-thousands-of-dollars price tag? I fell back on my comfort zone as a journalist. I needed more information. And reassurance. That's what I really wanted. It was time to find more resources—individuals, companies, doctors—to help me feel confident, before I went through with it, that freezing my eggs was the right decision.

9

The Femtech Revolution

~~~~~~

Egg Freezing, Commodified

It was just after 6 P.M. on a Monday at Kindbody, a women-led fertility start-up headquartered in Manhattan. Specifically, it was the company's flagship clinic in the Flatiron District, but "clinic" brings to mind a doctor's office, and the chic, welcoming space I'd just entered felt more like a West Elm—which is exactly how Kindbody wants it to feel for anyone walking through the doors. I was there for Fertility 101, one of Kindbody's educational events. As soon as I arrived, I had a flashback to the EggBanxx cocktail parties, which made sense: The same woman was behind both.

When Gina Bartasi, founder and executive chairperson of Kindbody, launched the venture-capital-backed company in 2018, it wasn't her first rodeo. Back in 2008, Bartasi had started FertilityAuthority, an IVF referral network. FertilityAuthority's spin-off egg freezing company, EggBanxx, contracted with physicians to offer lower egg freezing prices for patients and focused heavily on marketing. Then she founded Progyny, which manages fertility benefits on behalf of employers and operates similarly to a health insurance company.*

---

* EggBanxx, which was an arm of FertilityAuthority, was absorbed into Progyny when FertilityAuthority was acquired and became Progyny. Bartasi is no longer involved with Progyny.

From there, she set her sights on building a national network of boutique fertility clinics that offered services without the premium price tag. With Kindbody, Bartasi removes the intermediary entirely, by selling directly to consumers and employers. Valued at nearly $2 billion just five years after it launched, Kindbody is her most ambitious vision and among her biggest successes yet.

It was the first day of spring, and the fresh faces and youthful energy of the fifty or so female—and two male—attendees gathered in the lobby reflected it. That evening, at least, walking into the future of fertility felt like walking into the living room of a friend who had a lot more money than me. Also better taste. Light wood floors, perky succulents, a gray couch with a soft blanket draped over one arm. Soft music played overhead. Books with their jackets removed sat on coffee tables. *Period Power. The Kinfolk Table. Ask Me About My Uterus.* Quiet chatter filled the room, punctuated by the occasional pop of a prosecco bottle being opened.

The event was led by OB/GYN Dr. Fahimeh Sasan, founding physician and Kindbody's chief innovation officer, who's been at the company's helm since day one. Two wool-hatted camera operators from CNN were there, filming a segment for National Infertility Awareness Week. Dr. Sasan stood at the front of the room, a mic clipped to her collar for the camera crew. The company's slogan, "Own Your Future," hung in whimsical cursive lettering on the white brick wall behind her. Splashes of Kindbody's signature yellow—"We call it 'optimistic' yellow," Bartasi told me later—were everywhere: the napkins, the fresh flowers, even Dr. Sasan's fitted sleeveless dress. It was a fireside fertility chat without the fireplace. The crowd was younger and more diverse than the EggBanxx parties, a reflection of egg freezing's changing clientele. Fewer wedding rings, too.

After briefly explaining the basics of male and female fertility, Dr. Sasan gave a rundown of egg freezing and IVF with Kindbody— what's involved physically, logistically, and financially. At this, I watched several women in the room smile and nod, as if to say, *Yes, this is why we came.* The sun was beginning to set, and I noticed the fluorescent yellow Kindbody sign in the window, facing bustling Fifth Avenue, shining brighter. Dr. Sasan answered questions from several attendees before ending her presentation with an ask—"talk about this with your friends, share some of the empowering information you learned tonight"—and an offer ("good for twenty-four hours"): $500 off any IVF or egg freezing cycle when you book an assessment with Kindbody.

Kindbody's reach in the femtech world is unparalleled. Along with its fleet of pop-up van clinics and retail products, the company owns and operates more than thirty brick-and-mortar fertility clinics across the United States, mostly in metropolitan areas. Kindbody also contracts directly with employers to provide fertility and family-building benefits to their employees, including companies such as Walmart, Lyft, BuzzFeed, Princeton University, even Disney and SpaceX.

Bartasi, now in her mid-fifties, is queen of the castle. She doesn't have a medical degree but has taken executive education courses at Harvard and went on to become a major player in the increasingly big-business fertility industry. What EggBanxx set out to do—sell the idea of egg freezing to women—is what Kindbody, the fastest-growing egg freezing provider in the country, now does better than anyone. With EggBanxx, Bartasi *marketed* egg freezing and connected women to fertility clinics where they could do it; with Kindbody, women fall in love with the idea and freeze right there. Scroll through Bartasi's Instagram account and you'll quickly get a sense of the company's reach and influence. There are posts announcing millions in venture capital dollars raised, babies garbed in yellow Kindbody onesies, and even a photo of Bartasi speaking on a panel with Gwyneth Paltrow, one of Kindbody's celebrity investors. (Two others: Chelsea Clinton and Gabrielle Union.) "The SoulCycle of Fertility Sells Egg-Freezing and 'Empowerment' to 25-Year-Olds," read one headline about the company. An article in *The Verge* began: "How do you build a cult following for an egg-freezing clinic?" For one, make an app. Use social media to announce signature boutique openings and where the next pop-up event will land. And launch an influencer program and provide egg freezing discounts to content creators.

Kindbody is predominantly run by women, and more than 50 percent of both the clinic and corporate teams are BIPOC, which is notable, considering the fertility industry has historically been white and male. The company's doctors don't wear white coats or hang their medical degrees on their office walls. They don't have offices at all, in fact; they meet with patients in exam rooms that have the same cozy, living-room vibe as the clinic's lobby. When Bartasi and her team designed the flagship New York City clinic, they purposely sought to avoid the cold and sterile feel of traditional medical exam rooms and instead took design cues from Soho House, the global chain of private members' clubs, and branding inspiration from Drybar and SoulCycle. Months from now, I'd step into Kindbody's Denver clinic and have déjà vu from my Manhattan visit; all Kindbody clinics, like all Starbucks stores, look and feel the same.

The day after the Fertility 101 gathering, I sat down with Bartasi in one of Kindbody's conference rooms, with floor-to-ceiling glass walls. She wore a blue sheer blouse and small silver hoops; glasses were perched atop her chestnut hair; her nails were unpolished, and she had on a hint of red lipstick. A can of seltzer and a rose-gold MacBook sat on the large glass table, where a few signature-yellow Kindbody pens lay scattered. I recalled that she'd had children via IVF and asked her if she wished she had frozen her eggs when she was younger. "I should've, could've, would've," she replied in her southern accent, lamenting that when she was in her thirties vitrification had yet to be developed and egg freezing technology was not yet reliable. "I'm an eternal optimist," she went on. "I think most entrepreneurs have to be. I try to always look forward and think, 'Okay, what train do I have to catch to be home for taco Tuesday with my kids tonight?' So I always think about the future instead of the past. No regrets." It's a mindset Bartasi has centered Kindbody around: help women live a life free of regret by helping them have children in their own time frame. Doing so means building brand loyalty with women in their mid-twenties who will come back at age thirty-five and forty-two and even fifty, offering a continuum of care from their first OB/GYN visit to the birth of their last child.

Elizabeth Holmes's Theranos was in Walgreens. Modern Fertility is in Target. Kindbody is near enough to your office building for you to pop by on your lunch break. The Kindbody educational session I attended may have moved on from the EggBanxx event I went to years earlier, but the hors d'oeuvres and low-grade anxiety filling the room sure felt similar. And the fanfare around eggs and fertility testing had skyrocketed.

By now, I'd spoken with several experts who expressed concern about women seeing egg freezing as a commodity. I'd learned about the new business models cropping up in the femtech sector. I'd taken in the alarming language being used in features written about the industry in general (*aggressively expand; target women; it's an insurance policy; it's control*) and the breezier verbiage of egg freezing articles in particular (*break free from your fertility; empowering, efficient, cutting-edge; it's like freezing time*). The headlines I read were eyebrow-raising: "Femtech Shows the Way to Billion-Dollar Opportunities" (*Forbes*), "The Race to Hack Your Period Is On" (*Elle*), "The Women Who Empty Their Savings to Freeze Their Eggs" (BBC), "Can Silicon Valley Get You Pregnant?" (*Fast Company*), "The Dawn of the Femtech Revolution" (McKinsey & Company).

The media hype reflects a new phenomenon: Egg freezing is a booming sector of the multibillion-dollar femtech industry. The influx of private equity and slew of venture-capital-backed start-ups have pumped a ton of money into what was not very long ago a niche area of ART. There are egg freezing concierge services, acupuncturists, egg hormone experts, and nurses who moonlight as on-call fertility coaches, going to people's homes to walk egg freezing patients through the injections. The target demographic of new companies specializing in egg freezing is women in their late twenties and early-to-mid thirties. In lieu of the typical medical experience, these companies offer sleek décor and top-notch customer service to help brand the procedure as a logical, savvy choice, not unlike researching mutual funds or charting a path from renting to mortgage. "Just like Uber, Seamless, Spotify, and Tinder," an article in *The Cut* read, the new egg freezing companies "cater to the millennial desire for infinite options and a user experience that's more stylish and efficient than the traditional clinic."

Dr. Joshua Klein worked at Reproductive Medicine Associates

(RMA) of New York, one of the country's most prominent fertility centers, before co-founding Extend Fertility, the boutique clinic I visited to see egg freezing in action. His move follows a trend wherein the few big prestigious institutions that dominated the fertility industry have splintered into small, nimble clinics able to operate—and flourish—without the associated overhead. Extend Fertility was innovative because when it opened in 2016, it was the first medical practice in the world to focus exclusively on egg freezing.* Until then, a woman could freeze her eggs only at one of the country's large fertility centers. At these bustling IVF-focused facilities, where egg freezing is certainly not the priority and often an afterthought, waiting rooms are typically full of couples there because they need medical help to have a baby. It is not a particularly welcoming environment for, say, a woman in her early thirties who is curious about the possibility of delayed childbearing or a transgender man interested in fertility preservation before beginning gender-affirming medical care. In terms of marketing, IVF patients want to see pictures of happy babies on the walls, diapered and smiling. Egg freezers, by contrast, are typically women sitting alone in those same waiting rooms, and they don't particularly want to see images of babies—not then. This subtle but important difference between consumers—one seeking a baby now, one seeking to preserve her ability to have a baby later—is the raison d'être for the popular egg-freezing-first clinics. These sleek facilities often tout the procedure as breezy and accessible, an investment in one's reproductive future, the fertility equivalent of a 401(k). But what egg freezing patients gain at these spa-like, picturesque clinics can sometimes, as we'll see, come at a cost.

"A Baby or Your Money Back": Paying for Egg Freezing

Speaking of which, fertility treatment of any kind is expensive, and financing it is beyond the realm of possibility for most Americans. So when it comes to egg freezing, cost can be a major barrier. For many

---

* The company now thaws eggs as well as freezes them; it's expanded to offer IVF and other standard fertility treatment services.

women, it's the most significant obstacle by far. I mentioned earlier that egg freezing in the United States costs an average of roughly $16,000 per cycle. The two major components: the cost of treatment and the cost of hormone medications. Each cost varies, by clinic and by patient. The clinic will likely charge the patient around $7,000 to $10,000 for treatment—including monitoring, the egg retrieval (with anesthesia), and vitrification—and the fertility meds, which she buys separately from a specialty pharmacy and injects herself, will cost around $3,000 to $6,000 or more.* Egg storage costs about $500 to $1,000 per year.† Keep in mind that these are rough estimates for *one* cycle of egg freezing. A fact that many fertility clinics and articles about egg freezing rarely mention: Most women undergo more than one cycle—on average, 2.1 cycles—so of course these costs increase if a patient does multiple cycles. The typical egg freezing patient in the United States is therefore looking at a total price tag of upward of $30,000. And that doesn't include the cost of using her frozen eggs down the road—which entails thawing and fertilizing the eggs, developing embryos in the lab and testing them for genetic abnormalities, then transferring them to the woman's uterus. All that's another $15,000 to $20,000, at least.

"Welcome to the fertility casino," *The New York Times* said in an article about the latest trends in fertility clinics' package deals. As more and more women want to freeze their eggs but balk at the prohibitive price tag, various business models have sprung up to help them afford the procedure, offering financing options and helping them coordinate coverage. I'll talk more in a moment about how insurance coverage, employer benefits, and self-pay options help people afford egg freezing, but first, let me set the scene of fertility financing's contemporary landscape.

---

* The amount of medications an egg freezer needs varies depending on how aggressively her ovaries are stimulated—that is, the protocol determined by her doctor. So, the total amount spent on fertility drugs rises fast if a patient requires additional meds. Many egg freezers feel that the high and separate cost of the fertility medications is not explained well by clinics.

† And they're going up; prices for egg, embryo, and sperm storage have risen sharply since 2019, largely due to inflation and supply chain pressures.

I first learned of fertility financing companies when I read a *Forbes* article topped by the headline "Meet Prelude Fertility, the $200 Million Startup That Wants to Stop the Biological Clock." Prelude is a lucrative private-equity-backed start-up created in 2016 by Argentine serial entrepreneur Martin Varsavsky. Soon after it launched, Prelude began aggressively acquiring fertility clinics around the United States, and is now one of the largest networks of fertility centers in North America. Varsavsky "envisioned a new norm for reproduction, one that would anticipate infertility rather than simply react to it. Young people in their reproductive prime could freeze their sperm or eggs in their twenties, live their lives, pursue careers, and then, when they finally met the right person, thaw their frozen gametes," a *New Yorker* article described. Varsavsky, who often touted the line "Sex is great, but not to make babies" while raising funds for the company, called his vision the Prelude Method. The aim was to own every step of a fertility patient's journey, starting with egg freezing in their twenties and ending with a baby in their thirties or forties.

Initially, the Prelude Method started at $199 a month for the four-step process: egg freezing, embryo creation, genetic screening, and embryo transfer. A patient could choose between two product plans and, after plunking down several thousands of dollars up front, pay a couple of hundreds of dollars each month, sort of like a car layaway plan. Now, the company directs potential clients to a fertility clinic in its network, then provides financing options via third-party companies for services a patient will undergo. In 2019, Varsavsky joined forces with T. J. Farnsworth, a healthcare entrepreneur, who was building a similar chain of fertility practices in Texas and Georgia. Prelude, which now owns more than eighty clinics in the United States and Canada, offers its fertility treatment packages via Bundl, the company Farnsworth started, which combines ART procedures and charges customers a package price. Bundl also promises patients a baby or their money back.

When I finished reading the *Forbes* article, I felt a little sick to my stomach. I was still coming to terms with egg freezing's high price tag; who has a spare $30,000 lying around to pay for this? Not me. I found myself calculating the cost of the egg freezing packages over the years one would need them, and getting a little panicky thinking about a near future where egg freezing and storage is just one of a young professional woman's usual fixed costs, like rent or car insurance. Which, it turns out, is exactly how Prelude wants women like me to think about reproduction—and that was another aspect that made me queasy. It was the "commanding every aspect of a woman's fertility" bit that bothered me about Prelude's business model and mission to dominate the market, along with its subliminal messaging: *Invest in your fertility now so you don't have to resort to buying your way out of infertility later.* "We are now targeting women in their 20s and early 30s," Susan Herzberg, then Prelude's president, told *The New York Times* in 2018. It's smart from a business perspective, of course: The earlier a woman freezes her eggs, the more money she'll shell out to keep them on ice until she's ready to use them. A convenient omission by companies like Prelude, however, is the fact that the vast majority of women who have frozen eggs to date haven't returned to thaw them.

The goal of helping people finance fertility treatment the way they might pay for a car, though, makes sense—even if it sounds icky—especially for millennials and Gen Zers who need help affording what for many of them is the largest out-of-pocket health expense they've ever encountered. That's what led Claire Tomkins to co-found Future Family, which offers sixty-month loan plans for IVF or egg freezing, including discounted lab work and medications, and a "fertility coach" to field questions and help patients navigate their treatment. Other fertility entrepreneurs have expanded into financial products to address cost barriers and appeal to the "buy now, pay later" mindset; their companies partner with fertility clinics to attract customers and offer payment plans similar to Future Family's to help patients finance treatment.

Fertility clinics now extend all sorts of finance options on their own to both entice patients and ease their minds. Some clinics offer egg freezing discounts for women with a medical diagnosis, for transgender men, and for women in the military. Some offer "freeze with

friends" deals: Southern California Reproductive Center ran a pro-
motion saying if three friends freeze eggs together, each receives
30 percent off; Ova, a clinic in Chicago, advertises on its website,
"The more friends in your circle who freeze together, the bigger the
discount!" There's an increasingly popular "freeze and share" hybrid
model, where a woman can freeze eggs for free or at a discount when
she donates half of her retrieved eggs to an egg donor program or to
prospective parents who can't otherwise conceive. There are also
package or "shared risk" programs for when patients return to use
their frozen eggs—this offsets the high risk of IVF cycle failure.*
Shady Grove Fertility, which has dozens of clinics nationwide, offers
a more-or-less "satisfaction guaranteed" program in which qualifying
egg freezing patients pay a flat amount for unlimited attempts to get
pregnant with their frozen eggs. At Spring Fertility, where Mandy
froze eggs, if a patient freezes at least twenty eggs before age thirty-
five or thirty eggs before age thirty-eight at one of the company's
clinics and doesn't get pregnant when she returns to use them, she is
refunded all of the money she paid to Spring for freezing and attempting to use her eggs.

Fertility clinics and for-profit companies they partner with are financially incentivized to sell egg freezing and IVF. They pitch programs and packages that go like hotcakes; many patients end up losing
money on them, while others save. That's the reality of fertility treatment's capitalistic backdrop. The way I see it: Fertility financing companies aren't the enemy, and many do a good service helping people
pay for incredibly expensive procedures. But while efforts to make
egg freezing more affordable are one thing, aggressively targeting
young women to sell them on a procedure they may not need, or that
may not pan out, is another. It's an aspect of egg freezing's bigger picture I would come to be increasingly troubled by.

The fertility financing scene is . . . a lot. But onward to the prag-
matics of paying. In lieu of or in addition to leveraging a shared risk

---

* In a preliminary national report from 2022, SART found that 43.1 percent of
women under thirty-five had a live birth after a cycle of egg retrieval. The number was 3.2 percent for women over forty-two.

program or fertility treatment loan, many women turn to other avenues to help them afford egg freezing, particularly their health insurance or employer.

When it comes to paying for egg freezing, we need to talk about three things: state insurance regulations, employer-offered fertility benefits, and self-pay.*

The short answer to the question *Does health insurance cover egg freezing?* is that it depends. In the United States, private health insurance, which includes employer-sponsored plans (known as group plans), is regulated at the federal level and more heavily at the state level, and laws often address which healthcare services must be covered by group and individual plans. As of September 2023, twenty-one states and Washington, D.C., have laws requiring insurance companies to cover or offer some variation of fertility testing, diagnosis, or treatment. But each of these states can define "fertility coverage" however it sees fit, and they vary considerably in their entitlements, including how long a person has struggled with infertility before qualifying for treatment, what sort of treatment is covered, whether same-sex couples and unmarried individuals are covered, and more.

The list of states that offer fertility treatment coverage has been growing steadily since the 1980s, though benefits vary widely. Here are a few state-specific examples (accurate as of this writing). Massachusetts, which has one of the most generous laws, requires insurers that provide pregnancy-related benefits to also cover infertility diagnosis and treatment, which includes IVF and egg freezing, among other procedures. Delaware, New Hampshire, and New Jersey have comprehensive infertility coverage, including for the pricey fertility meds. In New York and Colorado, certain patients are eligible for up to three rounds of IVF and are covered for medically necessary fertility preservation procedures, such as freezing eggs or sperm before

---

* For a few comprehensive resources pertaining to fertility insurance coverage laws, fertility treatment grants and financing programs, and getting fertility insurance coverage at work, see the top of chapter 9 in the Notes section at the back of this book.

undergoing cancer treatment. California does not require insurers to cover fertility treatment; if employers choose to offer it as part of their employee health benefit package, IVF isn't included. The opposite is the case in Texas, where insurers *must* offer IVF, and if employers elect to extend the benefit, patients must have a history of *five continuous years* of infertility or meet a long list of criteria to qualify for coverage. Also, the patient's eggs must be fertilized only with her spouse's sperm, rather than a donor's. The spouse's-sperm-only stipulation is also the case in Hawaii and Arkansas, once again effectively excluding same-sex couples and single people. Finally, some states place age limits on female patients who can access fertility benefits—a woman in New Jersey, for example, must be under the age of forty-six to be eligible; in Rhode Island, she must be between the ages of twenty-five and forty-two—and others place restrictions on marital status.

To put it bluntly, the United States has never considered any sort of fertility treatment worthy of widespread subsidized healthcare coverage. Most of the mandates stipulating that private insurers cover some fertility treatments are geared toward infertility, and in the majority of cases, as I've said, a person must have a diagnosis of infertility from a doctor in order to qualify for coverage.* This is problematic in that it doesn't apply to same-sex couples who aren't infertile; they're just not in a situation where they can achieve pregnancy via sex (more on ART access issues and how these laws affect LGBTQ+ people shortly). It also doesn't apply to healthy women wanting to proactively freeze eggs.† While some insurance mandates include at least partial coverage for fertility preservation due to medical conditions, there is no coverage for egg freezing without a medical reason or for proactive fertility testing (discussed in chapter 6) without an infertility diagnosis.

---

* Infertility, a disease of the male or female reproductive system, affects roughly one in six adults worldwide and is defined by physicians as the inability to conceive despite having regular, unprotected sex for twelve months or more if you're under thirty-five years old or for six months or more if you're thirty-five or older.

† I spoke to a few women who, to get around this rule, were given an infertility diagnosis by the doctor they saw at the fertility clinic—even though they were not at the time actively trying to get pregnant—so that they could have egg freezing covered by their insurance.

. . .

Employer coverage for fertility is a different story. Many private sector companies have changed their healthcare coverage plans to include ART for less limited reasons. Apple and Facebook, back in 2014, were among the first large firms to announce that their insurance plans would cover egg freezing for employees for non-medical reasons. By 2017, egg freezing was the hot new perk in Silicon Valley. At first it was mainly tech and finance companies that covered it; then new media companies, start-ups, and universities began extending the benefit, too. As of 2021, 19 percent of large U.S. employers offered egg freezing, compared to just 6 percent in 2015. No longer a nice-to-have perk, fertility treatment coverage in general has become a staple in many employers' healthcare packages: More than 42 percent of large U.S. employers, and 27 percent of smaller companies, offer IVF benefits.★

Back to Progyny, one of the largest publicly traded femtech companies, which partners with companies to manage fertility benefits for employees. An employer decides to offer fertility benefits to its employees; Progyny then manages all aspects of those benefits, connecting members to its network of more than 950 fertility specialists, covering fertility medications under Progyny Rx, and overseeing treatment. Each member receives access to a "patient care advocate," who helps the patient coordinate appointments, connects the patient to an on-demand nurse for help with fertility meds, and even offers emotional support. (Um, wow.) Progyny's more than 370 clients include Amazon, Google, Meta, and Microsoft.

Becca, while working at Google, froze twenty eggs thanks to the company's Progyny benefit, and doubts she would've frozen her eggs without it. When she froze, she was thirty-seven and single and didn't know if she wanted kids. "But I wouldn't want my fertility to be the reason I couldn't be with someone I fell in love with, if kids were very

★ For a good resource on family-building coverage offered by employers, check out FertilityIQ's Workplace Index. The report, which FertilityIQ publishes every year, analyzes industry trends and provides up-to-date employer fertility benefit information.

important to him," she told me when we spoke on the phone a few days after the procedure. To Becca's relief, the week of her egg retrieval was a relatively calm one at work. Becca's boss, who was male, knew she was freezing her eggs, but her colleagues—also mostly men—didn't. "There was a part of me that didn't want to make people feel uncomfortable," she said, adding that she also didn't want to draw attention to the fact that she was thirty-seven and unpartnered. "Almost everyone I know at work that's my age is married and has kids," she said. "The fact that I'm single at my age feels a little bit like a failure, like I've done something wrong. And so it's not something I like to highlight to the people I'm trying to instill confidence with." A year later, Becca told me that freezing her eggs helped her realize that having a kid isn't critical to her being happy in life. She also more confidently pursued things she wanted—a new job, a location change, and a partner. "There's so much more to life than whether or not you're fertile," she said, with a satisfied sigh.

How do people without insurance benefits or employer coverage afford egg freezing? Since I fell into that boat, I'd been mulling for months over how I would manage to pay for the procedure. Dr. Noyes had offered me a medical discount for freezing, since in the clinic's view my having one ovary was a sort of "condition," but I was having trouble getting my health insurance to agree.★ After I published my first story about egg freezing, my mother emailed me: *Great article! Maybe an egg freezing place will contact you to freeze your eggs at no cost!*†
Women often freeze their eggs in their mid-thirties, just as they enter prime wealth-building years. For some, that means depleting their savings, going into debt, and/or delaying goals such as homeowner-

★ I'd enrolled in an NYU-sponsored health insurance plan when I began graduate school, and when I called and asked them if and how I might have any kind of egg freezing coverage, I was told that without an infertility diagnosis I was out of luck.

† As I published more egg freezing pieces, I did receive offers of this nature from a couple of clinics and doctors. While the offers were enticing, journalism ethics make it clear that accepting free or discounted goods or services in exchange for press—even if, in this case, a fertility clinic doesn't explicitly ask for it—isn't okay.

ship in order to self-finance egg freezing. They take out loans, mort-gage their houses, borrow from 401(k) accounts, start GoFundMe campaigns, or take on second jobs in order to afford one or more cycles. Increasingly, many women travel abroad for a better deal; egg freezing is a fraction of the cost in countries like Spain and the Czech Republic. I would need to look into every possible way to get the dollar signs down, because the more I scrutinized egg freezing costs, the more clearly I saw it as a financial impossibility.

Remy paid for egg freezing by taking out a $20,000 personal loan and charging the meds to a credit card. She also sold her engagement ring—"extra cash for the eggs," she told me—and took on additional shifts at the hospital. Sometimes alimony can finance egg freezing; I read about cases in which women fought hard for egg freezing to be paid for by their ex-husbands as part of their divorce settlements—and won. There are nonprofit organizations that provide fertility treatment scholarships and grants. Often, families help, as Mandy's offered to. A few years ago, Valerie,* a Chicago woman who froze her eggs in her early thirties, began documenting her experience on a blog and a weekly podcast. When she started her project, her respondents were mostly in their late thirties. Now she hears from women in their mid-twenties whose grandparents want to help finance the procedure, as they might a down payment for a house. She also gets calls from parents with teenagers and college-age daughters, who see egg freezing as a future gift and are willing to foot the bill—the return on investment coming in the form of a grandchild down the road. Danielle, a thirty-nine-year-old in Dallas who did two rounds of IVF before getting pregnant, echoed this, telling me: "My husband and I are not going to pay for our daughters' weddings one day, but we will pay for them to have their eggs frozen when they're in their twenties."

"We pay too much for the things we think are precious, but we also start to believe things are precious if someone makes us pay too much," writes Jia Tolentino in her essay collection *Trick Mirror*. She was refer-

---

* A different Valerie from the fertility doctor Valerie I mentioned earlier.

ring to the wedding industry and trendy workouts like barre and the world of beauty and wellness in general, but when I read that sentence I immediately thought about a woman's eggs. A modern-day young woman learns her eggs are precious upon discovering they are something of a commodity. Her eggs are fragile, and every moment brings them closer to expiration. It makes sense, then, at least on an emotional level, that it costs thousands of dollars to freeze them, and thousands more down the road to use them. For many women, egg freezing is both exorbitantly expensive and the easiest money they've ever spent.

Dr. Lora Shahine, a reproductive endocrinologist in Seattle, summed it up to me like this: "I think of egg freezing as this incredible opportunity. It's very empowering, it's wonderful, but the way it's sold as insurance and a guarantee is really scary." If a woman works at a company like Amazon or Google, she went on, "egg freezing is a no-brainer. For them, the financial pressure is really eased. So that's a real win. It shouldn't change someone's family goals. But it can relieve a large burden and allow people to feel a little bit more free."

The people benefitting from egg freezing and being courted by fertility clinics, though, are a specific subset: predominantly white middle- to upper-middle-class professionals in their thirties. Prohibitively high costs make egg freezing and IVF impractical, if not impossible, for many people, especially those with lower incomes. And so, I realized, it isn't just that egg freezing is a new and complicated technology. Or that it's really expensive. When I began to learn more about the inequalities in access to treatment, I realized it was more about the ways in which fertility is a privilege, not a right.

Embryo Destruction Meets Anti-Abortion

A revolution of sorts might have been taking place in the femtech world, but elsewhere, the opposite was happening. In 2017, Donald Trump's administration, with evangelical Mike Pence at the helm as vice president, began to dismantle reproductive freedoms—and many other civil liberties—on its first days in office. Although the landscape changed under President Biden, reproductive rights remain fragile, and the abortion battleground is particularly inflamed. The year 2021 was an especially dark time for abortion access, with more than a hundred new restrictions passed. Americans gained a constitutional right to abortion in 1973. In 2022 they lost it when the U.S. Supreme Court, in its *Dobbs v. Jackson Women's Health Organization* ruling, delivered the most consequential abortion decision in five decades by overturning *Roe v. Wade* and striking down the nationwide right to abortion. The modern climate with regard to abortion access is anxiety-inducing, to say the least, but the more terrifying reality is that the laws in development threaten anyone with a uterus, and have implications beyond a woman's ability to not remain pregnant if she doesn't want to.

Women's judgment about our own bodies and futures cannot be trusted, politicians insist, so our reproductive systems must be controlled by lawmakers—overwhelmingly, older white men. The Court's ruling leaves it up to states to dictate abortion access, without requiring state bans to include exceptions of any kind. While some states are trying to make abortion access more robust, other states are aggressively pushing to limit the scope of when abortions can be performed. As of December 2023, twenty-one states now ban abortion or restrict the procedure earlier in pregnancy than the standard set by *Roe v. Wade.* Several states ban abortion after six weeks of pregnancy—which is before many women know they are pregnant.

The new abortion bans have had a less recognized effect—namely, creating confusion and legal questions about the practice of discarding embryos, which is a normal part of IVF. That's the nature of the technology; creating multiple embryos is the point. Those with the greatest chance of developing into a healthy baby are used first, and the excess embryos are typically frozen, until the person or people who made them decide to use or discard them. As long as IVF is here to stay, so too is the reality of leftover unused embryos on ice. But IVF and related fertility treatments may not, in fact, be here to stay.

The current configuration of the Supreme Court has already begun to impact the state of reproductive rights in the United States for decades to come; it has also called into question the status of legal rights for women undergoing fertility treatment, as well as their doctors. "The United States has a political debate about abortion that has spilled over into everything that has to do with embryos," Alta Charo, a retired professor of law and bioethics at the University of Wisconsin–Madison, told *The New Yorker* in 2023. The abortion bans could mean impaired access to ART. The concern is that as some states rush to pass fetal personhood bills, they may inadvertently or purposely ban IVF. Some states specifically exempt IVF from their abortion bans, but in others, restrictive "personhood laws" have been passed that use murkier language—such as specifying that life begins at fertilization, when an egg becomes an embryo, as opposed to the implantation of an embryo or a fetus being viable—and leave several stages of the fertility treatment process vulnerable to government interference, opening up the legal terrain for states to interfere with IVF and curtail patients' access to care. If the bans are interpreted as granting embryos legal rights and protections, a fertilized egg would have the same rights as a child. Yet even if the two are deemed legally equivalent, they are decidedly not biologically equivalent, and giving an embryo "personhood" status raises all sorts of questions about what can be done with embryos created outside the body.

Experts have been worried about the impact of abortion bans on IVF for years. Many anti-abortion activists object to embryos being destroyed due to genetic screening results or because people have finished building their families. Legal experts predict that the new state abortion bans could make it easier to place controls on genetic testing, storage, and disposal of embryos. Parts of the IVF process could become illegal; in some states, it could be banned altogether. In states where the law dictates that life begins at fertilization, frozen embryos could be defined as unborn children under law, and discarding unused or frozen embryos could be criminalized (although it's worth noting that even within the anti-abortion movement, this view of IVF and what's created through ART is considered extreme).

What could it mean practically if laws banning embryo destruction were to pass? Fertility clinics might choose to limit the number of embryos created per cycle to try to avoid having any "extra," but that could mean more expensive and invasive cycles until someone successfully gets pregnant. Doctors who perform IVF and discard unused frozen embryos in accordance with their patients' wishes may be prosecuted. Fertility patients in states where the use of ART is questionable might find it necessary to have their eggs and sperm collected in-state, then shipped to a clinic in a state where the legal climate is less volatile and their eggs or embryos won't exist in limbo—a workaround that adds another cost and burden to the already burdensome process of fertility treatment.*

So the *Dobbs* ruling not only threatens the health of pregnant people but also, ironically, may lead to fewer healthy babies being born to parents who want them. The downstream effects are unclear. Ensuing state policies could affect everything from how miscarriages are managed to how certain birth control is provided.† The impact of restrictive abortion laws on fertility treatment will likely come down to the legislation's language and the tenacity of individual prosecutors who are interpreting it. Time will tell how the impact of *Roe v. Wade*'s reversal on the U.S. fertility industry will play out—and if going after embryos will become the next frontier of the anti-abortion movement—but the operational and legal implications could be enormous.

In the meantime, as fertility technology forges ahead, reproductive rights are in many ways regressing. It's a disconcerting juxtaposition: We may soon live in a country where abortion is heavily restricted or illegal in most states but IVF and egg freezing are a guaranteed benefit at many private companies; where across America abortion providers are forced to shutter their doors while fertility clinics host "Cocktails and Cryo" egg freezing parties to drum up new business. That is, at least, if access to ART remains intact and until the legal definition of viability and the reproductive medical view that life does not begin at fertilization come to a head.

---

* After the Supreme Court ruling came down, fertility patients across the country immediately began contacting their clinics to arrange to move their eggs or embryos out of red states to avoid possible legal complications.

† In some states, this is already happening. One of many egregious examples: In 2022, public universities in Idaho stopped providing not just abortion referrals but contraception referrals, too—even going so far as stipulating that condoms are to be distributed only to prevent STIs, not to prevent pregnancy, and warning faculty members that they could face felony charges if they refer students to abortion services or "promote" abortion.

It's enough to make anyone's ovaries tremble. I had spent so much time thinking and asking questions about a woman's ability to get pregnant that, some days, it was easy to forget about the legal and political forces at work to, one, make her stay pregnant against her wishes and, two, not adequately help her if her pregnancy went wrong. The stark reminder that, in today's world, women's fertility, sexuality, and overall health are politicized in ways that men's are not prompted me to take a harder look at the systemic barriers and socio-economic disparities blocking people from accessing reproductive technologies.

Access Denied

Despite the incredible technological advancements surrounding re-productive technology in recent decades, there are still substantial roadblocks to having children for many people—infertile or not. Since the first IVF program opened in the United States in 1980, stigmatizing laws and entrenched social and cultural attitudes have contributed to significant disparities—dictated by state of residence, insurance plan, income level, race and ethnicity, and sexual orienta-tion and gender identity—that have made ART difficult to access. The result is that today systemic barriers prevent many people who are not white, cis, heterosexual, and upper-middle-class from pursu-ing fertility services.

Let's start with race. How race affects maternal and reproductive health in a more general sense is a larger conversation, but in essence: The reasons that Black women, overall, have poorer pregnancy out-comes and face more obstacles in accessing fundamentals such as af-fordable housing, healthy food, transportation, and good prenatal care are embedded in broader social disparities, a complicated matrix of external forces—including structural racism and income inequality—at play. This context is important to understand why, compared to white women, so few BIPOC women pursue fertility treatment, and the ways in which race in America gravely affects many Black women's fertility journeys, from both medical and emotional standpoints.

In the United States, about 12 percent of women ages fifteen to forty-four have trouble getting pregnant, and Black women are twice as likely to experience infertility as white women.* Despite these higher rates of infertility, Black women are less likely to access medical help to get pregnant, and if they do, they may wait twice as long before seeking treatment. Many women experiencing infertility face an uphill battle in getting care, but Black women face additional challenges, such as a lack of Black sperm and egg donors and prejudice from physicians in a medical space that is overwhelmingly white.† Several factors, including income, differences in coverage rates, and availability of services, affect access to infertility care. So does the history of discriminatory reproductive care and harm inflicted upon BIPOC women over decades.

Studies have shown that doctors may consciously or unconsciously make assumptions or possess biases about who deserves to be a parent or deserves treatment. Black women, for example, have reported that some providers brush off their fertility concerns, emphasize birth control over procreation, and dissuade them from having children. Or doctors assume they can get pregnant easily; misconceptions and stereotypes about fertility have often portrayed Black women as not needing medical help to get pregnant. Feelings of shame and isolation are particularly pervasive among BIPOC women with infertility: In a survey of more than one thousand women of a variety of races, Black women were more than twice as likely as white women to say that they wouldn't feel comfortable talking about their fertility issues with friends, family, a partner, their doctor, or even a support group. This is one reason it was a big deal when Michelle Obama, in her memoir *Becoming,* told the world about her miscarriage and undergoing IVF.

The egg freezing employer benefit discussed earlier raises deeper questions about race and class inequality regarding fertility care. The benefit affects employees at largely white-collar companies, who tend

---

* Black women also suffer from higher rates of uterine fibroids—non-cancerous tumors in the uterus that typically develop during a woman's childbearing years—and obesity, two conditions that can negatively impact fertility.

† The lack of ethnic diversity among donors leaves many intended parents without adequate options for building families that reflect their backgrounds.

to be highly educated, higher-income, and predominantly white—meaning the policy helps alleviate the financial burden for those already at an advantage. Historically, fertility treatments have been mostly marketed to and used disproportionately by white women of high socioeconomic and educational backgrounds, which is one reason Black women have been largely left out of the conversation around egg freezing. A few years ago, SART analyzed nearly thirty thousand egg retrievals and found that only 4 percent of women who undergo the procedure identify as Hispanic, while just 7 percent are Black. As it stands now, egg freezing is available to those (relatively few) who are aware enough to seek it out and can afford it. As reproductive freedoms continue to get chipped away at throughout the country, it is the lower-income, often BIPOC women who will end up the least able to attempt to buy back some of that reproductive autonomy with fertility preservation.

There is at least one aspect of access to ART that America does well—in theory, at least, if not always in practice. In the United States, egg freezing and IVF play a pivotal role in making the LGBTQ+-parent family as viable as any other family. This is important, given that availability of ART for LGBTQ+ and unmarried people is restricted in many places worldwide. In most countries, only married heterosexual couples with a diagnosis of infertility can access fertility treatment; it was only in the last few years that social egg freezing became legal for lesbians and single women in countries like France and Norway.* In the United States, virtually anyone who can afford ART can use it—a rare example of America being more progressive than its European peers.

For many in the LGBTQ+ community, especially lesbian couples, egg freezing can be, in some cases, a no-brainer. If a queer or bisexual woman or a nonbinary or AFAB (assigned female at birth) person wants to use their or their partner's eggs, as opposed to donor eggs, to create embryos, having eggs already frozen puts them a step ahead.

---

* Meanwhile, in China, egg freezing and IVF are largely available only to married women (even though the country's population has fallen for the first time in decades). On the other side of the spectrum, Japan and South Korea now provide subsidies for healthy women wishing to freeze their eggs for future pregnancies.

Egg freezing is also an option for transgender men; freezing their eggs before beginning gender-affirming medical care leaves open the possibility of having biological children someday.

But hurdles to receiving insurance coverage make it difficult for two groups of people in the United States in particular to undergo fertility treatment: LGBTQ+ couples and solo parents by choice.* Some states have revised language in their legislation in recent years to feature a definition of infertility that includes LGBTQ+ and unpartnered people. But most state insurance laws incorporate a definition of infertility similar to the one mentioned above: six to twelve months of unprotected heterosexual intercourse. And, again, some states only cover IVF if the couple's own eggs and sperm are used, stipulations that exclude same-sex couples and would-be solo parents. If it seems unfair that queer couples often cannot qualify for insurance coverage in order to have a biological child—and are discriminated against because they cannot "prove" infertility the way heterosexual couples having sex can—that's because it is.

Lack of fertility preservation coverage is also a major inequity issue for the expanding transgender population seeking hormonal therapies. While pursuing reproductive services is not the most pressing problem that patients seeking gender transitions currently face—that would be states restricting gender-affirming care for adolescents—it matters. Fertility preservation for transgender youth is, for the most part, understudied and underreported. Professional societies have published guidelines highlighting the need to establish standardized protocols for primary care doctors when counseling transgender patients as they consider sex reassignment, to discuss the potential risk of fertility impairment as well as fertility preservation options before a transgender person begins hormonal or surgical therapies. But it will be a while until such discussions become the standard of care.

If transgender youth do happen to receive counseling about egg or sperm freezing prior to undergoing hormonal interventions, the de-

* RESOLVE has compiled a helpful list of resources specific to family building for LGBTQ+ people: resolve.org/learn/what-are-my-options/lgbtq-family-building-options/.

cision about whether to pursue it isn't an easy one. Similar to BIPOC people, transgender individuals face barriers such as discrimination and refusal of services. And even if they overcome the hurdles and decide yes, the issue remains: How to pay? Few can afford the substantial out-of-pocket costs of fertility preservation of eggs for transgender men or—less expensive but still not inconsequential—fertility preservation of sperm for transgender women. And, of course, those price tags don't include *use* of the frozen eggs or sperm if and when the person wants to have children. As with cancer patients, the onus is often on transgender patients to prove to insurance companies that fertility preservation is medically necessary. It's hard to say for certain how insurance coverage would change the current low rate of transgender people who preserve their reproductive cells, but as Devin O'Brien Coon, medical director for the Johns Hopkins Center for Transgender Health, has said, "There's no question that transgender patients would preserve their fertility if insurance covered it."

There isn't a one-size-fits-all solution to overcome these limitations and make it easier for BIPOC and LGBTQ+ people to use ART to build biological families. A major step in the direction of progress would be including fertility treatment in all health insurance coverage, as with other health conditions and diseases affecting other major bodily systems, which would help address needs faced by low-income persons. Another would be to expand insurance companies' definition of infertility to ensure that same-sex, single, and transgender individuals are not precluded from coverage. Femtech's ability to help improve racial equity in reproductive healthcare offers some hope; solutions tailored for delivering culturally sensitive care to subpopulations are emerging. One, the digital platform Health in Her HUE, connects Black women and women of color to culturally sensitive healthcare providers, evidence-based health content, and community support. Another, FOLX Health, is the first major queer and trans venture-backed company to offer virtual care and prescriptions for hormone replacement therapy and sexual health. Still, until better policies are in place to help combat the economic, cultural, and social barriers at play, many people who need fertility services will remain unable to benefit from them, and egg freezing will remain a far cry from an equal-opportunity venture. Inequitable access to reproductive opportunity has plagued the fertility industry from its earliest days, but it doesn't have to define its future—something to keep in mind as the landscape of reproduction continues to quickly evolve before our eyes.

I finished graduate school with strong grades and several bylines to my name. The week of graduation was a happy time. I celebrated with my professors and fellow journalism grads, as well as my parents, best friends, and Ben. But I was beyond burned out. Somewhere between finishing my thesis and yet another internship and figuring out what I was doing after that final semester, I had lost fifteen pounds on my already petite frame and had dropped the ball helping a mentor complete research for her next book. I'd spent two years hustling, and I had published pieces and professional connections to show for it. I'd also acquired significant credit card debt and what seemed like permanent dark circles under my eyes.

Two days after graduation, I flew to Berlin for a journalism fellowship in Germany and Poland. Then I taught a high school creative writing program in the Czech Republic. Ben had taken a new job in Houston, and I'd decided it was time to leave New York for a while, mostly because I couldn't fathom how to afford continuing to live there as a freelance writer. In August, Ben and I packed up my Brooklyn apartment in a flurry of boxes and sweat. He went back to Houston and I went to Colorado, where my parents had bought a house in the mountains and where I had decided to catch my breath. When I arrived, my father took one look at me and said, "You look about twenty years older than when I last saw you. Please go eat something and rest." I slept for what felt like a week.

A few months later, I flew back to New York to meet Ben for a weekend; it was his birthday, and he wanted to celebrate in the city. We stayed at an Airbnb in Williamsburg. The morning of his birthday, Ben went out to get us food. "Hunting and gathering," we called it:

his love for bringing back breakfast on weekend mornings and my love for starting the day slowly and anticipating his walking in the door with delicious treats. We spent the day on the Lower East Side: drinks at McSorley's, a movie, a walk through Union Square. That evening, he wanted to stay out late, but I was tired and not up for the night he wanted to have. The cab dropped me off at the apartment and took him back across the bridge. When he crawled into bed hours later, I pretended to be asleep.

When it came to going out, Ben and I had always been pretty far apart on the spectrum, but lately the divide had been causing problems. He almost always preferred staying out late and partied harder than I did. When I visited him in Houston, I'd often opt to stay in or leave the bar early, taking an Uber back to the apartment alone. This became a pattern, and it bothered me. There were times we simply did not enjoy doing things together the way we used to, as if the bitterness that built up after several small fights dulled the easy joy we were used to sharing. At our best, we fell naturally into what it is to *be here now* with a person you love. Once, burrowed in sleeping bags at the bottom of the Grand Canyon, he thanked me for being in the moment with him, living in the present as opposed to the future, where my thoughts often dwelled. Murmuring something in reply, I leaned up to kiss him and a bug with long legs bit me. I yelped, he promptly ushered the bug out of the tent, and we fell asleep spooning under the stars.

Lately, though, that levity and natural ease felt light-years away. The next night in New York, we lay in bed, tension between us. We'd been talking about moving in together for several weeks. "I've been having some doubts," I said quietly into the dark. I asked him if he was sure he wanted me to move to Houston. "Ninety-five, ninety-eight percent sure, yeah," he said, his voice low. A moment later: "Are you hesitant?"

"Yes," I whispered. His arms were wrapped around me, but I felt far away.

Ovaries in Overdrive

~~~~~~

Lauren: A Bad Bout of Lupron

I never, ever thought I would live in Texas. I also never thought I would move somewhere for a boyfriend, but, well, the heart wants what it wants, which is how I came to be barreling south on Route 287 in early March, making the trek to Houston in my red Volkswagen. Moving meant trading in a long-distance relationship for the start of a shared life in an awkwardly shaped apartment in Montrose. It was a few blocks from the bayou. We had dubbed it The Bungalow.

Houston. The country's fourth-largest city; the most ethnically diverse place in America, according to an article I read in the *Los Angeles Times* a few weeks before I moved. I took it as a promising sign. I wasn't moving to *Texas;* I was moving to dynamic, colorful Houston. A port; a metropolis; a million different stories. A city known for its intersections: on roads, within communities, through politics. A city still trying to find itself, and yet, in many ways, so comfortable in its own skin.

My honeymoon with Houston lasted all of six weeks. There were cold beers at neighborhood watering holes and cocktails at bars with names like Little Dipper and El Big Bad. There were crawfish boils, food-truck tacos, and more barbecue than I'd ever had in my life. We took salsa lessons and biked along the bayou. We toured NASA and watched aggressive roller derby games at a local rink. We joined a CrossFit gym around the corner from the apartment and suffered through workouts together in the early evening heat. The city was funky and fun, and Ben was an eager guide, taking me to places he knew I would enjoy: Rothko Chapel, the rodeo, slam poetry open mic nights. I wrote in the early morning light while Ben slept. He'd turned a corner of the kitchen into a tiny office for me and gone out of his way to make space for my (many) belongings. When the afternoons turned muggy, I would itch for the workday to be over and was glad to close my laptop when Ben arrived home from his sales job. We'd cook simple dinners, take walks in the cool night air, or sometimes meet up with friends, almost all of whom were Ben's from before I moved in. I liked his friends but didn't have much in common with most of them except for our mutual fondness for Ben. When feelings of unease crept up about having uprooted myself to live with him, I channeled my anxious energy into work and down-the-road plans. Thinking about the future was easier than worrying about the present.

During one of my visits months earlier, Ben had surprised me with an all-day culinary tour, and we'd stayed in touch with a few of the people we met that day. That's how I came to know Lauren. We connected a few stops into the food tour, at an open-air market in a pocket of Houston I'd not been to before. I was wandering around the narrow rows of stalls and noticed one boasting an array of colorful spices and homeopathic powders. Curious, I stopped, then noticed Lauren, and we got to talking. She asked what sorts of things I wrote about as a journalist, and when I told her, her eyes widened.

"Do I have a story for you," she said, putting her hand on my arm in a *you're-not-going-to-believe-this* sort of way. She began to tell me about her experience freezing her eggs two days before her thirty-ninth birthday. As she talked, I looked more closely at the small, brightly colored signs sticking out of the dozens of bags of herbs arranged behind glass in front of us. They were not, in fact, food spices, but herbs for various illnesses and ailments, with handwritten labels in both English and Spanish, several misspelled: PROSTATE and KEDNYS, ASTHMA and ANEMIA, DETOX and RELAX/NERVIOUS, CANCER and CIRCULATIONS. "I want to know more about these ones," said Lauren, laughing as she pointed to three bags of herbs, each $40 per pound, labeled OVARIES/CRAMPS, HORMONES, and FERTILILY. As we walked back to the bus, I asked Lauren if I could interview her in more depth about what she'd told me as we stood at the market stall. She readily agreed. We would end up talking and texting frequently over the next few years, but at the time, I simply appreciated the coincidence of meeting someone who'd frozen her eggs in a place where I wasn't researching or reporting about it.

Many of her friends had children or were trying to get pregnant, but Lauren, who was single, wasn't sure how she would get to motherhood. Still, since turning thirty-five, she'd found her thoughts preoccupied by her biological clock in a way she'd never experienced before. When she turned thirty-eight, she decided to have a chat with her gynecologist about egg freezing at her annual exam. Conversations with friends and family members helped her decide that she did, in fact, want kids someday. Not now, but when she wasn't too old, either. Her gynecologist recommended a fertility clinic in town, and after briefly perusing their website, Lauren made an appointment.

As far as egg freezing stories go, the impetus behind Lauren's pursuit of the procedure was in line with much of what I'd heard from other women—but the similarities stopped there. What she remembers most about her first appointment at Houston IVF* was that the clinic had an excellent sales pitch. "They were really pushy, which made it hard to say no," Lauren told me. She did the usual blood work, and when the results came back, her doctor said, "Your body really wants to be pregnant." When Lauren heard that, it felt like being told she was validated as a woman. "If the doctor had told me on day one, 'You can't have kids,' I would've said, 'Fine.' I would've moved on. But the minute she said, 'You have really strong, viable eggs,' I was immediately married to it. I was *going* to have biological children at that point."

---

* Houston IVF was rebranded in 2018 and is now CCRM Houston.

Then everything started happening very fast. Lauren hadn't made time to research egg freezing before her appointment but now wishes she had. She doesn't remember having hesitations or concerns about the procedure at the time but thinks she would have if she had known what questions to ask. A few months after that first appointment, Lauren began the hormone regimen. She had sold stock to pay a pharmacy nearly $5,000 for the medications. Her experience at the bustling, urban fertility center was, in a word, terrible. "It felt like a sweatshop," she said, reflecting on what it was like to go in several mornings for blood work and monitoring. "They lined us up like cattle." At one of her appointments, she remembers a nurse used a pin cushion to demonstrate how to self-administer the shots, which Lauren did not find helpful. For the first few days, not knowing to change injection sites, Lauren injected the shot in the same spot; it started to bruise and hurt. She turned to YouTube for clearer instructions. Then, a few days after starting the medications, she began feeling strange—and not in the way she'd read was normal when starting fertility drugs. Her most immediate symptom was painful cystic acne, breaking out on her face and back. She also struggled with insomnia. At her next monitoring appointment, the nurse told her something wasn't adding up and sent her home, saying they'd be in touch. Lauren had difficulty getting direct answers from the clinic but was eventually told that she had been taking the wrong form of leuprolide, commonly known as Lupron. Lauren was instructed to stop taking all of the medications, effectively ending her egg freezing cycle.

It's not clear who was to blame for the issue with the Lupron that Lauren took. She went back and forth with the fertility clinic and pharmacy for weeks, trying to figure it all out. At this point she'd already paid more than $10,000—for nothing. Despite the distress from the first botched attempt, Lauren decided to try again. The pharmacy and the clinic continued to claim no responsibility for the mistake. "I told them, 'Y'all can fight about this as long as you want. But I'm still thirty-eight and I would like to get my eggs out—if I still have any.'" Her resolve had hardened—"I'm a really competitive person and was hell-bent on having thirty-eight-year-old eggs frozen," she told me—but she remained highly skeptical. On a sweltering day three months after her first failed attempt, Lauren went in for the egg retrieval. This second cycle was successful, yielding fourteen viable eggs. When she got the news, she sobbed with relief.

Two days later, Lauren turned thirty-nine. She celebrated with a birthday brunch at an upscale restaurant in downtown Houston with her mother, sister, and friends. She had felt bloated since early that morning, and when she arrived home from brunch, she felt much worse. She remembers weighing herself later that night and feeling shocked realizing she'd gained several pounds; her stomach had gone from being a bit puffy to looking nine months pregnant. She was so bloated she couldn't put on her elastic-waist pajamas. Frantic, she asked her mother and sister to drive her to the hospital. After waiting for hours in the crowded emergency room, she was taken back to an exam room and told that her ovaries were so big that they were touching each other, swollen to the size of oranges. The physician told Lauren she needed to have fluid drained from her abdomen right away but that the ER physicians didn't have the skill set to do the procedure. She left the hospital around 4 A.M. and later that morning returned to the fertility clinic to have the excess fluid drained from her belly.

What Lauren was experiencing was ovarian hyperstimulation syndrome (OHSS), the chief health risk that comes with egg freezing. I'll go more into detail about this in a moment, but in short, OHSS is a response to excessive hormones. The painful condition happens when drugs used in fertility treatment cause the blood vessels surrounding the ovaries to swell and leak fluid into the body. Though her paperwork shows she signed off on the procedural risks of her egg retrieval, including OHSS, Lauren doesn't remember hearing about the condition before she was diagnosed with it at the hospital or discussing it with her doctor. "The fertility clinic handed me a folder. The only thing they would walk me through was the money," she told me. The procedure to remove the fluid worked, and within a few days, Lauren's ovaries returned to their normal size, though it took another six months for her weight and body to return to normal. The cystic acne caused by the Lupron error left temporary dark scars on her face, chest, and back, which made her too self-conscious to take her shirt off at the pool that summer. She filed complaints with the Texas Medical Board and Texas Pharmacy Board and began preparing to pursue legal action against the clinic and the pharmacy.

Months after the whole ordeal, Lauren discussed the Lupron scare and OHSS nightmare with her OB/GYN. "I don't think these errors will do permanent damage, but there's really no way to be sure," her doctor said. Lauren, only half-joking, replied: "Can I have my eggs back? And I want a cookie." Lauren's dry humor is one of her defining traits, and she makes jokes about nearly everything—usually in a deadpan, *I'm-friendly-but-don't-mess-with-me* tone. Her first egg freezing attempt was a failure and her second landed her in the emergency room, and while she was able to freeze more than a dozen eggs, *so* much had gone wrong. Finding ways to laugh about the ordeal helped her feel less broken—which, to this day, is the first word that comes to mind when she's describing her egg freezing experience and how it made her feel. *Broken.*

Fertility Drugs: The Nitty-Gritty

Lauren's experience was among the most disturbing I had heard in all the time I'd spent reporting on and researching egg freezing. We mostly hear egg freezing success stories; it's rare to hear about egg freezing gone horribly wrong. I wondered how many other women out there had experiences similar to Lauren's. And I couldn't stop thinking about the shots and drugs. One afternoon not long after moving to Houston, I pulled out the file that I'd been keeping on the procedure's risks, which eventually led me to dive into the nitty-gritty science—and bits of quirky history—behind the hormones and medications used in fertility treatments.

As I read deeply into the history of infertility research, I noticed a repeating pattern: A person or people (white men, mostly) discover a previously unknown fact about the menstrual cycle or ovulation, and then someone develops a drug or medication that remedies in a woman what her reproductive system does not or cannot do on its own. One example is clomiphene, marketed as Clomid. First came the discovery that regular menstrual cycles were a good marker of ovulation in women. It was a major breakthrough for researchers focused on infertility as a medical issue and paved the way for what came next: In the 1950s, an organic chemist, Frank Palopoli, and his team of researchers began developing Clomid, which became one of the world's most widely prescribed fertility drugs. For women who don't develop and release eggs on their own, Clomid helps them to ovulate and then go on to conceive naturally or through intrauterine insemination (IUI) or IVF. It's particularly effective for women with PCOS. The drug works by blocking estrogen production, which tricks the brain—ah, that familiar story of synthetic hormones deceiving our brains—into compensating by producing more FSH and LH, the hormones that stimulate ovulation. The drug addresses an essential first step that many women struggling to get pregnant have: getting eggs into the fallopian tube. For more than fifty years, clomiphene—on the World Health Organization's list of essential medicines—has helped millions of women become pregnant.

Another example is Gonal-f, a fertility medication with a strange tale "involving the Pope's blessing and gallons of nun urine" (part of the title of the *Quartz* article where I first encountered this story). Piero Donini, a scientist working in the late 1940s for the Italian pharmaceutical company that would later be known as Serono, was the first to extract and purify FSH and LH, which can be found in women's urine. After experimenting with urine from pregnant women, Donini discovered the highest levels of the hormone actually were in postmenopausal women, who produce massive amounts of FSH and LH in a futile attempt to revive the ovaries, which stop developing eggs after menopause. "Donini called his new substance Pergonal, after the Italian 'per gonadi,' or 'from the gonads,' and speculated that it could be used to treat infertility," the article said. A decade later, scientists researching the use of human hormones to stimulate pregnancy learned of Donini's work.

Long story short: Ultimately, a man named Giulio Pacelli, an Italian aristocrat and nephew of Pope Pius XII, convinced Serono's board of directors to make enough Pergonal to run a clinical trial. Doing so would require obtaining thousands of gallons of urine from menopausal women, which, in a speech to the board, Prince Pacelli assured

wouldn't be a problem, explaining that his uncle, Pope Pius, was prepared to ask nuns living in convents to collect urine daily for a sacred
cause. The board hurried to commit money and resources. (As it
happened, the Vatican owned 25 percent of Serono.) Tanker trucks
began hauling the urine of hundreds of nuns from nearby retirement
homes to Serono's headquarters in Rome.* Then, in 1962, a woman
treated with Pergonal in Tel Aviv gave birth to a baby girl, the first
child born from the treatment. "Within two years, another twenty
pregnancies had been achieved with Pergonal," the *Quartz* piece explains, "and by the mid-1980s, demand had grown so much that Serono needed 30,000 liters of urine a day to produce sufficient
quantities of the drug."

The company began to synthesize the hormones in labs, and the
resulting treatment, Gonal-f, was first approved in 1995. The active
ingredient in Pergonal equivalents used as fertility medications today,
such as Menopur, is still obtained from the urine of postmenopausal
women. Also, the modern method of producing FSH for fertility
treatment comes from—equally bizarre, perhaps—cells derived from
Chinese hamsters, whose ovaries are injected with the DNA for FSH,
which tricks them into producing human FSH.† Millions of cells are
cultured in huge vats, enabling more FSH to be produced than can
practically be derived from urine.

So, one of the most important advancements in infertility treatment was the ability to put the ovaries into overdrive. That's not a
technical term, of course, but it's an easy way to conceptualize the
act of stimulating a woman's ovaries to produce a bounty of eggs by
way of medications she takes, which are made in labs and/or through
genetic recombination. Brief recap: During egg freezing, a woman's
ovaries are artificially prodded with hormone medications to prepare

---

* While the urine of any postmenopausal women would work, nuns provided
Serono with an extra advantage: Because hormones from pregnant women would
contaminate the batch, it was critical there be no chance any of the women were
pregnant. Working with nuns improved the odds.

† The ovary cells of this type of rodent are commonly used in biological and
medical research and are a cell line of choice for scientists because they produce
proteins that are similar to those produced in humans.

her body for treatment and to increase the probability that a plethora of viable eggs will be extracted from her ovaries. The cocktail of medicines involves drugs to stimulate the ovaries, drugs to prevent premature ovulation, and finally the trigger shot—usually hCG, the pregnancy hormone we discussed earlier—which causes the follicles to rupture, allowing the doctor to collect the eggs during the retrieval.*

It's remarkable, really, how scientists discovered and how doctors use synthetic hormones to manipulate the reproductive system. Ovaries in overdrive can yield an arguably invaluable return—a baby—but the powerful rewards go hand in hand with alarming risks, which aren't talked about nearly as much as they ought to be. Lauren's story made that clear, and her saga took me down an unsettling new side road of research.

Much of the concern around egg freezing stems from these self-injected hormones. The medical risks associated with egg freezing fall into two categories: short-term knowns and longer-term unknowns. Hyperstimulation is the common short-term risk most egg freezers are warned about. Other short-term knowns include pelvic infection and bladder and bowel damage. Less serious but still unpleasant side effects of the hormonal fluctuations caused by fertility drugs are similar to PMS symptoms and include headaches, insomnia, mood swings, breast tenderness, and bloating. Some women have a pretty awful time during the several days of hormone shots—their abdomens feel like bricks; the emotional volatility is overwhelming—while others experience mild discomfort. It's uncommon to experience issues during the egg retrieval itself; the chances of pelvic infection, significant bleeding, or serious anesthesia complications are quite low.

OHSS, one of the most common and potentially most severe complications, occurs when a woman's ovaries receive more stimulation than her body can handle, and then the final trigger shot acts like a

---

* For a helpful resource on all fertility treatment medications, see resolve.org /learn/what-are-my-options/medications/types-of-medications/.

flame igniting a kerosene-soaked woodpile. OHSS typically hits within a week of the patient taking the trigger shot and undergoing the egg retrieval, as it did with Lauren. The condition is diagnosed by a physical exam, an ultrasound, and/or a blood test measuring hormone levels. OHSS symptoms can be anywhere from mild or moderate (nausea, bloating, diarrhea) to severe (extreme abdominal pain, persistent vomiting, blood clots, shortness of breath, and rapid weight gain of more than ten pounds in a few days), with acute cases of OHSS causing abnormal enlargement of the ovaries and sometimes ovarian cysts and torsion. As many as one in three women experience mild OHSS during IVF or egg freezing; fewer than 2 percent will develop a severe case. Women who freeze their eggs in their twenties or early thirties are at more risk for OHSS because larger egg supplies can cause hyperstimulation; the more eggs a woman has, the higher the chance that the medication she takes before her egg retrieval will stimulate a higher-than-desired number of ovarian follicles. For the same reason, women with PCOS are also more at risk for developing OHSS.

Determining how much medication an egg freezing patient needs to safely stimulate her ovaries isn't an exact science. Monitoring the patient's hormone levels throughout the days of self-injected shots allows the doctor to make necessary dose adjustments. The initial assessments and blood work help the doctor ascertain a baseline level of hormones and determine a treatment regime, as well as assess for any risk of OHSS at the outset while considering existing risk factors.[*] Individualizing treatment regimens is typically the best way to prevent OHSS. If a doctor does this properly, severe OHSS shouldn't develop. But if a doctor prescribes an overly aggressive medication protocol or insists on pressing forward with stimulation in the face of mild to moderate OHSS, that's when things can get dangerous.[†]

---

[*] In addition to young age and high egg count, other OHSS risk factors include having low BMI, having high AMH, and having a very high estrogen level during treatment.

[†] While it's true that most fertility doctors act in the best interest of their patients, it's also true that some are incentivized to give patients more intense hormone regimes in order to harvest as many eggs from them as possible, which can lead to spikes in OHSS.

For all the colorful stories behind the development of several fertility drugs, troubling unknowns surround a few of the major ones. Take Lupron, a medication commonly prescribed during fertility treatment to prevent premature ovulation during the ovarian stimulation process.* Except it's not FDA-approved for that use; its use during egg freezing and IVF is considered off-label. Lupron is approved to treat prostate cancer; it's also approved for and used to reduce the size of uterine fibroids, treat endometriosis symptoms, and block early puberty. For all the good it does, the drug has a dark side, too. Most drugs do, but Lupron, the use of which among women has been linked with bone density loss, severe joint and muscle pain, and memory loss, is particularly harrowing. The FDA has received thousands of adverse event reports for Lupron products in the past decade† and people have petitioned Congress for further investigation into the drug's side effects; there's even a website called Lupron Victims Hub.

Why are Lupron and other off-label drugs permitted to be used in ways they were not intended to be used? Because while the FDA has the authority to punish drug companies for marketing a drug for a use that it has not approved, regulating the *practice* of medicine is outside its jurisdiction; the agency doesn't oversee where and how off-label drugs are being used. Fertility doctors, like doctors in other fields of medicine, can only prescribe FDA-approved medications—but the purpose for prescribing isn't tracked. So, unless a case clearly violates ethical guidelines and safety regulations, physicians can prescribe drugs like Lupron for off-label uses without fear of consequences. I remembered something Remy's doctor said to her: "A lot of these drugs are not FDA-approved for what we do. The pharmaceutical companies don't spend the money getting things approved for fertility. So a lot of times there's a black box warning on the meds . . . but don't worry about it."

---

* Yet, the Lupron label warns of birth defects in rodents and advises against using the drug when one is considering pregnancy.

† A list on the FDA's website, noting Lupron's potential serious risks, says the agency is "evaluating the need for regulatory action."

What I took away from my deep dive into hormone injections was this: Fertility medications are both powerful and somewhat frightening, and OHSS is clear evidence that bodies can respond badly when pumped too full of hormones. When undergoing fertility treatment, everyone's baseline hormone cocktail is different. Every body is different, and a person's reaction to the drugs falls across a wide spectrum. Reproductive endocrinologists have to find the sweet spot for their egg freezing patients as they try to successfully stimulate the ovaries to produce eggs. Not too many, but not too few. Dial up, dial down, get the most eggs possible without endangering a woman's life or ovaries. *Holy shit, this is complicated,* I texted a friend one day while I was absorbed in my research. Avoiding overstimulating the ovaries and causing conditions such as OHSS was clearly a complex skill that involved an artful interpretation of the science. Egg freezing's price tag, it now occurred to me, seemed a bit more justified. And the stakes? Much higher than I'd realized.

"There Are No Known Risks" and Other Half-Truths

I turned to the second category of egg freezing's medical risks: longer-term unknowns. While the short-term effects of injecting lots of hormones to stimulate the release of multiple eggs at once are known, I discovered that there's almost no information on potential long-term harm, because research is so sparse. Hormone therapy typically raises a patient's estrogen levels, and estrogen can abet the growth of, specifically, ovarian and breast cancers. Studies examining the relationship between fertility drugs and the risk of hormone-sensitive cancers show mixed results. For the most part, they conclude that the medications used during fertility treatment don't appear to increase a woman's risk of cancer. That's the good news. But as I dug into the limited data, I learned that the validity of these findings may be affected by confounding variables such as small subject numbers, as well as specific characteristics of the populations being studied: women who have been diagnosed with infertility versus women—typically younger—who have not. I also happened upon dark stories, many deep in reddit threads, and read studies that *do* indicate that the high doses of hormones used during fertility treatments may increase a woman's risk of cancer. What I found as I tumbled down rabbit holes on the internet was some of the most worrisome stuff I had encountered since first learning about egg freezing.

Around this time I listened to an episode on *Reveal,* an investigative reporting podcast, on egg donors. It was a short but shocking story about a young woman, Jessica Wing, who by age twenty-five had donated her eggs three times and who died from colon cancer when she was thirty-one. Jessica was an undergraduate at Stanford when she saw an ad recruiting students to donate their eggs. She called her mother, a doctor, to ask her about it. Her mother had only one question: *Is it safe?* Jessica said she was told it was, and decided to do it, using the money to help pay for her college education. The eggs she donated resulted in a pregnancy. According to Jessica's mother, this made the fertility clinic deem Jessica a "proven" donor, and the clinic offered Jessica twice as much money to donate again. Through Jessica's egg donations, five healthy children were born to three formerly childless families. Four years after her third donation, Jessica learned she had metastatic colon cancer. Doctors also found tumors in her ovaries. There was no history of any early cancer or colon cancer in her family, and twenty-nine is a young age for such a diagnosis, especially in a health-conscious woman like Jessica. To this day, her mother wonders if the extensive hormone treatments her daughter had undergone as an egg donor might have stimulated the growth of the cancer.

The reason Jessica's story stuck with me—besides its objectively tragic nature—was because I knew how similar egg donation is to egg freezing. Egg donation, a multimillion-dollar and poorly regulated industry, has been around a lot longer than egg freezing. The processes of donating eggs and freezing one's own eggs are exactly the same up until the last step: An egg donor is compensated for her eggs, which are used for research or to help another person or couple have a baby, while an egg freezer's eggs go into a cryotank and remain hers. But egg freezers undergo the same hormone treatments as egg donors do. And like egg donors, egg freezers often cycle more than once if not enough viable eggs are obtained on a first attempt.*

You would think that after more than forty years, we'd know more about long-term effects for women who use ART. But in fact large gaps in our knowledge persist. Part of the problem is a dearth of follow-up data, especially in our fragmented American health system, which lacks national medical records. While organ registries exist for many kinds of organ donation in the United States, there is no egg donor registry. Because of the anonymity of egg donors, there are no other databases from which to cull numbers. The rationale is that not having a registry protects egg donors' privacy. But not monitoring an egg donor's health after the fact means not knowing anything about the potential long-term risks of egg donation—which, in turn, means knowing little about the long-term risks of egg freezing. Egg banks have rules about women donating more than a few times, but because the government doesn't maintain an egg donor registry, there isn't any centralized tracking of who has donated eggs and where and when.[†] It's easy for a young woman to donate eggs at different clinics and be a repeat donor as many times as she wants; once she walks out of a facility's door, she's lost to medical history.

Another difficulty arises when subsets of patients are treated alike even when they're not. Most of the research conducted on egg retrievals has focused on women undergoing IVF—the first half of which, you'll recall, involves ovarian stimulation, as do egg donation and egg freezing. And so, similar to how much of the limited data that exists on egg freezing success rates relies partially on data extrapolated from IVF (discussed in chapter 8), the health risks to women who freeze or donate their eggs have been extrapolated from research on IVF patients—but the populations are different. Most women undergo IVF because they are struggling with infertility, which can be a symptom of other health problems. Egg donors, by contrast, are cho-

---

* Many egg freezers I interviewed had done three or four cycles.

[†] When I went looking for hard data on the number of egg donors in the United States, the closest statistic I could find was the number of IVF cycles that used frozen donor eggs, which increased to 22,563 in 2020 from 7,733 in 2011.

sen precisely because they have zero health problems (or at least, very few and not serious ones) and are not infertile. They're almost always younger, unlike most women undergoing IVF, who tend to be a good deal older. Egg donors are also typically given higher amounts of hormones to stimulate the production of eggs, and many undergo the procedure several times. So, OHSS rates among egg donors differ from those of IVF patients, too. The point is, using IVF patients to draw conclusions about ovarian stimulation's risks to egg donors and egg freezers is about as helpful as using kindergartners to draw conclusions about car seats for infants.

I read several cases about people who donated eggs and then developed cancer while relatively young. None of these egg donors had an apparent genetic risk for the disease. (Of course, cancer also develops in young people who haven't donated their eggs.)* In most of the reports, women hadn't been given any information about the long-term risks of egg donation—in part because no such information exists. More studies on egg donors in the United States, which a national egg donor registry would help to facilitate, would give us more to rely on than anecdotal evidence of women who served as egg donors and later developed cancer, struggled with infertility, or experienced other health issues. Without such long-term follow-up data, it's impossible to gather information to estimate the prevalence of cancer in egg donors or draw conclusions about the possibility of an increased risk compared to the general population. In a statement to *Reveal,* the CDC said, "Better understanding the long-term outcomes of fertility treatments for donors . . . is a priority within the field." Is it, though? The CDC collects data on IVF. It or the Department of Health and Human Services could also collect data on egg donors that would help shed light on the potential link between hormone treatments and increased risk of cancer and other health issues in patients donating or freezing eggs.

The pessimistic take is that there isn't any incentive for anyone to

---

* Also, though, while there's no single cause of, for example, gynecologic cancers, there are many risk factors that could contribute to their development—such as the use of fertility drugs, especially if used repeatedly over the course of multiple egg retrievals.

study the health risks to egg donors because the system as it stands now seems like a win–win–win: Fertility clinics get business, egg donors are well compensated, and infertile couples have a better chance to conceive a baby. An embryologist* I spoke with who manages the lab of a well-known fertility clinic on the East Coast told me: "In the early days of IVF, everybody talked about the concerns of the drugs putting women at risk for certain cancers. Now, it's just so swept under the rug. And before the question even comes out of people's mouths, REIs [reproductive endocrinologists] say, 'There's absolutely no clinical evidence to suggest it,'" the embryologist continued, referring to the potential long-term health risks associated with fertility medications. "The question isn't even allowed in the room anymore."

The bottom line is this: The absence of information on egg donors has led to inadequate attention to potential health risks in egg freezers. And both groups aren't appropriately counseled about the nature of that absence of information. Which brings us to the issue of informed consent. In the United States, the informed consent agreements that fertility clinics give to egg donors include minimal information on long-term risks. And the information they do provide is based on studies of infertile women rather than egg donors—and doesn't include the crucial fact that this is a different group.

There are no known risks. That's how most fertility clinics characterize the possible association between fertility drugs and health concerns, particularly cancers.† The problem is with the word "known": Can we really say there aren't any long-term adverse effects associated with hyperstimulating ovaries unless such effects have been systematically researched? A 2020 *New York Times* article titled "What We

---

* They asked to remain anonymous out of concern of pushback from their boss and colleagues in the field.

† Sometimes fertility doctors don't even hedge with the word "known." A 2023 episode on the podcast *This Is Uncomfortable* featured a twenty-one-year-old egg donor who, speaking about the clinic's doctors and nurses reassuring her about the procedure, said, "I specifically remember them saying, 'No study has shown that there are any negative side effects from egg donation.'" Shortly after her egg retrieval, she was hospitalized with OHSS.

Don't Know About I.V.F." summed up the issue well with a quote from an NYU School of Medicine professor: "We have no idea what this level of hormonal stimulation at this time in a woman's life might be doing to her body." All women who take fertility medications and undergo ovarian stimulation, especially more than once, should be told that such risks amount to a big fat question mark. But they're not. Instead, patients are told there is no evidence proving harm, when in fact there remains considerable uncertainty about the true extent and severity of ovarian stimulation's potential long-term health risks—especially to egg donors and egg freezers.

The podcast episode about Jessica wasn't the first cautionary tale I had heard about the potential correlation between fertility drugs and cancer, but it was the most alarming—until I met Lesley. A nurse in Colorado, Lesley froze eighteen eggs when she was thirty-five and going through a divorce. She was driving to work one morning when, on the radio, she heard an interview with a Google employee who had frozen her eggs and used the company's fertility benefit to pay for the procedure. Lesley felt like biology might be passing her by, and egg freezing sounded like a good idea. "It seemed harmless," she told me. Lesley mentioned it to her mom, had a consultation at a fertility clinic, and afterward thought, *Why not? Kind of expensive, but seems worth it.* Using some of her savings, money from her parents, and some help from insurance (they covered a portion of the medications), she froze her eggs. Eighteen months later, she found out she had breast cancer.

Lesley's biopsy showed that her cancer was highly hormone-driven. When she brought up with her radiologist and fertility doctor the possible connection between the egg freezing medications she'd taken and her cancer diagnosis, "they wouldn't even open the door to go there. It was a hard stop. It's really something that seems like it's not talked about at all even though, logically, there seems like there would be a correlation." While undergoing thirty rounds of radiation and a radical mastectomy—meaning the whole breast, lymph nodes under the arm, and the chest wall muscles under the breast are removed—Lesley met several other women battling cancer who also had been through fertility treatment. She learned more about how bodies have varying abilities when it comes to blocking estrogen receptors and metabolizing harmful toxins, which can make someone more susceptible to disease.

"I think we're all these hormonal Frankensteins," she said, sounding almost in awe of something she'd long known as a nurse but now understood in a much more personal way: the major influence hormones have on our bodies and our health. "Looking back, I probably had a ductal carcinoma in situ"—cancer cells present in her breast's milk ducts, meaning non- or pre-invasive breast cancer—"that probably would've stayed dormant for forty years . . . and then I go and pour fuel on the fire by pumping myself up with all those hormones." Lesley, now remarried, does not plan on using her frozen eggs. "I feel disillusioned. The trust has been fractured. And then I think, what would having a baby mean for my chances of a cancer relapse? I don't want to have a baby and then not be there to raise it." Looking back at her egg freezing experience, Lesley told me: "I have these eggs now that I paid a fortune for, but it doesn't seem like it was worth it." Her biggest regret is not doing more research beforehand. Ultimately, she told me, she wishes she hadn't done it.

Learning about the longer-term unknowns of egg freezing that are rarely discussed between fertility doctors and patients made me frustrated—a bit angry, even. Concerned, too: I already worried when I felt a small cramp that it was another cyst on my ovary, that I was going to lose the ovary. Now I was afraid if I froze my eggs in the next few months I'd just be trading that fear for this other paranoid fear in which I'm just hoping I don't develop a random cancer. I reminded myself that the journal articles and studies that did indicate a link showed correlation, not causation, between fertility medications and cancer. But the disquieting lack of long-term safety data, and the unsettling personal stories I'd absorbed, gave me serious pause—more than anything else I had encountered thus far on this journey.

Even though I now lived in Houston, I had decided I would fly back to New York to freeze with Dr. Noyes. I had forgotten to tell the fertility clinic I had moved, though, and it had been a long time since our last communication. The ball was in my court; if and when I was ready to freeze, the next step was working with the clinic's nurses to schedule the process around my menstrual cycle, including going off the Pill, before starting the injections.

I dug around my desk in The Bungalow looking for my notes from my egg freezing orientation at the clinic. The two-hour session had been similar to the one Mandy had attended, with a handful of other women and couples. Diligent student that I was, I'd scratched out notes until my hand ached, circling the parts I'd need to figure out later, which was most of what I wrote down. The nurse talked quickly as she flipped through the slides. I turned to a fresh page in my note-book and began writing a list of to-dos. *Contact patient coordinator one month prior to date of egg freezing cycle to confirm medication protocol and cycle schedule. Do online injection training. Get red sharps container from pharmacy and take needles to doc's office. Think about disposition of eggs re: custody in event of death—donate for research or discard or . . . ?* I remem-ber feeling flustered as I sat in the dim conference room that morning, scribbling names of drugs and medication protocols that might as well have been in Latin. In the months that followed, some of my confu-sion would abate as I learned more about egg freezing's science. But my apprehension would only grow. I'd felt uneasy at the egg freezing orientation because much of it felt foreign. Now, reviewing these notes, the uneasiness was because it felt much more real—because of my trying to decide about whether or not to freeze my eggs, but also because of Ben.

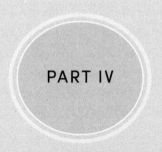

PART IV

The Retrieval

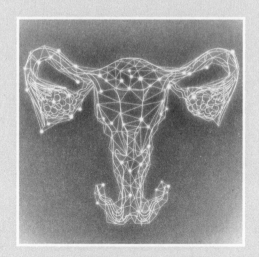

Scar Tissue

~~~~~~

Marrying Eggs to Sperm

By this point, I had arrived at the darker side of egg freezing. The deeper I went, the more questions I had about some of my unsettling discoveries. At the same time, I was much clearer on the process of vitrification, egg freezing success rates, and financing the procedure (I understood the avenues to paying, at least, even if I had no idea how I would afford to do it myself). I knew, too, that for all of the horror stories like Lauren's and Lesley's, egg freezing goes perfectly right most of the time. Now I was ready to turn to another facet of fertility preservation: the healthy debate over egg versus embryo freezing. Anyone considering freezing reproductive cells should consider the trade-offs between the two.

Egg freezing entails cryopreserving eggs for future fertilization. Embryo freezing is cryopreserving eggs that have been fertilized with sperm. To create an embryo, an embryologist fertilizes one or more of a woman's harvested eggs with the sperm of a partner or donor, then observes the embryos as they develop (remember attrition rates?) in a petri dish over several days. Then, using vitrification technology we discussed earlier, the embryologist freezes the embryos. Mature, chromosomally normal eggs help to make good embryos (the quality of the sperm, of course, matters, too), which is why the younger a woman is when she freezes eggs, the more likely she is to freeze healthy eggs. Clinicians can tell if eggs are mature when they freeze them, but they can't know if the eggs are genetically normal—that is, viable—until they thaw and fertilize the eggs, then test the resulting embryos.

It's not currently possible to tell whether eggs are good quality at the time of freezing. This is egg freezing's biggest weakness. Eggs, you'll remember, are trickier to thaw than embryos. An egg is a single cell, whereas a developing embryo contains more than one hundred cells, each of which is less vulnerable to damage. Frozen eggs are less sturdy than frozen embryos; more than 95 percent of embryos typically survive the thawing process, compared to 80 to 90 percent of eggs.* So, a major advantage of freezing embryos over eggs is that embryos that develop successfully can be biopsied and tested for the presence and correct number of chromosomes—forty-six—giving the person or couple more information about each embryo's likelihood of leading to a successful pregnancy and a healthy child. Embryos can also be screened for a specific gene, which is especially helpful if one or both of the people providing the eggs and the sperm are known to have a certain gene mutation or be a carrier of a genetic disorder. (More on genetic testing in chapter 15.) In short: A benefit of freezing embryos is that you have a better idea of what you have in the freezer.

A downside of freezing embryos is that it costs a few thousand dollars more than egg freezing; on top of that, preimplantation genetic testing is another $4,000 to $6,000 or so, depending in part on the number of embryos tested. Another con is the possibility of creating excess embryos that the couple may never need in the future, after they've attained their ideal family size. This can pose a practical dilemma—the ongoing cost to store them, hundreds of dollars per year—as well as an ethical and more personal one: Many couples who have leftover frozen embryos after they're done having children struggle with whether to discard them, donate them, or pay to keep them

---

* These percentages can vary among labs, which is one reason why choosing a fertility clinic that has a reputable laboratory and well-trained embryology staff is important—really important. More on this in chapter 14.

on ice even if they never plan to use them.* Still, the fact that frozen embryos are sturdier than frozen eggs and can be genetically tested have contributed to embryo freezing becoming an increasingly popular option: Between 2015 and 2020, procedures to freeze embryos rose nearly 60 percent.

Ben remained supportive of whatever I decided to do about egg freezing. His encouragement and steadiness when it came to my work as well as my more personal endeavors had been a dependable constant of our relationship. But it was still surprising when one evening he walked into my quasi-office in the kitchen, his frame filling the doorway and a twinkle in his eye, and said, half-jokingly, "So, are you saying you would like some of my sperm? Wanna make a zygote?" He had overheard some of the phone conversations I'd been having as part of my research, like with Mandy, when during one of our long phone calls I had pressed her about her decision to freeze embryos with her husband, an option she learned about after she'd said yes to egg freezing. I laughed—what is it with men and their feeling macho about their sperm readying for a mission?—and unfolded my body from its hunched-over, deep-in-work-mode position to go hug him. He wrapped his arms around me and I relaxed into our familiar, comforting embrace, smiling into his chest.

Though Ben had been half-joking in that moment, I thought about the proposition more seriously in the context of my egg freezing plans. Marrying my eggs to Ben's sperm would be a big biological and legal commitment. I learned that some women do half-and-half: fertilize some of the retrieved eggs to make embryos, but leave the rest, resulting in both eggs and embryos on ice.† If I froze my eggs, I

---

* Frozen eggs and sperm, on the other hand, do not independently have the potential to initiate a pregnancy, which makes the choices surrounding the disposition of stored gametes less fraught. More on egg and embryo disposition decisions in chapter 14.

† A major benefit: By fertilizing half of my retrieved eggs and hopefully getting a few high-quality embryos, I'd have a sense of how good my remaining unfertilized eggs were likely to be.

could theoretically mix half of them with Ben's sperm to make embryos—our future children—and leave the other half unfertilized, just in case. The rest of that sentence that I didn't want to say out loud was: *in case we break up.* If Ben and I froze embryos and broke up, our embryos would belong to both of us. But my eggs would still be just mine.

It was time to make another list:

Pros of freezing just eggs:
Retain sole control and optionality over whose sperm to fertilize with
Fewer issues surrounding ownership
Fewer up-front costs
In short: fertility preservation autonomy

Pros of freezing embryos:
Ability to do preimplantation genetic testing
Better and more info regarding whether frozen embryos will lead to a healthy baby/babies
Reduce risk during the freeze-and-thaw process
In short: more data to work with

When it came to marriage and kids, Ben and I didn't feel any rush, but our conversations about a future together had been real and present since our early days of dating. And as our relationship became more serious, I wanted things to progress with intention, which I'd communicated to Ben. A couple of weeks earlier, during a long weekend in Colorado with Ben's parents, who'd flown in from Florida, and mine, his father had made a few lighthearted comments about Ben buying me an engagement ring. Being in a relationship and debating freezing eggs versus embryos casts a spotlight on the big questions: How serious is this? How likely are we to really, truly have kids together? The thought experiment of egg freezing, already difficult to conceptualize, becomes trickier. All in one basket, or all in with one person, or something in between? I was clear on the science: Freezing eggs affords more choice. Freezing embryos offers better odds. But when you're doing the latter with a partner, matters of the heart require some degree of certainty, too.

Over the next few weeks, as Ben and I joked about and then more seriously discussed fusing our sex cells to create embryos, I kept thinking about the day we drove from Colorado to Texas, moving me and a car full of my things to The Bungalow. I'd had my first panic attack that day, as we traversed bad weather that made driving conditions treacherous. A few hours into the long drive, high winds whipped up and we noticed a few semi-trucks teetering on the two-lane highway we were barreling down. The truck in front of us, its trailer empty, swayed and then began to tip sideways. I started to cry and couldn't catch my breath. "I think I need you to pull over," I said, anxiety rising in my throat.

"You're fine. Just breathe," he said, concentrating on the road. As he moved into the left lane to attempt to pass the wild truck, I didn't understand why the car wasn't slowing to a stop, or why I was having such a strong reaction.

When I realized we were gaining speed, not losing it, I tensed my arm against the passenger window, as if to steel against the crash I felt was imminent. "I really need you to pull over," I repeated. I don't remember what Ben replied, but he did not pull over. Maybe it wasn't safe to slow down, but I hated that he sped up. I looked to my right—so close to the swaying truck trailer we were now parallel to that if my window had been down, I was sure I could've reached my arm out and touched it—and then lurched forward when Ben hit the brakes, unable to pass. We were now both scared, but I began having flashbacks to other frightening close calls I'd experienced in cars, and I struggled to control my breathing. This was my first full-on panic attack, though not my first time feeling very panicked, and I recognized a specific kind of fear in the deep center of my chest, so sharp I put my palm against my breastbone to quell it.

The winds eventually died down, and though we were almost in an accident and later witnessed other empty semi-trucks nearly careen off the highway, we were okay. But it was the first time I knew, in my gut, it might not work out between us. Just as quickly as the thought came, I willed it away, refusing to allow it to crystallize. I told no one. I did not write about it in my journal. I told myself it was misplaced fear after the stressful drive, an overreaction to an unnerving day. I tried to convince myself that my panic attack had nothing to do with my deciding to move in with Ben. It was raining by the time we pulled into a motel parking lot in Dallas hours later, and the thought had faded, or I'd managed to stuff it away, or both. We would get some rest, and when we woke in the morning to finish the drive, my bones would no longer ache the way they had been since we'd left Denver at dawn. I composed these wishes as facts because I needed them to be true.

But now those thoughts and memories of that day were resurfacing. The reason I kept revisiting that distressing day, amid my wondering about freezing embryos with Ben, was because, pleasant zygote discussions aside, we had been fighting. A lot. Since moving to Houston, I had cried myself to sleep more times than I could count. Our differences had begun to go beyond his partying and my projecting. We disagreed more than seemed normal for two people in love. We even disagreed about whether the things we disagreed about were a big deal or not at all. Driving. Drugs. Cooking. Monogamy. God. I'd become nagging and controlling, and Ben had begun to distance himself from what he sometimes called my "roller coaster of emotions"; "you're too much" was a criticism he often leveled at me, and it cut straight to my core. The hard parts of our relationship were not the right kind of hard, the misalignment more serious than when car tires go awry and the steering is no longer properly calibrated. Something fundamental was missing—I didn't know what, exactly, but I knew it was essential—and that made it difficult to see past the trivial stuff, to compromise, to keep believing it could work. But when these thoughts bubbled up I would berate myself for feeling unsure, for conflating work and personal life. After all, it had been my choice to move to Texas and live with Ben when he asked me. I was here now, digging my heels in, swatting away red flags that popped up. I had—we had—invested too much to undo things now.

So this was a pretty big hang-up. Embryo freezing made sense for women in committed relationships, or who otherwise knew whose sperm they wanted to mix with their eggs. And the truth was, I realized with an ache, that I was not deep-down certain I wanted to freeze embryos with Ben. As much as I wanted to believe he was the person with whom I wanted to and would have children down the road, I was no longer sure.

No Place to Be

An early August evening in Houston. One hundred degrees outside. I am at Walmart buying plastic bins. I am pretty sure I am moving out and that Ben's and my relationship is over.

The breakup had happened slowly, then all at once. I had been clinging tightly to the idea that we had just been having trouble adjusting to living together. But our differences had become irreconcilable, and we'd come to a point where most days we just weren't happy. Where we were in complete agreement: We were tired of fighting and tired of trying so hard to make it work.

A couple of nights earlier we'd biked to Blanket Bingo, a monthly summertime event downtown. We sprawled out on the grass among groups of friends and families and attempted only light conversation. It was humid and sticky. After, Ben asked if I wanted to get a drink at a nearby bar he loved before biking home. I didn't, really, but I'd felt as if we had been walking on eggshells around each other for days and was afraid my not being up for this would start another fight. We sat at a high-top table near the bar. Ben ordered a cocktail; I asked for ice water. His phone buzzed, and I watched him look at it lighting up. "I'm going to take this," he said. It was a work call. He launched into an animated conversation with a colleague about renewable fuels and I sat there and waited.

I watched Ben as he laughed and talked, sipping his drink between sentences. I considered this person I had fallen in love with. This man who loved old-fashioneds and the Green Bay Packers, playing the drums and chatting up interesting strangers. Who had lived in the same house for most of his childhood and whose Midwestern niceties had made him charming and sweet. Who lit up and said *oh, golly* when he saw a road sign announcing a Friday night fish fry. Whose high school years as a soccer player and star running back had made him so physically sturdy. Who hadn't gone to the dentist in a decade. Who avoided conflict like it was poison. I looked at this man who knew my secrets, who rubbed my feet on long airplane rides, who texted me things like *Come be the queen of my bungalow and I'll love you madly* and *I want our lives together to be as colorful as your breakfasts.* Who more than once bought me a big bouquet of flowers and said, "Because I love you. And because you should have flowers like this every single day." My ice water was sweating, leaving dark rings on the wood table. Ben, still on the phone, got up and paced, drink in hand. I stared at the water rings, feeling more ignored and resentful by the second. *What am I doing here?* I thought. I stood up from the table, grabbed my bag from the back of the chair, and left.

I was halfway to where we'd locked our bikes when I felt Ben's hand on the back of my shoulder. I turned to face him. "Where are you going?" he asked. He was still on the phone, holding it against his ear away from his mouth. "Back to the apartment," I said. He turned the phone and told his colleague he was going to need to call him back. Then he looked at me, his light eyes stormy. I asked why he'd taken the call; he said something about being bored.

"Bored with me?" I asked.

"The thrill is dead," he said coldly, and my already queasy stomach lurched, his words a punch to my gut.

"What does that even mean?" I said.

It didn't seem like we were talking about what had just happened in the bar anymore. He said something about it being my job—or did he say both of our jobs? My memory fogs here—to keep things interesting. Then:

"So captivate me," he said. "If you want to be talked to, captivate me." I froze, then felt my face flush with anger. It was one of those ugly sentences that slips out during a fight; Ben seldom spoke to me this way, which is why it stayed imprinted. More final than the packing bins and boxes, than the uncomfortable silence that had come to fill the apartment like stale air. A wave of dizziness washed over me, blurring the twinkly bar lights above the street corner we stood on. A memory came hard and fast: the first night we met, a different city, a different street corner, a different bar. Two years and a lifetime ago.

Inside Walmart, I blinked back tears in the home storage aisle and debated buying the cheap bins or the sturdier ones. When I had moved in with Ben half a year earlier, I'd convinced myself I would never move out. It was my first time living with a partner. I thought settling in together and hanging art on our shared walls would make me feel pinned securely to my world. All I knew now was that I was scared to leave but more scared, in a soul sense, to stay. I piled several of the sturdier bins into my cart. I felt drained, already overwhelmed by the prospect of packing—again. Too much life packed into plastic containers.

Back at The Bungalow, fruit flies fluttered around the kitchen sink. Sunlight streamed through a window, settling on an unassembled shoe rack, a placemat, a pile of mail. When I was done carrying the storage bins in from the car, I kicked off my sandals and caught a glance of myself in the mirror that hung next to the front door. I forced myself to face my reflection, the realization ringing in my ears: Commitment does not always mean staying. Sometimes, to commit is to leave. Leave the person you thought you'd always remain alongside. Leave a place you tried hard to make your home. Leave even if you're not sure how to let go or what comes next or if you'll be okay.

A few days later, I was sitting in a corner in Terminal A at Houston's international airport, about to board a flight to Seattle. From there, I would rent a car and drive to Banff, Canada. A ten-day trip to celebrate my birthday—a trip Ben and I were supposed to take together. We'd planned to camp and stay in hostels sprinkled around national parks, the Icefields Parkway, the famously blue Lake Louise. It was out of a sort of stubborn pride that I didn't cancel the trip as soon as Ben and I broke up. But even if I had admitted to not being sure I wanted to take the trip without him, he would have insisted I go solo.

I had been packing since dawn. The day I returned to Houston from Banff was the day I would move out. It had made sense when Ben and I discussed it—it was going to be painful no matter what, but this was the most logistically feasible option—but now that I was about to board, I was finding it difficult to get on the plane. I called

Ben from a corner of the gate area. He was driving back from Dallas; he'd been there for work for the past few days, so at least he wasn't there to watch me pack. "You don't sound good," he said. He was right. I felt depleted. Empty. Numb. I did not want to spend the next ten days alone in one of the most beautiful places in the world. I wanted to stay curled up in a corner at Gate A16, hiccup-crying into the phone to the person who at that moment still felt like my person. I hoped that hearing his voice might calm me down enough to get me on the plane.

"We're doing the right thing—right?" I said weakly. "I need to hear you say it."

Ben made a sound that I'd never heard him make before, a mournful half-groan, half-sigh. "Natalie. It's so hard to hear you ask that. But yes. I think deep down we know we need this space. A break."

I closed my eyes and held on to those words, even though I knew this was not, would not be, just a break. I knew he knew that, too. It doesn't make sense to rip off half a Band-Aid, but it hurts less that way. Before we hung up, he shared a few heartfelt sentiments, the kind that always made me feel better when he said them—but this time they made me feel worse.

I got on the plane. He sent me a text I read just before I switched my phone off: *Felt an unfamiliar ache during that call which I haven't felt in long time. This is gonna be ok. This trip should be ideal for you. Be there. Be in it all.* I wrapped one arm around the other, hugging myself, and took a deep breath. I felt irrevocably alone. As the plane lifted off the tarmac, I pressed my nose against the tiny window and looked out and down, trying not to think about the empty seat beside me.

In Seattle, I forgot to buy a map before driving into Canada. When my cell service went out just across the border and Google Maps was no more, I used road signs and a helpful gas station attendant's directions to wind my way to Banff. I drove for hours on the Trans-Canada Highway, nestled between impossibly beautiful mountain passes. I tried to ground myself in the stunning landscape, the dizzying views of sharp, rock-faced mountains and deep green trees, but the sadness from the past few weeks and my fears about what came next felt like a weighted blanket, smothering.

Banff is a small ski town in western Canada surrounded by dense alpine woods with lots of trails. There are glacial lakes and steep mountains protruding above the treeline. The morning of my twenty-eighth birthday, I woke in a bunk bed at a hostel. I ate pancakes in the hostel's small restaurant and, connected to their Wi-Fi, scrolled on my phone and replied to a few birthday messages. Then I bought a packed lunch and headed to a lake nearby that I'd been told had fewer tourists and even brighter aqua-blue water than Lake Louise. It was the first time I could remember celebrating a birthday alone. I needed this solitude. Needed space, and sky, and hiking to heal, and gulps of mountain air to make me believe I would be okay again. I sat on the edge of the water, watching canoers gently paddle the length of the lake. The late morning sun blanketed my face. A few friends and relatives had mailed birthday cards to Houston, which I'd packed before leaving. I reached in my bag for them and opened them one by one.

Ben did not call or text me on my birthday, and though I knew he rarely texted anyone on their birthdays, I tried but failed to not take it personally.

The next day, I set out to hike to the Plain of Six Glaciers Teahouse. From Lake Louise's inlet, I began to climb, eventually emerging from a forest to a deposit of glacial moraine. Rain fell steadily as I neared the small, historic chalet. I huddled with others to stay warm and slurped an overly high-priced bowl of steaming soup. On the hike back down, I sat for a while in a meadow surrounded by spectacular glaciated peaks. I had decided that when I left Houston I would go back to Colorado, stash my bins of belongings at my parents' house, and move to Denver or Boulder. I tried to find the bright spots. One was that starting over could be an adventure, a chance to plant my feet firmly in a new city I would learn to call my own. The chilling part, the reality I was finding it painful to stomach, was that I had no place to *be*. I had choices of places to live, but nowhere I belonged.

When the rain eventually let up, the meadow glistened. The sun began to peek out from behind the clouds and I stood to go, feeling a familiar, curious tug of fullness and regret. I paused, then did something I hadn't done in years: put my palms on the earth and kick my legs up. After a few more handstands, feeling better, I pulled my jacket tight against the wind and walked on.

Mandy: Resilient Ovaries

Several weeks before my personal life started to crumble, I had planned out a reporting trip to San Francisco. The Bay Area was an incubator for the future of fertility; I wanted to interview some of the doctors and entrepreneurs at the center. And visit Mandy, and see Fertility-IQ's Deborah and Jake. In mid-September, a few weeks after leaving Houston, I flew to San Francisco. I arrived at my Airbnb, dropped my bags, and promptly lay down on the carpeted bedroom floor. I thought my heart had settled enough to get back to work reporting, but anxiety sat like a pile of rocks on my chest, the post-breakup heavy sadness still lurking. I started to cry, taking gulps of air between sobs, then turned to look through the sliding screen door at the sliver of ocean blocks away, willing the sight of water to calm me some. Many minutes later, a distant ice cream truck and its cheery, annoying song helped bring me back. I forced myself to stand up and make a plan. I decided to walk to get my nails done because a female graduate school professor had once commented on my messy, short nails, admonishing me to never conduct an interview with chipped nail polish. I threw my hair into a bun, grabbed a scarf, and headed out into the drizzle.

A few evenings later, I visited Mandy at her home in Oakland to have dinner with her and Quincy. I was eager to ask her more about her embryo freezing experience, especially now that it was over and behind her. The meetings I'd had since arriving in San Francisco had been mostly with doctors, and while helpful, they hadn't been all that, well, interesting. It was talking with women like Mandy, who had experienced egg or embryo freezing themselves, that revealed the most about the process. When I knocked, she greeted me with a warm smile. We sat at the kitchen table, catching up a bit. I'd last spoken with Mandy before I moved out of The Bungalow. She asked me how life in Houston had been going. I wasn't prepared to talk about my personal life. After all, I was there to ask Mandy more questions. I was there as a reporter. But for months now, she had been sharing intimate details of her life with me. She'd cried on the phone, laughed, and gotten angry. And she'd sometimes ask me about my egg freezing decision. She knew I was in a relationship and was exploring freezing embryos instead. I didn't want to deflect or dodge her question. So I explained about the breakup and moving out.

"Oh my God," Mandy said. "I'm so sorry."

My throat felt thick, as if the feelings I'd been trying to shove down for weeks were clawing to come out. "He was always so supportive of me possibly freezing my eggs," I heard myself say. Hearing Mandy talk about her relationship with Quincy reminded me of that. When their teaching program in China had ended, Mandy moved back to Los Angeles and Quincy back to Boston. They were in their early twenties. Did they want to move for each other? They broke up, then got back together, then broke up again. The cycle continued until they realized they kept coming back to each other for a reason. Quincy moved to the Bay Area and the two of them started fresh, beginning a committed relationship that led to their getting married.

I expected Mandy's next question, and sure enough, she asked it. "So, are you going to do it now? Freeze your eggs? Or are you still torn?"

I hesitated. "Well," I said, "I'm grateful I'm still relatively young. It's not weighing on me in that way quite so much. But in some ways I feel like I'm back at square one." The truth was, I had no idea how to think about egg freezing in personal terms anymore. With Ben no longer in the equation, my thoughts reverted to my sole ovary. It felt almost harder to decide yes or no because my ovary was fine—for now. But I didn't know for certain that I was fertile. No matter what doctors predicted for me, there'd be no certainty until I became or tried to become pregnant. And now that seemed further off than ever. "I don't want anything to happen to my ovary," I said. "But a part of me wishes that something would happen that would make the decision easier for me." Mandy nodded. She understood that, in a way most people couldn't.

Mandy had been forced to make a decision about egg freezing because of reproductive surgeries that had left her with partial ovaries. She'd decided to do it, but her next step, a consultation at a fertility clinic, had not exactly been comforting. A reproductive endocrinologist told her he agreed she should freeze her eggs, but that it wasn't very likely she'd be able to freeze a good number of them. *Don't get your hopes up,* he told her. One of her ovaries was virtually inactive, meaning it very likely wouldn't produce any eggs; the other one looked okay, but not great. The doctor predicted Mandy would freeze ten eggs at most. So she'd sped home and opened her laptop. *Chance of having a baby from ten frozen eggs,* she typed into Google. Then she remembered the doctor recommended she freeze embryos, since she and Quincy were married. *Chances of ten eggs becoming embryos,* she typed. The answers she found were all different, and dozens of clicked links and opened tabs later, Mandy felt dizzy. The ins and outs of embryo freezing and success rates were a lot to digest. She'd been keeping a list of questions to ask at her next appointment at the fertility clinic, and every day, it seemed, the list grew longer.

For Mandy, the egg freezing orientation had been one of the most difficult parts of the entire process. Injecting a cocktail of synthetic hormones, in particular, made her feel as if she was doing a science experiment. That she *was* a science experiment. She had gone alone; Quincy was working. A young nurse ran the training, showing Mandy and several couples how to prepare and inject the shots. The room was stuffy. Most of the couples held hands. A sense of sadness hung in the air; Mandy looked around and realized most people looked miserable. They looked older, too, and she felt a mix of sympathy and awkwardness, imagining they were there because they were having trouble conceiving and so were going through IVF. Mandy had felt so out of place. She wasn't even sure she wanted kids. What was she doing there, learning how to pump herself full of fertility drugs? Did she really want to be doing all this instead of just trying to get pregnant now? Quincy, who hated needles, still managed to administer all of Mandy's shots in the days leading up to her egg retrieval. He'd been stunned by how complicated it all was. She had watched hours of YouTube videos to make sure she understood how to unbox the thousands of dollars' worth of meds that arrived on her doorstep, check the inventory, and prepare the injections, carefully calculating how much liquid she needed for each shot.

"It was the longest month of my life," Mandy told me. She cried during every injection and never got used to the pain.* After the first few shots, she told her doctor they felt like torture. "Is that normal?" she asked. "Yeah, I've heard it stings," he replied. She returned to the internet and took comfort in online forums where other women shared about how much the injections hurt for them, too. Even Mandy's mother, who was thrilled that Mandy was taking action with regard to possibly having children someday, grew concerned during Mandy's several days of injections.

"We didn't know it was going to be like this," she told her daughter.

"Like what?" Mandy asked.

"Very . . . unnatural," her mother replied.

In darker moments, Mandy vacillated between wishing she would accidentally get pregnant and wishing she'd just discover she was infertile. She wanted to be free from worrying she was making the wrong decision—or would, or already had. An accidental pregnancy or infertility diagnosis would mean the decision had been made for her: She would accept the reality and that would be that. No more "figure out my fertility" as an item on her someday to-do list.

Finally, after all the visits to the clinic and the days of shots, it was time to harvest her eggs. Mandy's egg retrieval resulted in twenty eggs extracted from her ovaries, which were then fertilized with Quincy's sperm. They had successfully frozen eight embryos—which was a lot. The doctor told them that the chances of having one healthy child from their frozen embryos was extremely high.

Mandy accepted that being forced to consider her fertility at an early age meant always knowing that having biological children might not be possible for her. Most of her friends who knew they someday wanted children hadn't given their fertility much thought. Mandy, at least, felt somewhat mentally prepared. The cyst her doctors had dis-

---

* Icing the area before can make the shots more bearable; ice globe roller balls, the kind some people use to depuff their eye areas, work well.

covered that changed everything for her now felt like a blessing in disguise. Even so, despite having a medical reason for freezing, Mandy never really felt solid about her decision. *Shouldn't we just get pregnant now?* a voice in her head kept murmuring. But she and Quincy hadn't felt ready to be parents. It wasn't until the day she got the final results that the voice quieted down.

With the experience behind her, Mandy focused her thoughts on what it had all led to: her and Quincy's eight embryos on ice and the peace of mind that gave her. "It was really hard, and really expensive," she tells her friends when they ask. "And it's going to be more involved than you think. But I'm really glad I did it." Going back to regular life felt strange at first. For a while, it had felt as if fertility was all Mandy thought about. *Just freezing my eggs* had unexpectedly turned into months of contemplating motherhood and starting a family with her partner. Unaccustomed to dwelling on the future, she used to cringe when the subject of having kids was brought up. All those years she spent actively protecting *against* pregnancy meant that almost by default she had put off all thoughts of possible parenthood. But all that shifted while she was going through the many steps of egg freezing. She began to imagine what it would be like to have a family, how many kids she and Quincy might have, what he'd be like as a dad. Getting pregnant had, for so long, been the worst thing that could happen. Egg freezing changed all that. Having frozen embryos made motherhood seem more manageable; now, she felt she had more of a choice of when it would happen.

And if it didn't? She'd at least know she had done everything she could.

Our ovary sagas brushed up against each other in small but striking ways. It was almost as if where mine left off Mandy's began, and where mine lulled hers returned. We both had had two surgeries for ovarian cysts eight years apart: mine at ages twelve and twenty, Mandy's at twenty and twenty-eight. We both had fewer than the normal two healthy ovaries most women have, and before we met each other we'd never known someone with an ovary situation like ours. We both grew paranoid anytime we felt cramps or a sharp pain in our lower abdomens, thinking it was an ovary dangerously twisting on itself again.

I saw myself in Mandy's experience: her fragile ovaries and history of painful operations, the confused guilt she felt about the cyst that threatened her fertility, the ache in her voice when she said, "I should have known better. How did I let this happen again?" I empathized with how, for so long, she'd had low expectations about her ovaries' capabilities. Did they work? Would they one day help her conceive? She had harbored little hope over the years. Mandy was the sort of person who thought twice about a lot of things and often felt anxious about the future, quick to spiral into a thick fog of *what if* and *what then*. I understood this deeply. My doctors had painted a rosier picture for my one ovary, but no matter what any doctor ever said, I always wondered—and always knew the wondering would stop only if and when I became pregnant. For Mandy, freezing her eggs turned the wondering down to a low hum. I envied her that.

As we sat in the fading light of her kitchen, I realized I had been subconsciously hoping Mandy's journey would inform my decision. This truth had been simmering inside me for a while, and in that moment it welled up like a confession: A part of me wanted to let Mandy and the other women I had spent hours talking with over the past many months make my egg freezing choice for me. I had done my homework, but they had done the actual thing itself. I had uncovered some answers—some illuminating, others inconvenient—but they had *decided,* they had *experienced* it, and what truths, what answers, are more powerful than that? I could make my egg freezing experience look like theirs, couldn't I?

As I was getting ready to leave, Mandy repeated in almost an off-hand way a comment one of her doctors had made at one of her early egg freezing appointments: "Ovaries are really resilient, you know."

Heartbreak, Hormone Shots, and a Change of Plans

My last night in California, I holed up in the basement of a friend's apartment in Oakland. My half-open suitcase sat wedged between two large racks of Burning Man garb. During the week's meetings and interviews, I had compartmentalized my grief, cosplaying a put-together reporter instead of being a person with no idea how to start over.

My decision to freeze my eggs no longer felt sturdy. I wanted to Velcro myself to the facts. I was a reporter; facts were the bricks of gold paving the path to Knowing, to the Right Decision. I was nearing thirty and fresh out of a breakup. Egg freezing made more sense now than ever, at least on paper. But I still had questions about the fertility drugs and about the fact that I was a "cyst-former" with a history of my body overreacting to just natural hormones. The journalist in me had concluded that egg freezing was a striking, if presently overhyped, technology with powerful potential—but I wasn't sure I could live with the risks. As for the woman in me: My research into freezing eggs versus embryos, plus my recent visit with Mandy and hearing about her frozen embryos, had me close to convinced that freezing embryos was smarter than freezing just eggs. But now Ben—and his sperm—were gone.

I lay back on the bed, feeling weary. I closed my eyes and pictured going through with it by myself, injecting drugs into my abdomen late at night until the skin came to resemble a dartboard. It was getting more and more difficult to imagine putting myself through the hormone shots unless a doctor told me I was infertile and couldn't get pregnant without them. Harder to admit was that for now, at least, it was difficult to imagine going through any major life event without Ben.

As more time passed, I realized that I had been using my relationship with Ben to distract myself from actually making a choice. In both cases, to some degree, I'd been hedging, brushing aside many of the doubts and hard questions. I worried that I'd wanted things with Ben to work out so badly that I had lost the ability to tell if I was still happy. Now it sometimes seemed I'd begun looking at egg freezing with the same rose-colored glasses. As if the more I wanted it to be right for me, the less able I was to tell if it was a smart choice. But whether or not to freeze my eggs had been my decision to make before I met Ben, and it was mine to recommit to now that I was once again single. It was—still—just me and my ovary. That thought used to bring me comfort; now it made me feel profoundly alone.

I had wanted a straight line to what had felt like the right decision: to freeze my eggs. I *wanted* to be sold on egg freezing. I longed for the wave of relief I had been assured it would bring me if I went through with it. I'd already been counting on how sensible it was for me, the woman who'd always been certain about having biological children, the woman with one ovary who knew she wanted kids later but not now. Instead, on top of my achy heart, I was angry about how ending my relationship with Ben had thrown a wrench into my egg freezing plans. I worried Dr. Noyes had been right all along: The problem was that I knew too much. And that made it nearly impossible to stop vacillating, stop researching, stop chasing more data. Mostly I was afraid that I had no idea about anything anymore: where to live, how to write and do my job, how to move on.

"Freezing my eggs seemed like the best decision I could make with the information I had at the time," writes Sarah Elizabeth Richards, who spent $50,000 on several rounds of egg freezing more than fifteen years ago, in her memoir *Motherhood, Rescheduled.* Money aside— I'd never spent so much on anything—her statement made complete sense to me. But, unable to distinguish what I knew, or couldn't know, about the drugs' risks and shaky success rates from how I felt, which was lost and heartbroken, I had arrived at a fraught in-between place with egg freezing: I was afraid to do it and afraid to not do it.

I didn't know where to begin with confronting all this personal fear. I could, however, continue to channel my reporter energy in pursuit of more balanced answers and perspectives. Dr. Noyes was wrong, I decided: I didn't know too much. Not yet, at least. To recommit to freezing my eggs, I concluded, I needed to reassure myself I could live with the risks attached to the hormone injections—risks to my ovary as well as to my long-term health. And I wanted to learn more about the powerful peace of mind that Mandy, and many other egg freezers I'd interviewed, had gushed about.

That night, I fell asleep with Mandy's words echoing in my head: *Ovaries are resilient.*

Fertility-Industrial Complex

~~~~~~

The Lovely Louise

It was just after eight on a Monday at the convention center in San Antonio, Texas, the site of the American Society of Reproductive Medicine's annual meeting. Every year, the ASRM—the governing body that oversees most reproductive medicine and technology in the United States—holds a large conference for the industry's doctors and researchers. I wanted to see the world of fertility technology in action and put faces to names of the physicians at the forefront. So I reached out to the ASRM press office and obtained a media pass for the four-day event. Then I packed a bag and flew to Texas.

I stood there in the convention center, marveling at how huge it was. Thousands of fertility experts attend ASRM each year, with nearly one-third of them coming from outside the United States. The large hall echoed with the *click-clack* of women's heels and deep male voices. I shuffled around in a black dress and shoes that gave me blisters, getting the lay of the land before I made my way to one of the ballrooms for the conference's opening plenary. It was going to be a long day, and I was glad; being back in Texas just a couple of months after leaving Houston and Ben was painful, a dull ache and sharp sting all at once. The buzz of the conference, I hoped, would take the edge off.

"It is every woman's right to decide when, how, and with whom she wants to have a baby," ASRM's president at the time, Dr. Richard Paulson, said in the opening keynote address. He looked a lot like Tom Selleck. "This includes the ability to access not only family planning services, but also fertility promoting services."

That evening, I attended a talk titled "Louise Brown: My Life as the World's First Test Tube Baby." Louise, I knew, was the poster child for IVF and assisted reproductive technology. She was conceived in a petri dish—not a test tube, although the "world's first test-tube baby" moniker has stuck—and with her birth, the idea of making embryos outside of a woman's body became a reality. Louise Joy Brown came screaming into the world at five pounds twelve ounces on July 25, 1978, at Oldham General Hospital in England. When I learned that this year marked the fortieth anniversary of IVF and that Louise, the world's first IVF baby, would be speaking at ASRM's annual conference, I reached out to inquire about interviewing Louise in Texas. Her team said yes.

As I sat in the audience that evening, a huge telephoto camera was making *click click click* noises over my left shoulder. Rows of doctors held up their cellphones to take photos of Louise, seated in a chair on the stage next to Dr. Paulson. She wore glasses with square, slim frames. Her gray-blond curls shone with texture under the harsh stage lights. "None of us would be here without the lovely Louise," said Dr. Paulson. He beamed at her as they talked. The entire audience seemed to be beaming. I had read a lot about Louise and knew how significant her birth was within the field of reproductive medicine and beyond. Her birth had been an incredible breakthrough: Life could be created outside the body. But it wasn't until that evening that I realized how much of a legend and a celebrity she was to fertility doctors across the globe.

In ART's early days, embryos created through IVF were transferred to the uterus right away. This is how Louise, the first baby in the world made from fresh eggs, was born. Back then, IVF success rates were low; transferred embryos didn't often successfully implant in the uterine wall. IVF was originally intended to help a specific demographic—young married women—who were struggling to conceive. Louise's mother, Lesley Brown, had been unable to con-

ceive naturally because of a blockage in her fallopian tubes. IVF had
been designed to solve medical problems like hers.

Louise read to the audience from her memoir. Dozens of doctors
lined up to take a selfie with her. I'd read that some say her birth was
more monumental than a man landing on the moon. That struck me
as a bit outlandish until I remembered that since Louise's birth in
1978, millions of babies around the world have been born as a result
of ART—children who otherwise would not exist. After Louise's
birth, it took doctors six more years to perfect the freezing and un-
freezing technique. In 1984, the first baby from a frozen embryo was
born, in Australia; the embryo had been frozen for two months, quite
a brief period of time compared to how long embryos stay on ice
now. In 2022, healthy twins were born to a Portland, Oregon, couple
from donated embryos that had been frozen for thirty years—likely
the longest-frozen embryos to ever result in a successful live birth.

Revolutionary, indeed.

The next day, I arrived at the convention center early for my meeting with Louise. I sat on the floor in a side hallway and installed fresh
batteries in my recorder. Louise had given hundreds of interviews
over the years, and I knew there was probably very little I might ask
her that she wouldn't have been asked before. Still, I was excited to
meet ART's poster child one-on-one. Half an hour later, we sat in a
drafty room in a quiet section of the convention center. Louise wore
a white ruffled top with pastel hummingbirds, her gray-blond hair
loose. We started talking, and I forgot all about the questions for her
I'd written down. At some point I broached the topic of puberty and
asked her when she had first become aware of her body and self as a
young woman. I couldn't have been more delighted by her response.
"That's one I've never been asked before!" Louise laughed, before
launching into a story of menses-meets-fish-and-chips. "It was a Friday. I can't even remember what age I was, but on Friday evenings
we'd always have fish and chips," she said. But she felt too sick to eat
it. "My God, it's happened," she recalled thinking when she realized
it was her period. How did getting her period feel? I asked. "It put
me off my tea, put it that way."

As we joked and chatted, I thought about how, well, *normal* Louise was. After all I had read about her and her influential birth, I'd half-expected the first-ever miracle of reproductive medicine to present as the celebrity she was to fertility doctors and infertility patients across the globe. But she struck me as your average middle-aged woman. And that was maybe the point. Assisted reproductive technologies such as IVF symbolize an unconventional road that leads—some of the time—to a conventional end. Louise, now in her forties, lives in England with her husband and their children. She's had a few jobs over the years, from nursery nurse to postal worker to freight forwarder. She likes to sing karaoke—Madonna songs, mostly, and sometimes "Total Eclipse of the Heart." At eighteen she had her belly button pierced, and at twenty-one her tongue. At one point during our conversation she started talking about her tattoos and, one by one, showed them to me: a purple butterfly on her ankle; a Muppet in honor of her half sister who'd passed away; a rose and a heart with "Mum" and "Dad" written in; Tweety, from the Looney Tunes cartoons; Chinese characters that she'd forgotten the meaning of. She's also the mother of two boys. She and her husband conceived children naturally; she's never needed IVF.

"I'm pretty boring, really," said Louise, grinning. "Well, apart from how I was conceived and born." She said she'd grown used to being hounded by journalists and almost never answered her cellphone if she didn't recognize the caller. Her entire life, she's had to be careful about what she says in public. "As a teenager, I used to think, 'Why me?'" she said, explaining that she was at once proud to be the world's first IVF baby and eager to assert herself as normal. "Now I'm quite proud of it."

Money, Marketing, and Medicine: A Perfect Storm

On the third day of the conference, I braved the convention center's Expo Hall, a sprawling high-ceilinged space, map in hand. I walked around in a slightly stunned daze. At one end of the hall, a giant sperm poised to fertilize an ovum, which was the size of a small

weather balloon, rotated above a booth promoting egg banking services. An enormous mobile composed of more sperm and eggs—this
time wearing eerie human faces—grinned down from the rafters.
When I found the restroom, I noticed posters for injections and devices plastered to the mirrors above the sinks.

Big banners and flashy signs announced the Expo Hall's different
booths. At first, I couldn't tell which were the names of pharmaceutical companies, or procedures, or something else. Good Start Genetics. Celmatix. Fairfax Egg Bank. Fertility Drug Calculator. Center
for Drug Evaluation and Research. Even Panasonic had a booth.
There was fresh popcorn, just like there was at that first egg freezing
event I attended years earlier in Manhattan. Another booth was
handing out stress balls with unmissable squiggly tails, while attendees crowded around an arcade game for the chance to win T-shirts
stashed inside—what else?—golden eggs. I wandered the maze, nib-
bling on popcorn and marveling at all the gimmicky gametes on
display. I paused next to something called the Simulation Pavilion,
where physicians could observe various virtual-reality procedures
simulating things like embryo transfers. At Prelude's booth, I picked
up mint-green paper cardboard squares with messages like LET'S TALK
ABOUT SEX in huge dark letters and, in a smaller font, AND THE ALTER-
NATIVES YOU HAVE IF IT DOESN'T GET YOU PREGNANT. A poster advertised a conference session titled "Fertility Preservation Patients: How
to Re-engineer Your Practice to Accommodate Them." It was being
conducted not by a physician with an MD but by someone with
an MBA.

Today, there are some five hundred fertility clinics scattered across the
United States—employing more than fifteen hundred reproductive
endocrinologists and seeing hundreds of thousands of patients per
year—all competing for business. Private equity companies are pouring money into the for-profit fertility industry, a trend in line with
what's been happening a lot in medicine since the 1990s. The ART
industry in the United States has two things investors like most: scale

and growth. Fertility clinics are very profitable and have high margins.* Many have doubled down on practicing and promoting egg freezing, with specialized egg freezing start-ups in particular receiving hundreds of millions of dollars of venture capital and private equity. Writing about the financialization of fertility in her book *Freezing Fertility,* sociologist Lucy van de Wiel, whose research focuses on reproductive technologies, says: "These investments materialize the promise of egg freezing as a growth technology that may increasingly be targeted at a wide group of younger, fertile women, who may or may not want to have children in the future—a far greater segment of the population than those currently accessing IVF."

As I stood in the Expo Hall, I realized I was witnessing a perfect storm: the confluence of ticking biological clocks, investor money, and a shaky foundation of reliable basics. I thought about Kindbody and Prelude, companies that want to be global brands, one-stop solutions for all things fertility-related. NYU Langone Fertility Center, where I'd had my first few egg freezing appointments, was now a Prelude Network clinic. Kindbody doubled its already massive footprint when, in 2022, it acquired Vios Fertility Institute, a large fertility network with several clinics throughout the Midwest. It also has its own genetic testing division, called Kindlabs, as well as its own gestational carrier agency and egg and embryo donor program. By bringing these major and typically outsourced ART services in-house, Kindbody was—and this is an impressive feat—well on its way to achieving its goal of delivering end-to-end care to fertility patients. Which, if you squint, resembles an empire.

And my former fertility doctor, Dr. Noyes, one of egg freezing's early and best-known pioneers and who had co-founded NYU's egg freezing program, was now at Kindbody. One of the most senior and experienced reproductive endocrinologists in the business now worked at an egg freezing start-up—one with a minimal track record

---

* The hefty profits are in part because many patients pay for treatment out of pocket. So clinics often receive cash directly, rather than seeking reimbursement from health insurance companies, which tend to negotiate down the costs of services.

and little data on pregnancy success rates.* A *New Yorker* article about new fertility entrepreneurs explains that Dr. Noyes "credits private equity and venture-backed firms with spreading the word about egg freezing and other fertility care, both in the media and in the employer market," where company-sponsored egg freezing remains on the rise. But when the profit model is "volume-driven," she said, "it's like driving a car faster and faster. Okay, you're going ten, you can go twenty, you can go thirty, you can go forty—but when is it not safe?"

Meanwhile, the market continues to soar, backed by millions of dollars in capital, creating an endless feedback loop between egg freezing and young consumers. The more money invested, the more marketing dollars are thrown at selling women on the procedure. The public, though, isn't aware of these financial machinations—mostly because no one involved wants to talk about them. During my reporting trip to California, I'd asked Marcy Darnovsky, executive director of the Center for Genetics and Society, about this when we met at her Berkeley office. "Because we're so queasy about talking about babies and commerce in the same breath, the commercial dynamics that are often at play escape our notice," she'd said. "We're putting young women at unnecessary risk. A combination of the marketing persuasion on the part of these companies and cultural and social pressures make women afraid they're going to be infertile." So, fear, in part, fuels the business of egg freezing. Another issue, to state the obvious, is misinformation. Studies in the United States, United Kingdom, and Australia have shown that fertility clinic websites tend to be more persuasive, rather than informative, in their language, emphasizing the benefits of egg freezing while minimizing the risks and costs. Some clinics even fudge the numbers somewhat when it comes to describing the success rates of their procedures.

* When I asked Kindbody about this in April 2022, a spokeswoman for the company relayed: "We've had ten oocyte thaw cycles from eggs that were frozen at Kindbody. Only one patient has had a transfer as of now and she is pregnant." (When I reached out in October 2023 for an update, the company's response was that the ten oocyte thaw cycles was the most current figure they could offer.) This doesn't mean that Kindbody, or any newer clinic, is less adept at freezing eggs, necessarily; it just means they don't yet have the pregnancy rates from women who've frozen eggs with them to point to as a proven measure of success.

Ours is a capitalist society; money is a driving force behind so many decisions. The fact that women are patients but also customers is an uncomfortable notion, even if it's the reality of capitalism. They are being sold to, and many believe they're investing in a procedure that guarantees a future baby. And the people doing the selling are savvy salespeople. I know this firsthand: Before I ever seriously discussed egg freezing with a doctor, I learned about it from a company eager for my business. It was so easy to drink the Kool-Aid at the fancy egg freezing cocktail parties I attended—marketing events focused on the importance of persevering fertility while women like me are still in our "prime." And it's still easy. Egg freezing is now spoken about less like a medical advancement and more like a new tech product. It's even being marketed as a form of self-care.*

Given the number of women who may never need to use their frozen eggs, fertility clinics and egg freezing companies are profiting hugely off of women who freeze eggs, while also—depending on how one assesses the paltry data—putting them at risk for future cancers. Arthur Caplan, the NYU bioethicist, argues that market forces are distorting our ideas about fertility in troubling ways. "The consumer doesn't know what's going on, and the provider has every reason to sell it to you and make a lot of money," he told me. "It's not a good market—the consumer is disadvantaged and often desperate to do something. And there doesn't seem to be any inclination to regulate any of this." He's right, and we'll unpack that shortly. The bigger, unsettling point here is that the lack of consensus on how ART is regulated in the United States means we've by default agreed to let the market drive how such technologies are used and who can access them. But a uterus isn't Uber. Letting the market decide—instead of, say, well-studied public policy considerations—is not the best way to make a fundamental shift in our species' procreative habits. And on a more personal level, it's harder for women to make decisions about their bodies when they are not thoroughly counseled—about the ac-

---

* One ironic example of this: Last Valentine's Day, I received an email from a prominent national chain of fertility clinics with a discount code for 20 percent off an egg freezing cycle. The subject line read: "Here's a special gift in honor of self-love."

tual need for the eggs they freeze or the actual success rates, both of which are difficult to quantify for a given woman—and when the doctor-patient relationship is too easily influenced by a profit motive. A large portion of fertility doctors' bonuses are directly tied to metrics like patient conversion rate—how many consultations they were able to convert into treatment. "[Fertility companies] want customers, and they'll advertise accordingly. But that's not necessarily appropriate for a sensitive medical area like infertility," said Caplan. "They make me nervous."

A very profitable marketplace has shaped up to provide egg freezing, even though there is no guarantee of success down the road. Demand is high and competition between clinics is fierce. The marketing drives women to the newer clinics, which offer a more inclusive and feel-good patient experience and tend to charge less for freezing eggs, but lack solid track records in thawing them. This should be a red flag to a woman considering fertility preservation, in my opinion, but it's tough to care about cost and quality equally; a lower price tag often trumps an established reputation. Several reproductive endocrinologists I spoke with worried that these rapidly expanding, egg-freezing-focused clinics—which face increased pressure to generate revenue—also don't have enough physicians with the necessary experience to perform the delicate procedure well and, in some cases, have implemented cost-cutting measures that affect lab quality as well as patient care.*

Their concerns, it seems, are valid. A major story about Kindbody published in *Bloomberg* in October 2023 found that, "Beneath the firm's Instagrammable aesthetic lies a bonus-driven business model, a number of understaffed clinics, and instances of inconsistent safety protocols that have plagued some operations and contributed to errors," according to three dozen current and former employees and patients. The article described how the company's efforts to make fertility treatment more accessible and offer services at lower price

---

* I was reminded of one of the reasons why ASRM was so reluctant to remove egg freezing's experimental label a decade ago—that it's quite challenging to freeze an egg.

points than its competitors led to difficulties running its labs at the level needed to safely handle eggs and embryos. "Kindbody's challenges underscore the risks facing an industry that, on one hand, focuses on expensive, painstakingly precise biological procedures while at the same time pursuing a growth path funded by investors intent on an eventual return on their money," the article said. One of the more harrowing incidents described was a flood at Kindbody's Santa Monica clinic that affected lab operations.* Since 2022, at least four of the company's senior lab directors have quit, more errors have started surfacing, and some of Kindbody's clinics are losing money.

The idea of women freezing their eggs no longer seems futile or dangerous, yet in truth a lot of the enthusiasm around the procedure is still premature. The marketing is ahead of the reality, and in some cases it's just plain deceptive, like calling egg freezing an insurance policy—which I'd like to say a final word about, in an effort to put this all-too-common comparison to rest. A 2020 *Fertility and Sterility* study stated plainly: "Data suggest that to virtually guarantee one live birth (97 percent likelihood), a woman would need to freeze about forty oocytes." That would require about three or four cycles, which is both incredibly expensive and would necessitate a *lot* of fertility drugs. The paper continues: "If a woman younger than 35 years were to undergo one cycle and retrieve an average number of mature oocytes, she would have a 75 to 80 percent chance at one live birth. Although these odds are relatively favorable, they do not provide the kind of guarantee that the word 'insurance' brings to mind."

The fact remains that egg freezing is still a technologically advanced process riddled with risks. And yet, even though more data on the risks and success rates has been slow to emerge, and concerns about the aggressive sales culture and operations at some of the glitzy, newer fertility clinics seem to be well-founded, the medical community—especially the thousands of fertility doctors at this conference—acts as confident as ever.

---

* Kindbody told *Bloomberg* that it reports, investigates, and takes corrective action if incidents occur, including in each example the article detailed.

. . .

I left the convention center around eight in the evening. A long day. I walked on faux-cobblestone streets to the Tower of the Americas, the sounds of late summer in Texas washing over me: chirping crickets, a large fountain, big cars starting in a nearby parking lot, children still outdoors playing. I looked up at the lights on the tower and remembered hearing that the observation deck was closed for a private cocktail hour hosted by Progyny. I recalled something a man from a digital marketing company had told me after a session earlier that day: "If you knew how hard these doctors partied at conferences like this, you'd never want them doing things to your ovaries." He was half-joking, but the underlying bit of truth pointed to the confluence of forces—money, medicine, marketing, motherhood—at play here. And it worried me.

Plot Twists and Tangled Webs

One evening, a month after the ASRM conference, I received an email from my cousin Bridget, who was living in Washington, D.C. Subject line: "Some bummer news." Breast cancer. She'd just found out. There was no history of it in our family. She was twenty-nine years old.

She'd discovered a lump, had a biopsy, and was diagnosed with an aggressive form of breast cancer, stage III. She would undergo chemotherapy, have surgeries, and dutifully do as her doctors said. She might also freeze eggs or embryos—she and her husband, Chris, newly married, wanted children. That's in part why she wrote to me, to ask about egg freezing and urgent fertility preservation. Her email concluded: "Please make a calendar reminder to do a monthly self-exam."

Then, an excruciating plot twist: Bridget was pregnant. When she went in for the biopsy, there were signs all over blaring TELL YOUR DOCTOR IF YOU'RE PREGNANT. She and Chris had recently started trying, and she hadn't gotten her period that month—she was expecting it later that week—so she informed the doctor doing the biopsy she might be pregnant. The doctor called the next day to tell Bridget she had cancer, and then said, "You really don't want to be pregnant right now." Bridget took three at-home pregnancy tests—all immediately positive—then confirmed it with a test at her OB/GYN's office. That night, after she hosted her book club—the shock propelled her into a discombobulating autopilot mode—she and Chris googled "pregnancy + cancer treatment" and cried. Theirs was a pregnancy that was planned and very much wanted.

I closed my computer screen. Elbows on desk. Head in hands. I was in upstate New York, about halfway through a ten-week writing residency. Most days, I wrote in the mornings, sifted through research and reporting in the afternoons, and spent the evenings trying not to think about Ben. My belongings were in Colorado, part of my heart was still in Houston, and every day I wrestled with concentrating on my work. The residency was an incredible opportunity, one I didn't want to squander with the nagging anxiety I felt about returning west to live with my parents until I figured out my next move. But all that felt trivial compared to what Bridget was going through: learning that she had breast cancer and that she was pregnant on the same day. Forty-eight hours after being diagnosed, Bridget was thinking not about her body but about her future babies. Babies she had always been sure she'd have. Cancer means chemotherapy and chemo threatens fertility. We take it for granted, all of it, until one day there's a lump and a biopsy and suddenly you are a recently married woman on the cusp of thirty, with a job you love and a cat named Nancy Drew and a pregnancy you're longing for, and cancer growing in your chest.

After getting the okay from Bridget, I called my mother and told her about Bridget's diagnosis. We talked about breast exams and how radiation can damage ovaries and scar the uterus. I felt a newfound personal appreciation for ART and the scientific capability that existed and that would, I so deeply hoped, preserve my cousin's fertility, her ability to have biological children, the family she had always wanted.

Bridget's oncologist recommended she start chemotherapy as soon as possible; triple-negative breast cancer grows fast. Bridget and Chris met with a surgeon, who explained that options for breast cancer treatment in the first trimester are limited. If Bridget's health was the top priority, she couldn't be pregnant when she started chemo. Then they visited a reputable fertility center and learned Bridget couldn't start the process of an egg retrieval until at least six weeks after ending a pregnancy, because it would take time for the pregnancy hormones still in her body to normalize. She and Chris made the devastating decision to terminate the pregnancy, and a week before starting chemotherapy, she had a D&C.*

Ultimately, Bridget wasn't able to harvest eggs from her ovaries before starting chemotherapy. Her tumor had already grown quickly; there wasn't time to delay treatment for several weeks. The awful irony is that if she hadn't been pregnant, she most likely would have been able to do an egg retrieval. But needing chemo right away meant she couldn't safely stay pregnant, and terminating the pregnancy meant she didn't have time to undergo fertility preservation before starting treatment.

A month after starting chemotherapy, Bridget's genetic testing results came back: She was BRCA1 positive, which made her more susceptible to getting certain types of cancer. Our family later learned that Bridget's father—my mother's brother—also had the gene mutation. He'd never had cancer, and neither had his siblings, but he urged them to get tested. The child of a parent with the BRCA1 mutation has a 50 percent chance of inheriting the variant, and having a mutated BRCA gene greatly increases a woman's chance of developing breast and ovarian cancer and a man's chance of developing prostate and male breast cancer. Our family was worried: If my mother tested positive for BRCA1, it would mean my siblings and I each had a 50 percent chance of having inherited the mutation, too, as Bridget had.

During those long weeks of waiting and worrying, I did another

---

* A dilation and curettage, a procedure to remove tissue from inside the uterus, is one method of ending a pregnancy.

egg freezing one-eighty. There was no question that I would freeze my eggs as quickly as possible if I learned I was BRCA1 positive. I was so relieved when my mother learned she didn't have the mutation. But the waves that Bridget's cancer sent reverberating through our family—the females, in particular—lingered, and in my case they forced me to think anew about egg freezing in the face of yet another potential threat to my fertility. Life went on, but a new realization crystallized: Fertility-related decisions do not exist in a vacuum. The journey to figure out and make decisions about my fertility was, it turns out, inextricably tied up with my love life, career, physical and mental health—areas of my life that, often despite my best intentions, cannot be neatly compartmentalized.

I remembered something Lesley, the nurse who was diagnosed with breast cancer not long after freezing her eggs, told me: how she wished she had dedicated more time to understanding the procedure in detail. "I didn't have any questions," she told me, "so I just went for it." But, barring an urgent medical need like Bridget's, egg freezing isn't always an easy or simple decision. That, at least, I now knew with certainty. I also understood that most potential egg freezers had neither the time nor the desire to spend months or years studying the nuances and underlying questions. For better or for worse, though, that's what I'd decided to do, and by now I had researched the whole process long enough to go well beyond its shiny surface. At the core of my analysis paralysis was the realization that the decision to freeze was wrapped up in a tangled web: motherhood, marketing, medicine, money, and, now, even mortality. I couldn't know what might happen in the future. Cancer. Infertility. More romantic disappointments. A career that sputtered and fizzled out. Never feeling financially secure. But I knew I wanted to have a say about a lot of it. I wanted to control what I could.

Great Eggspectations

~~~~~~

Remy: A Sleepless Night and Seventeen Eggs

At five-thirty the morning of her egg retrieval, Remy pulled into her driveway. It was Monday, close to thirty-six hours after she'd taken the trigger shot. She was coming off an overnight shift at the hospital and had been awake for almost an entire day. She needed to be at the fertility center in an hour. She threw the Tupperware from her night shift dinner in the dishwasher, fed Sophie the cat, and gazed longingly at her Peloton, which she hadn't been able to use for several days. She couldn't recall the last time she'd neglected her exercise bike for this long.

In the bathroom, Remy shed her scrubs and showered, rinsing off her shift. She remembered to remove her belly button ring but forgot to wash her hair. She dressed in clothes easy to pull off and on: leggings, a loose denim button-down shirt, the brown boots she wore when she wasn't at the hospital. She pushed her long blond hair out of her face, yawning. On a table off the kitchen sat boxes of leftover meds surrounded by crystals. Glancing at the table while she changed Sophie's litter box, she felt relieved there'd be no more shots.

She pulled out her phone to call an Uber. The clinic's instructions were clear: She wasn't allowed to drive herself home from the egg retrieval, and a responsible driver had to pick her up. The clinic wanted to know ahead of time who this person would be. This had been the only hiccup so far; with no family nearby and most of her friends working at the hospital, she didn't have someone to ask to accompany her to the retrieval and wait until it was over to drive her home. It was the only part of the egg freezing process impossible to do alone. Remy could've done all the injections herself if she'd had to, though she was glad she'd had Leah's help for the trigger shot. She'd gone to all the appointments solo. She was doing this on her own, freezing her eggs for her future self. But the responsible driver requirement, at the very end of the whole ordeal, dampened her spirits a bit.

Her phone buzzed. She gasped. The driver was eighteen minutes away. "This is not going to work," she groaned, then checked her phone again. "Come on, dude." Prickles of anxiety fluttered in her stomach. This was why she didn't like relying on people. She checked her watch. Then she canceled the Uber, grabbed her purse and car keys, and flew out the door.

It was a cool morning and the streets were quiet. In the car, she plugged her phone in and balanced the sheet of paper with driving and parking instructions on her lap. The sky was dark blue, the sun just beginning to come up. She raced through yellow lights. Braking hard for a red, she winced: Her breasts felt huge, and slamming on the brakes hurt. For days, she'd felt like she'd been swimming in estrogen. She'd experienced some mittelschmerz on her left side while on call the day before; she grimaced a bit at the thought of a long needle going into her vagina today. A wave of tiredness came over her. Fatigue felt different to her now; she realized she'd been masking it with coffee for years. Learning she could survive a twenty-four-hour shift at the hospital without coffee was a nice side benefit of all this. Remy held the steering wheel with one hand, her phone and the crumpled paper directions in the other. She'd followed the instructions the clinic had provided her carefully: nothing to eat or drink after midnight the night before; arrive at the clinic an hour before her scheduled procedure time; park in the indicated garage.

Inside the building, Remy was momentarily confused by the signs on the doors. She sighed, recalling how it'd never been easy to remember all the different names of the offices, labs, and companies involved in her egg freezing process.* She found the door for Ovation Fertility Nashville, greeted the receptionist, and followed a nurse into a small room with bland tan walls and closed blinds. She slipped off her tall brown boots and changed into a teal hospital gown. She tied it expertly, thinking about how strange it felt to be the patient today. Her legs and bare feet dangled from the end of the exam table. She shivered, then pulled on the thick blue socks she'd been told she might want to wear during the procedure. She sat and waited. Now that she was there, the stress of the morning behind her, she wanted to get it over with.

A nurse came in to take her vitals. "Tell me you haven't been googling 'egg retrievals' and reading what all the crazy people on the internet say about it."

"I haven't," said Remy.

"Good girl!" the nurse replied. "People come in scared to death about the crap they read online." She went over the post-op basics and explained that Remy would still be at risk for ovarian torsion for several days, until all the swelling went away. When the nurse got to explaining how Remy might feel later in the day after the anesthesia wore off, Remy nodded, as if she weren't already an expert on anesthesia and its possible side effects.

The nurse left. Remy reached for her phone to check her texts and send a quick message to her parents. A few minutes later, Dr. Lewis knocked and opened the door. Gray scrubs, same glasses and blond straightened hair. Remy put down her phone and sat up straighter on the table. "Hi!" she said brightly, relief in her voice. She trusted Dr. Lewis and always felt better in her presence.

"Alrighty," said Dr. Lewis. "Here we go—you ready?"

"Ready," Remy replied. "But it's so weird being on the other side of all this."

The reason I can tell you all this word for word is not because Remy remembers it all so clearly—which she doesn't; she was ner-

---

* Remy did her initial egg freezing appointments at a different center and location than the clinic where she underwent her egg retrieval.

vous, and the anesthesia meant she didn't remember much once it was all over—but because I was with her during every part except for the retrieval itself, during which I sat in the waiting room. When Remy's retrieval was over—it lasted thirty minutes—a nurse led me back to Remy's room. I opened the door and Remy looked over at me from her gurney, where she was waking up. I crossed the room to talk to her. "Thank you, Natalie," she said groggily, reaching for my hand and squeezing it. She was crying, tears streaming down her temples. "It really means a lot that you're here."

"Thank you for letting me be here," I said, looking down at our hands. It was a powerful moment, the slow-motion kind that you realize as it's happening you likely won't ever forget. I looked at Remy and didn't know which part of me was doing the looking: the journalist, the potential egg freezer, the woman. "I'm so happy," Remy murmured groggily. "Relief. I feel such relief." Her voice was raspy and low, thick with emotion. "I really want to know how many eggs I got. How many do you think? A lot. I hope it's a lot." She closed her eyes and sank back into the pillow, pulling the blanket up to her chin.

Several minutes later, the embryologist came in and introduced herself. When she told Remy seventeen eggs had been extracted, Remy gasped. "Awesome." Remy was instructed to call a phone number, a voice mailbox, later in the day to find out how many of her retrieved eggs were in suitable condition to be frozen. When the embryologist left, a nurse popped her head into the room. "Ready to try to pee?" Afterward, she gave Remy more sheets of paper. Discharge instructions, prescriptions, more phone numbers. Then she was cleared to go home.

Remy had asked Rachel, a fellow anesthesia resident, to drive her home after the retrieval. She knew Rachel had been on call all night and might not be able to. But then Rachel, who was nursing her second kid, texted: *On my way! Sorry if you get flashed. I'm pumping and have no shame . . . The valet guys might be concerned.* Remy hated having to bother a colleague, especially one coming off a long overnight shift. She was tempted to break the rules and drive herself home; her car was already in the clinic's parking garage, after all. But Rachel insisted. Two young doctors, very little sleep between them; one lactating, one post–egg harvest. In the car, Remy talked excitedly, telling Rachel about the morning and getting lots of eggs. They stopped at a gas station so Remy could get Gatorade, though what she really wanted was a smoked rosemary latte. Also, a long nap. She took a deep breath and let her shoulders sink back against the passenger seat. Except for the logistics stress and last-minute change of transportation plans the morning of her retrieval, her egg freezing process couldn't have gone more smoothly.

Relief: palpable, overwhelming relief. Remy had felt only nervous anticipation in the days leading up to the retrieval, but as soon as she woke up from the procedure, it rolled over her in a euphoric wave. Of the many emotions she felt today, in the days and months to come it would be this feeling of relief she'd remember most.

Later that day, she called the voice mailbox to learn the fate of her eggs. All seventeen of them ended up being mature and frozen.

Peace of Mind and the Illusion of Control

Remy had been single for the past seven months and had learned to love her alone time, to relish arriving home to her bohemian sanctuary, where it was just her and Sophie. No drama, no tiptoeing, no fights. She'd made many concessions with the partners she had dated long-term, and now she was no longer willing to give up who she was for the sake of connection. Which, she figured, meant it was going to be harder to meet the right person—and finding the right person was already hard enough. Still, she was excited to start dating again, and even more excited that egg freezing had freed her from the pressure she usually felt to be hyperfocused on finding a partner.

The statistics and current data, as we've seen, lead to the conclusion that you can't count on having kids with your frozen eggs. Nevertheless, many women see egg freezing as insurance for the future. Mandy, Remy, and Lauren certainly did. But frozen eggs are *not* an insurance policy. So if egg freezers aren't getting that guarantee, what exactly *are* they getting?

As an egg freezing patient, Remy was more in the know than most. But even she was confused about what happened when her eggs left her body and embarked on their tenuous journey. She hadn't been counseled on attrition rates or the inverted pyramid detailing the multistep process involved in turning thawed eggs into viable embryos and then a healthy baby. Yet she wasn't concerned. Remy may not have been clear on the scientific intricacies behind egg freezing, but she was quite clear about what egg freezing would give her. "I just don't want to settle," she'd said to me more than once, referring to dating. "And now I don't feel like I have to." That's what egg freezing was really about, I realized. Not the guarantee of frozen eggs producing healthy children in the future. Not actual insurance, but *assurance*.

I considered Remy's certainty. I hadn't heard her express doubt, not even once, about her seventeen eggs on ice becoming babies.* Just as strong was the sense of relief—which she'd felt immediately after her egg retrieval—at being able to step away from her romantic future as a project she had to actively work on. I wanted to know if Remy's experience, particularly her strong emotions post-freeze, were in line with those of other women freezing eggs for non-medical reasons. I asked Jake and Deborah if FertilityIQ had this sort of data. They didn't, but they agreed to conduct a survey to help me learn more.

Nearly half of the survey's seventy respondents said the decision to freeze eggs caused them to change their timeline and delay childbearing. In other words, they were giving themselves more and better options moving forward. When asked if they'd still be glad they froze eggs even if those eggs never led to a baby, nearly three-quarters of respondents said yes. Later, I found more data on the psychological benefits—which felt like a small win after my slog with the paltry data on success rates. In one survey of 224 egg freezing patients, 60 percent reported feeling less time pressure while dating after they'd frozen their eggs, with many patients saying they felt "more relaxed,

---

* Some of Remy's conviction, I should mention, had to do with the fact that she is a crystal-carrying physician who believes in astrological signs and the hormonal swings associated with full moons (her menstrual cycles, she told me, have always been synced to the full moon). "I'm definitely part hippie, part scientist when it comes to something like egg freezing," she'd said to me the first time we met. "In the big scheme of things, it's just more fun to believe in this kind of magic."

focused, less desperate and with more time to find the right partner."
A whopping 96 percent said they would recommend egg freezing to
others. A study published in 2020 that surveyed women who underwent egg freezing between 2008 and 2018 found that 91 percent of
egg freezers reported no regret, even if they got pregnant without
having to use their frozen eggs.*

A study in the *American Sociological Review* provided context for all
these stats. The authors, sociologists Eliza Brown and Mary Patrick,
found that egg freezing helps women manage anxieties surrounding
the demands of biology and time in part because it helps them disen-
tangle the notion of finding the right partner from the notion of having children. By temporarily separating romance from the biological
clock, egg freezers in the study "hoped to bracket long-term childbearing goals, change the experience of their partnership trajectory,
and signal to prospective partners that they were not 'in a rush' to find
a long-term partner and have children," the sociologists wrote. Single
women, this and similar ethnographic studies show, see egg freezing
as an aspirational technology, allowing them to imagine future motherhood while also giving them the time to find and fall in love with
the person with whom they'll have their future children. Valerie, the
Chicago woman who started an egg freezing blog after her positive
experience, put it to me like this: "It's like I'm thirty again," she said
of the decision. "It's like I was given an additional seven years to date
to try to find the right person."

So perhaps we should be asking a different question that focuses on
the freezing instead of the thawing: Were women happy they froze?
In a word, yes. Frozen eggs make many women feel more empowered
in terms of their fertility, whether they ever use them or not. And
that's significant. Egg freezing can change how a woman dates—for
quality instead of speed—and, perhaps most powerfully of all, can
protect against regret down the line. Simply having a backup option—
even a shaky one—shifts how a woman considers the demands of

---

* Twenty percent of the patients in this study had successfully had a baby or were
pregnant at the time of the survey; half had conceived naturally and a quarter had
used their frozen eggs.

biology and time, and can transform her personal life in profound ways by offering a sense of independence here and now, as well as a feeling of assurance about the future.

The primary benefit of egg freezing, it turns out, isn't a baby—it's peace of mind. It's a considerable chunk of change to spend on a backup you hope not to use, and that might not work if you do, but taking the edge off the biological clock is hard to put a price on. And so, for many women, egg freezing provides a sense of hope that is well worth the physically taxing process, the exorbitant costs, and the uncertain chances of success.

A few months after her egg retrieval, Remy texted me: *Those precious frozen egg babies of mine helped snap some sense into me & end this past relationship (which I had hoped hoped hoped would be "the one") without the pressure of having to settle,* her message read. *He would have made GORGEOUS babies. But he would have driven me insane. In the back of my mind those eggs are the best insurance policy against settling.* The text ended with a string of emojis: ♥ 💪 🧊 🥚 👶 💪.

In Colorado, I'd moved into a small apartment in Boulder, nestled at the base of the Rocky Mountains. I tried to settle down some, find my footing amid the light and space and snowcapped peaks. One afternoon, I sat on the floor of my living room with a thick green folder that belonged to Remy. To undergo fertility treatment of any kind requires a certain grit—and a considerable amount of patience for paperwork and phone calls. Remy and I had talked about this, and when I was in Nashville she had referred several times to a folder she'd been keeping that contained every scrap of paperwork from her egg freezing journey. After her retrieval, Remy mailed me the folder. I opened it now, spreading its contents across the carpet. The tab of the folder was labeled *Eggs.* Almost every inch of the folder itself was covered in Remy's neat, all-caps handwriting. There were phone numbers and reminders to call the phone numbers. Credit card receipts. Sticky notes with prices, scratched-out math, and so many dollar signs. Signatures galore. Printed-out Google Maps directions. Retrieval Day instructions, folded up and creased as if they'd been read over many times. "Custody and transportation of reproductive materials—client's initials," a line from the sheet read. Question marks on insurance documents. Notepaper from Freedom Pharmacy with the slogan "We're very transparent." Printouts about needles, ice packs, overnight shipping. Notes Remy scribbled to herself: *Anti-mullerian hormone # = how many eggs in bank. Infertility does not apply to max out of pocket if . . . Be mindful w/ physical activity b/c big juicy ovaries.* Images of her follicles, captured in eight black-and-white ultrasound printouts. The terms "out-of-pocket" and "deductible" written everywhere.

Sitting with Remy's handwriting, noticing her extraordinary attention to detail, and seeing these dozens of documents took me back to our first meeting. How we'd talked excitedly over rosemary lattes in Nashville, where her warmth and pep lit up the small café. Nearly every time I was around Remy, I'd notice her energy, her self-assuredness—and sitting now with her egg freezing paper trail was no different. The green folder says, *I've got this.* It says, *I am in control of my fertility.* There are phone numbers to call, bills to pay, medicines to receive by mail and refrigerate, precise instructions for shots. Figure out the prices, stay on top of the where and when, read every paragraph carefully because she is a doctor, after all, a whip-smart, career-driven, independent woman accustomed to taking matters into her own hands, to sacrificing time, money, and emotional energy for her future family. This is matter-of-fact mom mode, and there is a process, a clear plan, and a personalized protocol for women like Remy to go about this. Whether it was Remy's training as a doctor or her training as a woman—or both—didn't matter as much as what taking action *did* for her. At the beginning, the only unknown was how well egg freezing would work, which is to say, how many eggs would be frozen. She'd gotten seventeen. Any future unknowns—whether her eggs will survive the thaw, whether they will fertilize successfully with the sperm of the man she'll marry, whether she will use them or never see them again—are for later. *Later.*

In her book *Don't Call Me Princess,* Peggy Orenstein writes that the existence of IVF "has created a new drive, as profound as either the biological or psychological: call it the techno-medical imperative, the need to exhaust every 'option,' to do 'whatever you can' to have a baby—regardless of the cost to self, marriage, or pocketbook—or feel that you have not done enough. It is now possible to remain hostage to perpetual hope for years." She goes on: "How will you know unless you try? And if you don't, will you be left always wondering what might have been? The uncertainty is agonizing." Egg freezing purports to protect against this agonizing uncertainty, but it also moves up the starting line from which women begin years of chasing these techno-fertility dreams. Some egg freezers, like Remy, have names for their future children picked out. Others, like Mandy, relish the way that egg freezing offers a *break* from thinking about someday kids and starting a family. What all egg freezers are buying into is the notion that fertility is not stagnant but an active state with its own narrative. The prospective, forward-looking manner underlying an egg freezer's motivations is perhaps the most important facet of the technology's story. "I just want to know that I did everything I could," Mandy had told me. It's a sentiment that explains why many find the process liberating, though it's easy to see how a young egg freezer's do-whatever-you-can mentality would later feed into the drive that Orenstein depicts, obsessively pursuing IVF and exhausting every avenue to ensure that one's frozen eggs, and ART in general, delivers on its promises.

"It's the best thing we have to help people delay fertility, but it's far from perfect," Dr. Lamb, the reproductive endocrinologist in Seattle, had said when we discussed egg freezing being misconstrued as an insurance policy. "My biggest hope for patients is for them to not have to use their frozen eggs."

Whoa. In spite of everything I'd already learned, to hear a fertility doctor tell me this blew me away. She was boldly declaring an irony that I find frustrating and, at times, overwhelming: Trust egg freezing technology to preserve my ability to have biological children, but don't rely on it so much that I alter my life choices or avoid seriously considering other options, like adoption or not having kids at all. Is this self-delusion at best? Egg freezing optimists would say no—at least for now. Even if it's not guaranteed, the *possibility* of agency over one's biological timeline is still worth it to most women. So long as they don't ignore the reality of the success rates and limited data that are currently available.

·   ·   ·

The illusion of control alters our perspectives. We like to think we have much more of it than we do. I thought about this often after Ben and I broke up. In time and with therapy, I would come to see how I had spent so much time and energy looking for egg freezing answers in part because I did not want to confront the difficult, in-my-face issues in my relationship. I had wanted to remain in the driver's seat, commanding the narrative—and avoiding our problems helped me do that, until, of course, it didn't.

But I became tired of trying to control it all, know it all, check all the boxes. And I was tired on behalf of all the women trying to do the same. Anxiety bubbles up in every corner of our lives, and it is exhausting how we attempt to secure everything while trusting in so little, how we don't allow ourselves the Right Now because we're so caught up with the Future. In my egg freezing journey and in my life, it felt as if I'd been spinning around in dizzying small circles across a wide field for a long time, trying to get my bearings. I wanted to loosen my grip, to feel things come into focus. I wanted to quit pretending everything—my ovary, my heart, my fertility—would be fine.

Maybe egg freezing was a way to reclaim some control. But I wasn't sure I wanted it.

The Economics of Parenthood

When I was young, I'd sometimes wait for my parents to arrive home from work, my nose pressed against the glass of the front door. They always looked the same walking up the driveway: my father in a dark suit, briefcase in hand, and my mother in her camouflage uniform and patrol cap. My parents, although two very different people, were a team—with a heck of a romantic meet-cute story—who had been married for seven years before having children. For most of my childhood, my entrepreneurial father managed his own business while my military mom managed a battalion and then a brigade. Our father nursed our playground cuts and bruises and taught us how to ride bikes. Our mother cheered us on at weekend sports games and read out loud to us at bedtime. Our parents' teamwork formed the rhythm of our lives, and my brother, sister, and I grew up assuming this was how the world worked, a close-knit family led by two full-time working parents who loved their jobs.

For the mid- to late twentysomethings of my parents' generation, a job was a major, stable part of your identity. If you landed a good one, you'd stick with it until retirement. Entering your prime childbearing years, you knew with a good deal of confidence where you'd be and what you'd likely be earning ten years down the road—as long as you showed up on time, made your bosses happy, and continued progressing up the totem pole. Maybe you didn't plan to continue working after you had children, and that was possible because your partner had one of these jobs and that sort of security. Today, it is only the rare, exceptional young adult who can count on any of these things. In the past, having this kind of stability made it inestimably easier to make long-term decisions. But while millennials earn more money than any other generation has at their age, they hold much less wealth, largely because the cost of living has outpaced wage increases.* For the most part, young women today are not simply capricious, commitment-phobic dreamers who want to delay childbearing until the last possible second in the name of career ambition or total equality with men. They—and the men, women, partners they love—are embarking on adult life on far different terms than their parents did.

I have always planned on being a parent someday. But especially lately, I've wrestled with ideas I have about the level of financial stability and career success I should attain before starting a family. I am incredibly privileged to have spent my twenties in school and on airplanes, studying and traveling while working. I attended a private liberal arts college. I earned a graduate degree without being crippled by student loans. I want these things for my future children, too, and it's easy to convince myself I'm being responsible by waiting to have kids until I have at least *some* savings. But waiting would also mean feeling burdened by timeline pressures, gnawing worries about my

---

* As a 2021 *Business Insider* article astutely notes, "Two recessions before the age of 40 and student debt haven't helped matters."

eggs expiring, and pursuing my career while stressing that I'm sacrificing my parenting prospects.

I'm not alone. A rising share of U.S. adults who are not already parents—44 percent—say they're unlikely to ever have children, according to a recent Pew Research Center survey. A few years ago, *The New York Times* asked: Why are young adults in America having fewer children than their ideal number? They surveyed 1,858 men and women ages twenty to forty-five. Most of the respondents said they delayed or stopped having children because of concerns about not having enough money or time.* Financial insecurities are altering the choices of today's generations, and money is a major factor affecting fertility decisions. Another is climate change. In a 2023 survey of about one thousand parents in India, Mexico, Singapore, the United States, and the United Kingdom, more than half of parents— 53 percent—said that climate change affects their decision about having more children. And a 2022 survey by Modern Fertility of nearly three thousand American women—mostly Gen Z and millennials— found that 58 percent of women have adjusted their family planning because of concerns about climate change. The respondents said they are worried, in particular, "about the world [their] kids will inherit."

"Around the world, economic, social and environmental conditions function as a diffuse, barely perceptible contraceptive," writes Anna Louie Sussman in a *New York Times* opinion essay titled "The End of Babies." She expounds on how such conditions are inimical to starting families—"our workweeks are longer and our wages lower, leaving us less time and money to meet, court and fall in love"—and notes the pervasive anxiety that plagues many would-be parents when thinking about the sort of life they might provide for their children. A generation's economic opportunities impact pretty much all of life's fundamentals: work, sex, love, family. The economics of modern parenthood are, in a word, brutal. Millennials and Gen Zers are the most educated generations ever, a distinction that perhaps should but does not make us rich or secure. And adulthood, it seems to me, is about

---

* Their reasons: "childcare is too expensive" (64 percent); "waited because of financial instability" (43 percent); "no paid family leave" (38 percent).

achieving security. Career, relationships, housing, healthcare. Some of my friends have 401(k)s and paid-off mortgages; others have credit card debt and crushing student loans. For women, add fertility to the list of their financial worries. While it is a luxury to be able to worry about fertility at all, many women do, in addition to everything else on our minds.

As young women lean into their ambitions and burgeoning careers in their twenties and thirties, many begin to sacrifice their fertility—whether they realize it or not. For those who are aware that the aforementioned "motherhood penalty" means they'll lose professional and economic power after they have kids, egg freezing looks like an empowering solution. The increasing number of companies offering fertility benefits has been one of the biggest developments in egg freezing's story over the last several years. But company-paid fertility preservation is not the next great equalizer many hoped it would be, and in some ways it distracts from true solutions that working women need, such as publicly funded, high-quality childcare and moderate-length paid parental leave. Ideally, employers would offer fertility benefits while simultaneously addressing the factors that drive their female employees to postpone starting families. As it is, egg freezing is advertised as one more tool in a woman's tool belt, when actually there should be more support given to women who have children and less pressure on women to have them if they don't want to.

People across all salary brackets choose to delay or forgo parenthood for a variety of reasons—career, travel, relationships, money, climate change, or perhaps no reason at all. Our assumptions about what shapes and motivates the lives of women are so hardwired that the notion that some women do not want children can be difficult for others to wrap their minds around. According to a 2023 CDC report, nearly half of U.S. women between the ages of fifteen and forty-four don't have biological children. This is in part because waiting to have biological children can increase the likelihood of not having them; delayed childbearing—having a first child at age thirty-five or older—has been associated with the decades-long trend in which the number of births in the United States has been declining. But it's also because many women simply choose not to have children. It should go without saying—but it doesn't, frustratingly, so I'm saying it—that for women, parenthood is not the only or the primary role from which they derive meaning and identity. When it comes to being child-free by choice, Gloria Steinem summed it up well: "When I was much younger I assumed I had to have children. I assumed everyone had to have children. But someone said once that not everyone with vocal chords [*sic*] is an opera singer. And not everyone with a womb needs to be a mother. When the Pill came along we were able to give birth—to ourselves."

The Little Ovary That . . . Could?

For a few years now, I had been struggling to articulate the reasons for and against freezing my eggs. The lists of pros and cons no longer cut it, but they were all I had. I tried to balance egg freezing's positives—the peace of mind, the diminished pressure when it came to the biological clock—with the success-rate unknowns, the potential health risks, and the hard-to-swallow price tag. But while the money and potential dangers of fertility medications were significant deterrents, they weren't the whole story. The decision point is different for every individual. And the sticking point for me, the one determinant that seemed as if it would tip the scales when it came to deciding yes or no about egg freezing, was my ovary.

I remained afraid that if I chose to move ahead with the process of freezing my eggs, something would happen or not happen that would leave me living in a constant fog of regret. If I went through with it and any one of the worst-case scenarios came to be—I lose my remaining ovary; I get only a few eggs, nowhere near enough to feel confident about their chances of producing a baby, then live with the low-level anxiety brought on by the possibility of health issues down the road caused by the injections; I freeze a ton and when I go back to use them in my late thirties, they don't work—it could be my comeuppance. I would blame my body but I would also blame my brain, because I had chosen to freeze my eggs after several years of learning about the very real upsides and benefits while disregarding the very real facts about the risks and potential downsides.

But *not* freezing my eggs also left the door open for deep regret, and this was something I came to understand only late in this journey. When I interviewed reproductive endocrinologists and fertility experts, the fact that I had one ovary and personal reasons for investigating egg freezing sometimes came up. And so I'd ask them their opinion, always with the disclaimer that I understood they were not my doctor and thus couldn't offer me specific medical advice. After telling Dr. Natalie Crawford, a reproductive endocrinologist in Austin, Texas, and host of the popular podcast *As a Woman,* about my history of reproductive surgeries and desire to have biological children someday, she said that if I froze my eggs, I'd need to be very careful about the risk of ovarian torsion, but that "it's extremely unlikely for someone with one ovary to get OHSS," which I was surprised and *so* relieved to hear. "You don't have room to spare," she said, referring to my sole ovary, telling me I may well want to "buffer this risk by getting some eggs or embryos in the freezer."

Dr. Crawford and other fertility specialists I spoke with about my personal situation weren't pushing egg freezing on me and had nothing to gain if I decided to do it. Given my medical history, they simply saw a compelling reason for me to freeze.

Amid all these conflicting thoughts, I caught up with Mandy, Remy, and Lauren. I wanted to know what life looked like for them now and if their thoughts about egg freezing had changed.

Mandy was approaching her mid-thirties and going through a job transition. When we spoke on the phone, she told me that she remained grateful that she froze her eggs when she did and didn't succumb to the pressure to start a family when she and her husband weren't ready. The feeling of bought time still mitigated her anxiety. "I did everything I was supposed to do, what my doctors told me to do—but it turned into a feeling of more not knowing," Mandy told me. "If you have lots of resources and things go really well, it seems like egg freezing is a no-brainer. But if your resources are limited and your path isn't as smooth, this can be such an emotional and confusing journey." She and Quincy were contemplating starting a family soon. "Thinking of conceiving brings up all these feelings again about egg freezing," she told me. "I'm back to over-googling and overanalyzing. What if it takes me a long time to conceive? How long should I try before using our frozen embryos? What's it all going to cost?"

When I talked to Remy over video a few weeks before her thirty-fifth birthday, she'd just gotten home from work. She wore blue scrubs, her long blond hair gathered to one side. She had recently moved to a studio apartment in North Carolina and was completing an OB/GYN fellowship at Duke University. I asked Remy what had been the most challenging part of the whole process, from when she first decided to freeze her eggs until now. "Number one, no caffeine. Number two, money," she replied. "The hardest part was the financial stress, figuring out and navigating how to pay for it." Remy was still paying annual fees to store her eggs, on top of $640 every month toward the loan she'd taken out to pay for the procedure. She told me egg freezing never really felt financially feasible for her, even though she'd managed to do it. Still, she said, "freezing my eggs was one of the smartest decisions I've ever made." Her mom brags about it to her friends who have daughters Remy's age, saying, "They should freeze their eggs like Remy did!" When the subject of kids is broached on dates, Remy tells men that because she froze her eggs, she's not in a rush to start a family.

As for Lauren, well, life looked very different indeed. One humid afternoon before I left Houston, I visited Lauren at her house. Bentley, her twelve-year-old bulldog, greeted me at the door and followed us into the living room, where we sat and talked. Lauren had chosen not to go back on birth control after freezing her eggs; she felt more levelheaded and even-tempered off the Pill and decided she felt better not taking it. She'd been on the Pill since she was fourteen and, until now, bled every month like clockwork—every fourth Tuesday at 9 A.M., to be exact. She had no idea how long her normal menstrual cycle was and had never tracked period symptoms. If she had, what happened next might not have.

Right around the time of Lauren's second egg freezing attempt, she went to dinner with the man she'd long ago lost her virginity to and he, in fact, had administered her trigger shot. "I was like, 'Can you give me this shot in my ass? Great to see you again,'" Lauren told me with a wry smile as she recounted the story. They rekindled a romance that night and began to date. A few months later, Lauren unexpectedly got pregnant. She was so shocked she had accidentally conceived naturally that she took five pregnancy tests before accepting it was real. Now she was eight months pregnant with a healthy baby boy. She had told me she was pregnant before I'd come over to hear the story, but seeing her now—reclined in a rocking chair, huge and glowing, her bare feet resting on an ottoman—I almost couldn't believe how egg freezing had changed her life in such an unexpected way. "If he's anything like he's been inside me—he's been partying for nine months—this kid is going to be a blast," Lauren said. "I accidentally got knocked up, and since the moment I found out I was pregnant, I've been happier than I've ever been in my entire life."

By the time Ben and I had been broken up for a year, I'd gone back and forth on my egg freezing decision what felt like a hundred times. I wanted to believe that if I froze my eggs it would go as well as it did for Mandy, Remy, and the many women who came out all smiles, more or less, and with a bounty of eggs. Or even if I experienced significant complications while freezing my eggs, as Lauren did, maybe egg freezing would be the catalyst for a journey into motherhood I otherwise couldn't have imagined, like it was for her. The factor of my sole ovary loomed large. Mandy, with two partial ovaries, was lucky to have beaten the odds as well as she did; no one, not even her doctors, would have predicted she'd have twenty eggs retrieved and eight chromosomally normal embryos frozen. I believe in my little ovary with all my heart, and I believe it would be up to the task of doing double duty to pump out as many eggs as it possibly could. But I had to face it: I couldn't be sure I'd be as fortunate as Mandy if I decided to freeze.

The truth—that I was finally starting to allow myself to inhabit—was that I never wanted to make the decision. I wanted it to be made *for* me. I wanted my body to decide: *Ovaries gone; it's too late now* (although at the same time I of course didn't want anything bad to happen to my ovary). I wanted my heart to decide: *He's the one; time for babies.* Most of all, I wanted my head to decide, because after all this time reporting, researching, and poking at this question with every sharp object I could find, I should have been able to logically determine the right choice.

"I'm the kind of person who tries to prevent regret, to control life in a way that optimizes the best outcome," Mandy had told me once. "That's what my embryo freezing decision was: a way to prevent the worst from happening." That resonated with me deeply. I saw myself in Mandy's rationalizing, the way her fear of the unknown prompted action. More than at any other point in this journey, when I imagined freezing my eggs now, I pictured the future me I'd be doing it for: years from now, trying so hard for a second or third child, regretting more than I've ever regretted anything not freezing my younger eggs when I'd had the chance. I felt caught between the promises and risks of egg freezing, the remaining gaps in our knowledge, and the pressure to protect against future regret. I was about to be reminded, however, that taking concrete action now is never a guarantee of future certainty.

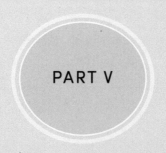

PART V

The Freeze

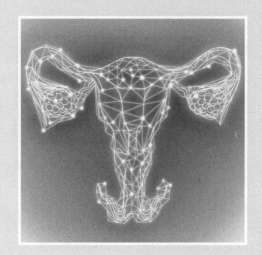

Unviable

~~~~~~

Tank Failures and Hidden Risks

Soon after lunchtime on March 3, 2018, temperatures rose inside a cryogenic storage tank inside a laboratory at University Hospitals Fertility Center in Cleveland, Ohio. The liquid-nitrogen-filled tank held more than four thousand frozen eggs and embryos belonging to nearly one thousand people. It was a Saturday, and the clinic's lab workers had left for the day forty minutes earlier. At 5:06 P.M., an alarm on the tank went off. Anyone within earshot would have heard it and immediately discovered that the temperature had risen to −156 degrees Celsius, forty degrees above normal—but the lab wasn't staffed on Saturday evenings. No one heard it. It would be many hours until anyone knew the tank had malfunctioned, damaging all the eggs and embryos inside.

The next day, 2,500 miles away, a cryotank inside a lab at Pacific Fertility Center in San Francisco also failed, compromising about 3,500 eggs and embryos and impacting nearly four hundred individuals and families. And so, over a single weekend, an unprecedented disaster had hit fertility clinics—twice. Despite the eerie timing, the incidents were not related.

The nightmare began in earnest for the Ohio patients when, four days after the incident, University Hospitals Cleveland Medical

Center—which oversees the fertility clinic—sent letters to patients informing them that "an unexpected temperature fluctuation" had occurred in the tank where their eggs or embryos were being stored. In this case, "fluctuation" is putting it mildly; an uncontrolled rise in temperature can have catastrophic consequences for frozen reproductive cells. In Pacific Fertility's case, the liquid nitrogen levels inside Tank 4 dropped too low, destroying the thousands of eggs and embryos inside. Tank 4 housed up to 15 percent of Pacific Fertility's total cryopreserved tissue. No alarms or phone alerts notified the clinic's lab staff of the malfunction; the problem was discovered by an embryologist during a routine walk-through at the end of the day. The California clinic began informing patients about the tank failure seven days later.

Two months after the cryotank failure in Cleveland, a memorial service was held on Mother's Day for families whose gametes and embryos had been destroyed. In mid-May, I flew to Ohio to cover the service. I had spent the better part of a month investigating University Hospitals Fertility Center's tank failure, speaking with several of the women and couples who found themselves facing an incalculable loss. When I called around to hear the disaster put into some context, the response was grim. "In my thirty years, I've never heard of this ever happening," said Cindee Khabani, embryologist and laboratory director at Pacific Northwest Fertility in Seattle. Other seasoned lab directors told me the same, expressing their shock and horror. For days, fertility doctors across the country answered calls from worried patients: *Are my eggs okay? Our embryos are safe, right?*

It was every fertility clinic's nightmare. Cryotank failures of this magnitude were a new kind of uncertainty, one not even I had considered. Most U.S. fertility clinics have backup systems to handle technical failures and make sure frozen specimens stay frozen. Embryologists I spoke to relayed the sorts of protocols they have in place—and hurriedly triple-checked when the news of the tank failures broke—in their labs: multiple backup cryotanks, freezers checked by staff members daily (at a minimum), specialized alarm systems that monitor tanks and their internal temperatures, and more. The breakdowns at the clinics in Cleveland and San Francisco both involved temperature and liquid nitrogen levels inside storage tanks, the details of which I'd soon glean. Both clinics were well known and reputable, their cryotanks and lab safeguards believed to be foolproof. But their systems had failed, resulting in the biggest such losses on record in the United States.

Kate Plants was thirty-one the first time she almost lost her fertility, upon learning she had ovarian cancer. *Thank God I still have a uterus,* she thought when her left ovary had to be removed. Kate and her husband, Jeremy, had been trying to conceive when she was diagnosed. *Thank God I can still get pregnant.* The second time Kate almost lost her fertility was two years later, when she learned the cancer had spread to her uterus. At the doctor's office that day, the look of horror on her mother-in-law's face said it all: This was bad, and Kate was in trouble. Three months later, doctors removed her uterus. *Thank God we still have our embryos,* she thought after the hysterectomy—she and Jeremy had frozen five before Kate underwent surgery. Kate had no chance of ever becoming pregnant, but she was comforted by the fact that a gestational carrier could carry the baby created by one of the embryos she and Jeremy had frozen. Then, the following year, the couple learned that their embryos, along with thousands of others, had been destroyed. And with this news, Kate's fertility was gone forever.

In Cleveland the day before the memorial service, I visited Kate in the single-story mint-chocolate-chip-colored house she shares with Jeremy and their two kittens. We sat cross-legged on the floor of the nursery. The room had never been used, and now might never be, but being in it comforted Kate. She likened it to a sanctuary, a place where she sat and thought about children. "I don't know what it's like to see your own flesh and blood walk around and know how fulfilling that is," she said, reaching for a hat she had crocheted for a baby she didn't have. Her head hung low, strands of red-orange hair framing her pale face. Then, her voice softer: "I don't think I want to admit to myself how badly I want a family."

The nursery's changing table dresser had been Kate's own when she was a baby. Raised by a single mother, Kate had wanted children for as long as she could remember. Growing up, she'd pretend to cook for her younger half sisters while they all played with dolls. Stroking a kitten that had climbed into her lap, Kate told me how not being able to have biological children has made her feel as if part of her identity as a woman has been taken away. She was still struggling to process it all—her cancers, the destroyed embryos, the loss of her fertility—and most mornings woke feeling a mix of red-hot anger and deep sadness that left her exhausted before she even climbed out of bed. *Protecting our eggs and embryos was their job,* she thought. *They're the experts. That's what they're paid to do.*

The service took place at a cemetery in Middleburg Heights, outside the city. The overcast sky made for an unusually cold spring day, even for Cleveland. An inscribed granite bench had been created to serve as a permanent memorial. *In memory of the unborn / Before I formed you in the womb, I knew you,* part of the bench read. *Dedicated to the memory of the lost eggs and embryos of 2018.* As it began to drizzle, I held the end of my umbrella with the inside of my elbow as I scribbled notes while interviewing patients at the service. They ranged in age from twenty-two to early forties. Some had frozen eggs and embryos prior to undergoing medical treatments that would render them infertile. Others had done so after going through IVF and having a child; their embryos on ice were their child's future siblings, in safekeeping until they wanted to grow their family. Hearing their stories, I recalled something Dr. Alice Domar, a reproductive psychologist at Boston IVF, had said when we spoke a few days before I traveled to Ohio: "To lose embryos through what looks like human error just feels really unfair. And for the cancer patients, this is a catastrophe on top of a crisis."

Halfway through the memorial service, the sky opened and huge raindrops fell on the crowd. "What we lost will not be forgotten," Jeremy Plants said, speaking to the couples and families, multiple generations, huddled under umbrellas. For the Plantses, it was a day to put to rest, once and for all, their last chance at having a biological child. Jeremy's voice broke as he continued: "There is a place for you to come, always." A husband pulled his crying wife in close; a grandfather gripped his granddaughter's hand while she stood quietly, draped in her father's suit jacket. Those gathered had each received a glass memorial candle and they held them now, the flames flickering in the rain.

That night, I curled up in my hotel room and skipped dinner. I was on deadline and needed to file my story about the memorial service to an editor in New York. It had been a gut-wrenching day. I wrote late into the night, the sounds of my keyboard clicks mixed with the sound of the rain pattering against the windows. *Grief—like forgiveness, like love—can be slow, hard work,* I wrote. *It is a characteristic of being human to honor the dead, but rituals sometimes have to take unusual forms.* Equipment failure, deactivated alarms, in an instant, thousands of gametes and embryos destroyed. I had stood inside embryology labs like the ones in Cleveland and San Francisco where the nightmares occurred. What I hadn't stopped to consider until now was what the tanks of liquid nitrogen inside those labs contained, really: fragile hopes, fervent desires, a thousand fraught conversations about preserving fertility—the whys, the hows, the what-ifs. Despite weeks of reporting, I struggled to grasp the magnitude of these families' loss.

Reproductive Negligence

The Ohio and California incidents made it clear that the vulnerability of the storage process was another hidden risk of fertility preservation. Those twin catastrophes had led me down a new rabbit hole. Back home in Colorado, I spent weeks speaking with more experts— embryologists, lab directors, reproductive endocrinologists, lawyers— about what had happened, pressing them about the broader nature of regulation within the fertility industry.

Thanks in large part to the fact-finding efforts by reporters at local news outlets and state health department investigations, answers began to surface. The calamity in Cleveland was the result of both human error and equipment glitches. University Hospitals Fertility Center had known for several weeks prior to the incident that its cryotank that stored eggs and embryos wasn't working properly. The clinic had been working with the tank manufacturer to correct the problem. The issue was the tank's autofill valve, which controlled the liquid nitrogen level inside.* While the autofill function was down, lab staff had been manually filling the tank for weeks by connecting it via a hose to a liquid nitrogen reserve container. But for several days before the failure, they couldn't fill the tank using the hose—because the clinic had run out of reserve liquid nitrogen containers. Instead, as a workaround, lab technicians manually filled the tank by pouring liquid nitrogen directly into the top of it, rather than into the reservoir where the liquid nitrogen is normally pumped by the hose. As it happens, the top-of-tank manual pouring is an improper filling technique, and in this case it is likely what caused the temperature inside to rise to critical levels.

Additionally, a remote alarm system on the tank should have alerted a lab worker about the tank's rise in temperature, but the remote alarm had been turned off. Had it been in use, someone likely would've been able to get to the cryotank and potentially fix the problem before the eggs and embryos inside were damaged. But no one was alerted. When the first employee arrived at the embryology lab early the next day, the tank's local alarm was still blaring. By that point, the temperature inside the tank had risen to −32 degrees Celsius, destroying everything inside. In an investigation, the Ohio Department of Health found that, in addition to the clinic having issues with keeping records of its tanks' temperature and liquid nitrogen levels, the fact that the clinic had only one designated point of contact for problems related to the tanks was also an issue. The health department determined that what happened at University Hospitals Fertility Center was largely preventable.†

---

* The nitrogen in cryotanks continuously evaporates at a slow rate, requiring it to be replenished on a daily basis. "It's standard in the egg and embryo storage industry for facilities to equip their tanks with auto-filling mechanisms to refill the liquid nitrogen when the system detects that levels are low," lab director Cindee Khabani told me.

† Ultimately, hundreds of affected patients settled claims with University Hospitals Fertility Center. The lawsuits included nondisclosure agreements and did not disclose settlement amounts, but it's likely the payout for those who sued was in the millions.

Explanations for the shocking news out of the California clinic were slower to materialize and predominantly came from subsequent legal proceedings. In 2021, a California jury awarded nearly $15 million to be shared among five people—three women who lost eggs and a married couple who lost embryos—in the tank failure, laying primary blame on the tank manufacturer. The jury determined that the storage tank had an equipment defect—a controller that was supposed to send alerts when the tank's liquid nitrogen levels dropped—that was to blame for the liquid nitrogen level inside the tank falling too low. The jury found the tank manufacturing company 90 percent responsible and Pacific Fertility 10 percent responsible; about two weeks before the March 4 incident, the clinic's lab director had disabled the tank's controller because it had started malfunctioning, which caused it to send out false alarms.

Pacific Fertility Center was not a defendant in the three-week trial, having won a motion to send its claims to private arbitration.* Neither was the clinic's parent company, Prelude Fertility—the same Prelude we talked about earlier. Prelude added Pacific Fertility to its nationwide network of clinics in September 2017. Five months later, the incident occurred. Prelude's ownership of Pacific Fertility went virtually unmentioned in the slew of news reports, but I immediately wondered if the major femtech company's recent acquisition had influenced the clinic's procedures and equipment quality and had any bearing on the tank failure. A few reproductive endocrinologists, also familiar with Prelude's grabs, speculated, too. "When you're about to be bought, you don't invest in new tanks and lab equipment," one told me. Her comment brought me back to the connection between the rapid expansion of the fertility industry's retail-purchase model and the private-equity-backed deep pockets that spur such growth, the concern being that in the fertility and ART sector, as in other areas of medicine, private equity can lead to cutting corners and cutting costs any way a company can, while quality of care and appropriate clinical staffing levels fall to the wayside in favor of the bottom line.

---

* Hundreds of plaintiffs filed claims against the tank manufacturer, Pacific Fertility, and Prelude.

Prelude owns Pacific Fertility's laboratory, storage facility, and tanks. It owned Tank 4 at the time of the incident. The employees responsible for performing daily monitoring and maintenance of the tanks were Prelude employees. It remains unclear why the clinic didn't have a functional autofilling mechanism to replenish the low liquid nitrogen levels or secondary monitoring, alarm, and response systems that would have detected the tank's dangerous temperature rise. Backup systems and monitoring protocols are standard at most fertility clinics in the country. And while at most clinics it's common to store frozen eggs and embryos belonging to hundreds or even thousands of patients together, some clinics spread individuals' reproductive tissue across multiple tanks to avoid putting all eggs in one basket, so to speak.*

I called up Dr. Michael Alper, medical director at Boston IVF, for more context. The reality is, he told me, that "any activity that involves humans and machines is associated with a failure or error rate." Malfunctions happen; equipment breaks. Misdeeds and misconduct in the fertility industry are rarely intentional. But while some of the mistakes aren't preventable, many are, especially those caused by human error and carelessness. I was troubled to learn that while mass incidents are rare, catastrophic errors in fertility clinics occur much more frequently than the public realizes. In addition to lost, discarded, or damaged frozen gametes, there are horrific cases of IVF mix-ups in which clinics have accidentally switched specimens so that women gave birth to someone else's baby.† Some of the mishaps make jaw-dropping headlines, but most do not. Sparse reporting requirements and the reluctance to disclose errors make it difficult to know just how frequently reproductive negligence takes place.

One study, published in 2022, determined that there have been at

---

* An article about the 2021 Pacific Fertility jury trial noted: "After the March 2018 mishap, Pacific Fertility Center made several changes to its protocols. The facility now has backup monitors and alarm systems for each storage tank. The lab also stores patients' eggs and embryos in separate vessels to ensure that one tank failure won't wipe out a patient's entire stock of reproductive tissue."

† One recent example: a *New York Times* story titled "'We Had Their Baby, and They Had Our Baby': Couple Sues Over Embryo 'Mix-Up'" in which a couple spent months raising a child who wasn't theirs and endured a painful custody exchange after DNA testing.

least nine major tank failures in the United States over the past fifteen years that have affected more than 1,800 patients. According to FertilityIQ, nearly 30 percent of all fertility patients will experience a clinical or clerical error at any given clinic. And a 2008 survey of U.S. fertility clinics—while not recent, it's among the most comprehensive studies of its kind—found that more than one in five clinics misdiagnosed, mislabeled, or mishandled reproductive materials.* Examples of what can cause frozen eggs to be damaged, be destroyed, be lost, or fail to develop, thus rendering them unviable, include power outages; mechanical or equipment failure, including loss of nitrogen or other tank failures; dropped materials, including vials, straws, and other containers used to freeze and store specimens; labeling errors; patient-specific differences in tolerance of gamete freezing; inventory record loss; natural and human-caused disasters; sabotage; and transportation or shipping accidents.

Millions of people rely on reproductive technologies to have children, and ART patients harmed by these sorts of accidents, errors, and negligence are often left without clear recourse. Victims often decline to sue. Those who do often settle out of court with undisclosed terms and nondisclosure agreements, keeping reproductive errors and lawsuit outcomes in the shadows. If a fertility clinic and/or its parent company are sued for losing or mishandling eggs and embryos, they are often shielded from liability because of the clauses in contracts patients have signed. It's a stark contrast to the shiny marketing and visibility the Preludes of the world typically portray.† Who,

---

* I gleaned what these statistics looked like in practice when I learned of a 2019 Accenture study that gathered data over two weeks in four IVF labs. The fifteen hours of recorded footage showed injuries (an embryologist was even sent to the hospital for a severe liquid nitrogen burn); a cane (a long piece of plastic, you'll recall) containing several embryos dropped on the floor; alarms repeatedly ignored; and liquid nitrogen spilled and mishandled. The footage also showed that about one in twenty-five specimens (embryos/eggs/sperm) were not where the inventory indicated they were stored.

† "It was absolutely devastating," a senior Prelude executive with direct knowledge of the tank failure told me. "We did everything we could to deal with the situation in the best possible way for the patients." As for the timing of Prelude's acquisition of Pacific Fertility, he likened it to "buying an airline, and then one of its aircrafts falls out of the sky."

then, is in charge of ensuring that fertility clinics and the companies that own them act ethically and responsibly?

Businesses often learn their strengths and weaknesses from a disaster that spirals out of control. The tank malfunctions offered a rare point of entry into the fertility industry's uneven regulations, but it wasn't the pivotal moment it could have been, and the historic verdict in 2021—the first time a jury has awarded damages in a case involving the destruction of eggs and embryos—didn't have far-reaching consequences. The lawsuits that played out in the public sphere weren't nothing, of course, but as Dr. Shahine, the Seattle fertility doctor I'd spoken with a few times, put it: "You can sue as much as you want, but you can't get your fertility back."

An industry that creates and maintains potential life, and which has become quite a lucrative market in the process, has invited a great deal of responsibility upon itself. My next obvious order of business was to peel back reproductive medicine's layers of oversight—or lack thereof.

Since the early 1970s, the United States has had policies in place that restrict federal funding for research involving human embryos. While that might sound like a clear illustration of strict regulation in the fertility industry, it's not. Federal regulation tends to follow federal funding. Absent the funding, there's no clear national guidance on this controversial area of research. Instead, states are left to develop their own policies, which range in their consistency, and privately funded fertility facilities operate without much consumer regulation or ethical oversight.

The complicated landscape surrounding human embryo research is emblematic of regulation in the U.S. fertility industry: at first glance fairly solid, but actually not great. Reproductive medicine in the United States is regulated by a complex patchwork of federal and state laws and self-oversight by the clinics.* On the federal level, regulating ART falls

* In contrast, several other countries have national ART regulatory agencies. The best known is the Human Fertilisation and Embryology Authority, the United Kingdom's independent regulator overseeing the use of sperm, eggs, and embryos in fertility treatment and research.

mainly to two agencies.* The CDC, which has jurisdiction over disease, collects and publishes data on ART procedures and birth rates but shirks other direct regulatory opportunities. Every year, clinics are required to report the outcomes and basic details of each ART procedure to the CDC; if they don't, all that happens is the CDC puts them on a list of "non-reporting" clinics. The FDA limits its ART oversight to its general regulation of drugs, devices, and donor tissue; it does not regulate the actual procedures clinics do. Much of what takes place in an IVF lab falls outside the FDA's purview, including, for example, the operation of the cryotanks that clinics use to store reproductive tissue.†

What we have, then, is a few big-name governmental players that oversee aspects of ART, but with several caveats to their regulatory responsibilities, including enforcing standards. As for the more local level, most states don't regulate ART to any substantial degree. This means that ART is largely self-policed, with some oversight from professional organizations. SART writes reports and opinions on various ART-related topics. ASRM sets forth best practices—including that fertility clinics should have policies in place regarding disclosure of medical errors involving gametes and embryos to patients as soon as such errors are discovered—but its recommendations are voluntary and sometimes ignored.‡ The College of American Pathologists

---

* There's also a murky third: the Clinical Laboratory Improvement Amendments (CLIA), passed by Congress in 1988 and administered by the Centers for Medicare and Medicaid Services (CMS). CMS, FDA, and the CDC have joint responsibility for the law, which requires that all diagnostic lab work performed on humans (in a fertility patient's case, semen and blood testing) adhere to quality standards. But CLIA doesn't extend to embryology, which involves the retrieval of eggs, their fertilization, and the transfer and storage of eggs and embryos. These procedures do not fall under CLIA's mandate.

† The tanks are considered medical devices, which the FDA does regulate—but it doesn't regulate the *use* of the tanks. The agency does not, for example, ask clinics to disclose how often tanks malfunction or how many specimens have been accidentally destroyed.

‡ ASRM acknowledges that if fertility clinics and doctors were required to follow ASRM guidelines, it "might improve the uniformity of practice nationwide." Even so, ASRM maintains that ART is highly regulated in the United States. But the examples it points to supporting this assertion all have caveats—the ones I've dug into here.

(CAP) visits fertility clinics every year or two to assess embryology labs for accreditation, which is optional in most states. Embryologists I interviewed respect CAP and its thorough checklists, and they care a great deal about their labs having CAP's stamp of approval. But fertility clinics can choose whether their labs are accredited or not—again, not a requirement in most states. (The good news is, most are; to be a member of SART, a clinic's embryology lab must be accredited by either CAP or the Joint Commission, another accrediting healthcare body.)

I was on the phone with a reproductive endocrinologist—who was on her Peloton at 6 A.M., her daily workout ritual before seeing patients—discussing the industry's checks-and-balances processes when I got it: The reason fertility clinics can withhold mix-ups and errors is that they are accountable to no one,* at least not in any official capacity. There is no repository for clinics' incident rates. No government agency or authority seriously polices reproductive negligence. No central agency oversees fertility procedures. And the organizations the industry mostly listens to, such as ASRM and SART, lack the power to enforce their guidelines in any consequential way. Most of the time, the industry does a good job regulating itself. But when it doesn't, the repercussions, as we've seen, can be enormous.

This is the moment in the darker parts of egg freezing's saga where you and I both would like me to introduce an in-the-works solution, evidence of the fertility industry's regulation failures and legal snarls working themselves out. The best I can do is this: The loosey-goosey regulation isn't a complete nightmare, and while the negatives of the lack of oversight can be significant, there are positives, too. One is the risk of regulation coming in a form that's really not wanted, such as anti-abortion legislation and unhelpfully strict embryo-destruction laws that could get fertility clinics in trouble, as discussed in chapter 9. In a post-*Dobbs* world, the inflammatory politics of conception and

---

* Save for their patients, which nearly all of the fertility doctors I spoke to in the course of reporting this book consider an important responsibility.

abortion have, as we've seen, already begun to encroach on ART and the ability of fertility doctors to do their job. Stricter regulation from lawmakers with anti-ART agendas could make the landscape far worse.

Another positive is freedom. Fertility doctors being allowed to do what their clinic and lab data shows offers the best chance of success for their patients is important. There aren't uniform standards for freezing and maintaining eggs in the United States, unlike in most of Europe's fertility clinics, and while the lack of micromanagement has its downsides, one benefit is that it encourages innovation. Reproductive medicine is a rapidly changing field, one that's, ironically, often characterized by not having as much exact science as one might think. As embryologist Cindee Khabani, the lab director in Seattle, explained to me, the acronym for assisted reproductive technology, ART, is appropriate in a metaphoric sense: "The field of fertility has gotten better because people around the world have come up with new and better ways to do things that work for them," she said. "And advances happen because of that." The industry needs better maintenance standards and more transparency, but hopefully not at the expense of responsible scientific development or patient outcomes.

Your Eggs on Ice

The reproductive negligence rabbit hole the tank failures took me down was a wake-up call regarding the fertility industry's regulatory vacuum. It also brought home the reality of eggs on ice and after the thaw, and had me considering the disposition decisions a woman freezing eggs or embryos has to make. Such decisions entail three options: preserving them in storage, discarding them, or donating them (whether to another couple trying to conceive, to science for research purposes, or, in the case of embryos, to an embryo donation program).

It can be incredibly difficult for a woman to decide when to *stop* storing her eggs or embryos. A question that therapists specializing in infertility often hear: Once you've invested in artificially extending the period in which you can decide to have a child, how do you go about deciding to end it? Even after having two or three healthy children, many women have a hard time deciding to pull the plug. With no easy answers when it comes to deciding to donate or discard, many patients simply stop paying for storage. Clinics will try to reach patients for years, after which they deem the eggs or embryos abandoned. If rent hasn't been paid, so to speak, clinics still usually shy away from destroying abandoned reproductive tissue, even with signed consent forms from patients indicating what is to be done with their frozen specimens in the event of death, divorce, or nonpayment of storage fees.

One area where the issue of embryo disposition comes up often is in divorce cases, when couples must confront the tough question of what to do with their embryos. Often, legal disputes ensue. Say a wife and husband freeze embryos before the woman undergoes chemotherapy. A few years later, they divorce, and she wants to use the embryos, but he sues to prevent her from doing so. A judge upholds the agreement they signed at the fertility clinic, which said that the embryos could be brought to term only with the consent of both partners.* Another scenario: A husband sues his ex-wife over frozen embryos the couple created together, seeking to make her a biological parent of his kids against her will.

The legal responses to such scenarios, and egg and embryo custody rights in general, vary from state to state. Most states recognize a fundamental right to reproductive autonomy when analyzing embryo disputes, with judges often ruling in favor of the person who does not want the embryo(s) used. But not always: In some states, the answer to the question "Who gets the embryos?" is "Whoever wants to make them into babies." Back in 2018, Arizona passed a first-in-the-nation law stipulating that custody of disputed embryos must be given to the party who intends to use them for reproduction.† The law explicitly

---

* Most clinics require that couples sign a contract prior to creating embryos that states their agreement about the fate of any remaining embryos after undergoing IVF.

† Reflecting on how Arizona's law gives the court guidance on how to award frozen embryos when there's a dispute during divorce proceedings, Cathi Herrod, president of the Center for Arizona Policy, said: "Just like a judge will decide

instructs a divorce court to overrule any prior agreement made by the couple in favor of the spouse who wants to make use of the frozen embryos.* In a 2023 ruling that drew criticism, a Virginia judge relied in part on a nineteenth-century law that defined enslaved people as property in a decision to allow a divorced woman to pursue using embryos that she shared with her former husband. Louisiana has a law defining embryos as "juridical persons" with the right to sue and be sued; women who undergo IVF cannot discard their unused embryos. It's not a new law; it was passed in 1986. While the law has had minimal effects to date and fertility treatments continue to be offered in the state, Louisiana's is the strictest embryo law in the country, and experts worry that it foreshadows what may be coming in many more states.

The legal gray area has grown more complicated since the fall of *Roe v. Wade,* but even before then, courts struggled to interpret laws regarding embryo custody and egg ownership. While it's unclear how many eggs are on ice, there are an estimated 1.5 million frozen embryos currently in storage in the United States, most being held for use by the couples who've created them. As the number of controversies involving human embryos increases and as the field of legal precedent surrounding frozen reproductive cells continues to emerge, future laws concerning the disposition of embryos will most likely also fall along the same pro-choice/pro-life lines. The evolving discussion of embryo rights, it seems, is really only just beginning.

One day, I came upon a "Shouts & Murmurs" piece in *The New Yorker* titled "Your Frozen Egg Has a Question":

> I live in a freezer now, with a dozen of your other eggs, and you don't. So I guess you are a "you" now, and I am a "me." But am I

---

when there are disputes over property, disputes over who gets the family dog— now, who gets the family embryos—will also be decided by a judge according to the law."

* The party/spouse who's against the reproductive use of the embryos is usually absolved of legal parental responsibility for any resulting children. But they're still being forced by the state to become a genetic parent against their will.

still thirty-five, like you? Will I continue to be thirty-five until you defrost me? And if we're going with that theory for a second—and I have temporarily stopped aging for the duration of the time that I am in this freezer, and am therefore currently in a state of suspended animation—does that mean I have temporarily ceased to exist? As you can tell, I'm freaking the fuck out in here. Not that that's your problem! Do your thing. I just figured I'd touch base to see whether you had a sense of a time frame for all this. Like, if you had to predict how long you'll be keeping me on ice, what would you say? Just a guesstimate is fine.

As funny as it was, the piece made me think about the process from a different point of view for the first time. I started wondering about all the frozen eggs on ice: How long could they stay there without going "bad," and in this case what did "going bad" entail?

Few studies have focused on outcomes beyond pregnancy. One, from a while ago, that has—the study reviewed reports published between 1986 and 2008 of more than nine hundred babies born from frozen eggs—found no difference in the rate of congenital anomalies compared to the rate for babies born with fresh eggs, meaning researchers didn't see a rise in chromosomal abnormalities or birth defects in children born from frozen eggs. A 2013 study found similar outcomes. Also, there's currently no evidence to suggest that eggs become less viable in storage, so, as far as we know, they can be frozen indefinitely. While most patients make disposition decisions about their embryos or eggs within five to ten years of freezing them, technically, in the United States, there's no limit on how long you can store frozen reproductive tissue.*

While it was reassuring to learn that, for now at least, there doesn't seem to be any compelling reason to worry about the safety of eggs on ice and potential health risks to children born from frozen eggs, it

---

* Most clinics require patients to sign a contract stipulating their frozen specimens be stored for a set number of years, and after that period of time patients can renew their contract.

wasn't lost on me that—once again—there isn't enough data yet to be fully confident.* Research with larger sample sizes is needed to reinforce this conclusion—and all of egg freezing studies' other conclusions. Experts have been saying so for years. The authors of the study on nine hundred frozen-egg-babies I just mentioned outlined the need for a systematic outcome reporting system, writing at the time: "A working knowledge of the actual number of babies born as a result of transferred cryopreserved, thawed-warmed fertilized oocytes, including fetal wellbeing, is an important step towards adequately judging the merits of this highly sought after technology." A worldwide egg freezing registry, they stated, "would help to assure the safest, most expeditious development of this technology." And yet, all these years later, no such registry exists, and there remains little information or follow-up from years of women having given birth using their frozen eggs. In time and with more robust data, we'll better understand possible risks of birth defects—if any—for children born from frozen eggs and how years of storage in liquid nitrogen may impact eggs.

In Ohio, I had witnessed the kind of permanent repercussion associated with ART that the public is rarely privy to. The tank failures were a distressing counterpoint to Remy's optimism and some of the rosier aspects of egg freezing I'd been immersed in. As I considered more seriously what happens after the thaw, as women return to use their frozen eggs, I found myself still wondering about individual cases of frozen eggs failing, and if women for whom egg freezing didn't work had been prepared for that difficult outcome.

In his book *When Breath Becomes Air,* Paul Kalanithi considers whether it is the medical expert's job to suggest what their patients should do or whether to simply provide information and sit back while patients and families figure out how to decide among their op-

---

* Especially when I zoomed out from frozen eggs and considered that there are studies showing that children born with the help of fertility treatments face various increased health risks. See the Notes section for examples.

tions. He writes that nowadays the second model is the norm, and so the proliferation of choices and medical possibilities just adds to stress and confusion. When it comes to fertility treatment, it's clear that walking patients through informed consent—the various disposition options, the reality of the success rates, the potential risks—is *so* important. Some doctors do a thorough job of this; others don't. I wasn't surprised to learn that there isn't enforced standardization of consent forms across fertility clinics; the several forms I reviewed varied greatly. SART has a detailed consent form on its website that SART-member clinics can use (and probably more should). Other limited guidance comes from ASRM's Ethics Committee, but their directives, as we've learned, exist merely in the realm of self-regulation. Proper informed consent entails collaborative discussions between physicians and patients about the technology's risks along with the limited outcome data, although as we'll see, such conversations are the exception, not the rule.

But the importance of fertility doctors helping to manage egg freezing patients' expectations, I was about to learn, was not something to gloss over.

All in One Basket

As I've said, more than 85 percent of women who have frozen their eggs have not attempted to use them. But some have, and their ordeals shed light on the precarious nature of the tightrope we walk with this new technology.

In the years since egg freezing became mainstream, accounts of it not working have increasingly been covered in major media outlets. Actor and writer Lena Dunham was a famous case. After nearly two decades of chronic pain from endometriosis, Dunham underwent surgery to have her uterus removed, and, eleven months later, her left ovary. In 2020, she froze eggs that her remaining ovary was still producing, in hopes that a gestational carrier could carry one of her fertilized eggs to term. But none of her eggs successfully fertilized. Reckoning with the end of her fertility in an essay for *Harper's Magazine,* Dunham writes: "I tried to have a child. Along the way, my body broke. . . . I had lost my way, and a half-dozen eggs sitting in Midtown promised to lead me home. Instead, each step took the process further from my body, my family, my reality. Each move was more expensive, more desperate, more lonely."

The rare instance of a cryotank failing is, obviously, one way in which frozen eggs don't lead to a baby. More common, though, are issues with safekeeping while eggs are being stored, as well as with the thawing and fertilization process when using eggs to make embryos. As we've seen, the problems can be mechanical, science-related, or the result of human error. Sometimes fertility doctors and embryologists ascertain why eggs aren't viable; sometimes they can't. Regardless, if a woman's frozen eggs or embryos are compromised and don't survive the thaw, patients are almost never given an explanation as to why. When Dayna,* a thirty-nine-year-old attorney who froze her eggs in New York City and later shipped them to Colorado after moving there, learned that her eggs had gone missing—only one egg arrived at the receiving clinic; both clinics claim not to know what happened to the rest—she hired lawyers and spent years trying to figure out what happened, to no avail. "When eggs die, there isn't a debrief," Dayna told me. It can be incredibly frustrating and dismaying paying thousands of dollars to undergo an intense procedure only to hear, "Sorry, it didn't work out. Maybe try again?" But that's usually all that's said.

Another headlines-making case was that of Brigitte Adams, who froze her eggs when she was thirty-nine. A marketing consultant living in San Francisco at the time, Adams was single and divorced when she froze her eggs. She'd learned about egg freezing from a friend who had done IVF using a sperm donor and figured with all the yoga she did and green juice she drank, her fertility was probably fine. But then Adams watched that same friend undergo multiple rounds of IVF, and the comments her friend made—*if you want to be a mom someday, you'd better get going now*—shook her. So she came up with a plan: freeze

---

* Name has been changed.

eggs now, meet and marry Mr. Right, have a baby before she turned forty (using her frozen eggs if need be), and never be a single mom.

Brigitte Adams would become egg freezing's de facto poster child. The 2014 *Bloomberg Businessweek* story about egg freezing and its exciting promises featured her on the cover. At the time, she felt somewhat excited about undergoing a new fertility procedure that was giving women more choices in, as the magazine noted provocatively, "the quest to have it all"—although she was also frustrated by the lack of resources on the procedure; neither doctors nor fertility clinic websites had much information to offer. That was why, while undergoing egg freezing, she had founded *Eggsurance,* a blog that grew into a robust community—the first of its kind—where people shared tips about the whole process. After the *Bloomberg* story ran, Adams was interviewed by major media outlets and appeared on morning talk shows, telling the world about the sense of freedom she felt after freezing her eggs. Many young women considering the procedure saw in Adams's story a road map for a happy ending. Her life had not followed the perfectly linear path she assumed it would, and theirs hadn't either. Egg freezing was a way to alter the course before the road disappeared entirely.

In late 2016, Adams was nearing forty-five and still hadn't met The Guy. Having abandoned her "don't ever be a single mom" thoughts from years earlier, she decided to start a family on her own. She excitedly unfroze the eleven eggs she'd put on ice five years earlier and selected a sperm donor. Then the horrific news started rolling in. Two eggs didn't survive the thawing process. Three more failed to fertilize. That left six embryos, of which five appeared to be abnormal. The last one, the single chromosomally normal embryo resulting from her frozen eggs, was implanted in her uterus. But, as we've learned, not all embryos that are transferred go on to develop. Then she got the devastating news that this embryo, too, had failed.

I met Brigitte in the fall of 2019. A few hours before our meeting, I listened to her speak to a ballroom full of fertility experts—the same ones who gather year after year at ASRM's annual conference. This year it was held in Philadelphia, and egg freezing was as hot a topic as ever.

"When I froze my eggs, I knew there were no guarantees," Brigitte told the audience. She wore a simple cardigan, black slacks, and low heels. "I'd researched the odds. But over the years my eggs were on ice, I began to think the rules didn't apply to me. I thought, 'Of course they're going to work for me.'" She clicked to the next slide on the movie-theater-sized screen behind her, then paused, looking up at it. The slide explained the path from frozen eggs to baby and showed the inverted pyramid, the one fertility doctors sometimes use to describe egg freezing's attrition rates—and the slide Dr. Zore showed me when she described how she counsels her patients. "This is the chart I wish I'd seen," Brigitte said, turning back to the audience, her voice sad but firm. "This slide should be laminated and given to every egg freezing patient." She'd been invited to speak at the large conference to offer a patient's perspective on egg freezing and explicitly address the doctors—and that's exactly what she did.

We met in an atrium on the top floor of the convention center. Brigitte had been immersed in the world of egg freezing for a decade and today, at least, it showed. "I'm tired," she said apologetically, looking deflated. She tucked a strand of her shoulder-length blond hair behind her ear. In a low voice, she told me what she now knows she would've asked about and perhaps tried to have done differently.

Freeze more eggs, for one. When a physician recently reviewed Brigitte's tests, they showed that her fertility was in more severe decline than expected for a woman her age, indicating that, based on her age and test results, she would have needed a lot of frozen eggs— many more than she'd had retrieved—to conceive. But no one had told her that. In addition to doing at least one more cycle, Brigitte would have frozen embryos instead of eggs. "And I would've stopped waiting for the perfect time in my career to become a mom. I would have embraced motherhood sooner," she said. When she described being told her eggs didn't work and the implanted embryo didn't result in a pregnancy, Brigitte's eyes filled with tears. I wanted to reach across the table and hug her. Instead, I thanked her for sharing her story. She didn't have to be at this reproductive medicine conference, onstage in front of thousands of fertility doctors explaining how their science and technology did not work for her. But here she was, talking about the cruel irony: how, for egg freezing's poster child, her frozen eggs ultimately failed. Brigitte didn't ask to be a character in the technology's saga, but she is willing to share what happened—how, egg by egg, all of it went wrong—because as the number of women freezing and thawing eggs continues to rise, Brigitte said, "I know more women are going to have my same story."

Brigitte's case is a quagmire of many of the possible flaws in this process. Much of what happened to her was not preventable—not yet, at least. But her story is one we can learn from. She insists we do.* Today, Brigitte continues to give talks and interviews about egg freezing, but her message has changed. Now she talks about the marketing hype and overpromises surrounding the procedure. And she encourages women to educate themselves about fertility basics because she knows that many who undergo egg freezing don't have a clear idea of the myriad components of the process, especially the reality of the success rates.†

Science can go only so far. Brigitte learned that when the crushing blow came that her frozen eggs had failed, which to some degree felt as if her clinic had failed her, too. It's frustrating to reflect on: Had more information been available at the time, had she known what to ask and then been diligent in asking more questions—she'd be thinking about all this quite differently. While she is still a proponent of egg freezing, Brigitte firmly believes women need to be better educated about the possibility of bad outcomes and that the industry needs to be more transparent. She remains frustrated about how egg freezing patients typically only see one-half of the story—the optimistic half. They need to be seeing both.‡

---

* Especially because, as she noted, the women freezing their eggs now are much younger than the first wave of egg freezers, of which she was part; they're also waiting longer before attempting to use their frozen eggs.

† Freezing eggs at an older age, it bears repeating, increases the likelihood of their being chromosomally abnormal, which is a reality of age and genetics. And, again, the freezing and thawing processes carry their own risks.

‡ A different and more pragmatic half that's also important to see: Brigitte pointed out the importance of considering and learning about actually using the eggs you've frozen. It's quite involved, as we've seen, and as she said, "If you're going

It was the bit about how important it is to figure out, as best we can, what questions to ask in the first place that resonated with me so deeply when I heard Brigitte's story. Also: how one of the worst things that happened to her ultimately led to the best thing that's happened to her. Brigitte remained determined to become a mom. After a dark period of mourning and soul-searching, she began IVF again, this time with a donor egg that had been fertilized with donor sperm to create an embryo that was then implanted in her uterus. In May 2018, when she was forty-five, she gave birth to her daughter, Georgie.

Ruthie Ackerman froze her eggs when she was thirty-five. She'd recently gotten married, but she and her husband had gone back and forth for years about having kids. Having eggs on ice felt like permission to take her time—to sit with the ambivalence she occasionally felt about motherhood, to figure out what to do about her marriage. She fully bought into egg freezing's oft-repeated marketing message: *Take your time. Your eggs will be here when you need them.* Fast-forward a few years: Ruthie, now divorced, met her current partner, Rob. They discussed the possibility of children, but because of her frozen eggs, she still felt no rush. Six years after undergoing egg freezing, Ruthie returned to thaw her eggs and learned that eight of the fourteen she'd frozen had survived. She and Rob used Rob's sperm to attempt to fertilize all eight eggs. Three eggs did fertilize, but none developed into viable embryos.

When I asked Ruthie what it felt like to go through egg freezing to no avail, she reflected on how her fertility doctor, in her view, didn't walk her through the informed consent piece thoroughly. "I wish somebody had said to me, 'Just so you know, I'm glad the science and the technology is here for you to be able to use it—but it may or may not work,'" she said, her tone a mix of remorse and

_____
to spend all that money on the first part—the freezing—you also have to know what goes along with that, especially cost-wise, to make a baby from those frozen eggs."

anger. "And so I waited. And I was willing to wait for Rob because I thought we had those eggs." I asked her about a line from an essay she'd published about her experience: *I felt less that my eggs had failed me than I had failed them.* She explained how she'd spent her twenties not doing the things her friends had been doing: taking certain jobs, meeting a certain kind of man, making a certain amount of money. "I felt like I was being punished for not being strategic enough," she told me. Punishment for not hustling to secure all she was "supposed" to as a woman, she explained. And the consequence—the price it felt like she paid for buying into the fantasy that she could have it all, on her own schedule, and for relying on a technology with no guarantees—was her eggs not working.

By this point in my journey, I'd met dozens of older women who had struggled with infertility. Most had gone through IVF, using their own or donor eggs; many ended up with a baby or two. When I told these women I was considering freezing my eggs, almost all emphatically expressed (unsolicited) advice: *If I was your age, I would run, not walk, to the nearest place to get eggs frozen.* They meant well, I knew, and spoke from a place of wishing they'd known about egg freezing or had had the opportunity to freeze their eggs years before trying to have children. But Brigitte's and Ruthie's experiences illustrated another part of egg freezing's story that's rarely acknowledged: its power to disappoint. Their frozen eggs hadn't led to babies, and by the time they learned their eggs weren't viable, their natural fertility was gone. In a stark contrast to what we often hear from our doctors, our social media feeds, and our friends at happy hour, their eggs are a chilling reminder that this far-from-perfect procedure remains riddled with mystery and heartbreak and unmet expectations.

Their stories also offer concrete bits of practical advice for anyone thinking of freezing eggs in order to have a baby later:

- Don't wait too long to thaw your frozen eggs, since you won't know if they will work until you attempt to use them.

- Make sure you freeze a lot of them, since most frozen eggs won't develop into chromosomally normal embryos.
- Do your homework, ask educated questions of your fertility doctor and clinic before you freeze, and insist on a thorough informed consent discussion.

On this last point: There are numerous factors to consider when a potential egg freezing patient is choosing a fertility clinic, but the two most important ones are a clinic's success rates and its embryology lab.* Inquire about rates of embryo formation and live birth, as well as success rates specific to your age group—and proceed with caution if the clinic isn't forthcoming about its outcomes or has few results to speak of. Ask about lab safety protocols. Embryology labs aren't created equal; almost every aspect of a fertility clinic's lab can be different from the one across the street. "You can take a brilliant reproductive endocrinologist and put him or her in a poorly functioning lab, and that fertility doctor is going to have very poor results," said Dr. Timothy Hickman, then president of SART, when I asked him about this often overlooked component. "The lab is really the key part of this whole enterprise." Also, look into credentials: You want your fertility doctor to be fellowship-trained and board-certified in obstetrics and gynecology as well as reproductive endocrinology and infertility. Finally, ask where, exactly, your frozen eggs will be stored.

Two years after the tank failures and a few months after the ASRM conference where I'd met Brigitte, a different sort of reckoning was about to occur—a catastrophe that would have a major impact on egg freezing, and, well, everything else.

---

* For more on choosing a fertility doctor and the importance of the lab, I recommend FertilityIQ's five-module course on the subject (there's a fee, but it's worth it): fertilityiq.com/the-ivf-laboratory/introduction-to-the-ivf-laboratory-and-course-plan.

Reproduction Reimagined

~~~~~~

Inconceivable

The beginning of the pandemic fell at the blurry line between late winter and early spring in Colorado. We didn't know anything about the coronavirus or how long we'd be hunkered down for. All we really knew, in those first months of 2020, was that a plague was up-ending the world. Covid-19 deaths mounted, the numbers unfathomable. New normals rearranged themselves in our homes, our grocery stores, our lives. We began wearing masks everywhere. We grew more afraid. We doom-scrolled. We settled in. I waited to feel anxious about spending so much time alone in my apartment. I thought I would resist the stillness, find ways to distract myself from quieting down. I'm good at drumming up noise when I fear solitude. Instead, as the weight of the days changed, as I felt time slow, I slowed with it. I learned the sounds of my neighborhood, the small slice of downtown Boulder I call home. I felt both opened up and tucked in; tender parts were exposed, but I wanted to keep them nestled. I walked the streets at dusk, struck by the hush, the empty sidewalks. I lay on the living room floor and hugged my legs to my chest, marveling at what it felt like to not be *doing* and *going* every minute of every day. I spent days with only myself and enjoyed it. I remember how that felt like a small miracle.

One thing I did not do during the pandemic that scores of other women did was freeze my eggs. In the context of a global pandemic, fertility preservation took on a new, urgent meaning. The number of women freezing their eggs had already been increasing year over year at fertility clinics across the country, and the uptick continued during Covid—despite the fact that most clinics were forced to shut down and suspend fertility treatments during the pandemic's early months. There was an overall 39 percent increase in egg retrievals compared to pre-pandemic levels and, interestingly, a notable increase in egg freezers under age thirty-five, as well as a significant decrease in time between patients' initial consultation and their egg retrieval. Between August 2020 and October 2021, Shady Grove Fertility, which has more than forty locations across the country, saw a 95 percent increase in women freezing their eggs compared to the same fifteen-month period pre-Covid. Kindbody quadrupled its revenue and tripled its number of clinics in 2021. NYU Langone Fertility Center saw almost three times the number of women—overall younger patients—starting egg freezing cycles in 2022 compared to 2019. And in the United Kingdom, where egg and embryo freezing cycles are the fastest-growing form of fertility treatments, clinics saw a 60 percent increase in egg freezing from 2019 to 2021, which experts said was in part prompted by the pandemic.

At first, I was amazed by the extent of the pandemic's impact on the egg freezing market. Then I spoke with a few reproductive psychologists and understood the larger context that such a seismic event had on how people thought about fertility and family. For many women, myself included, as life became quieter, our eggs became louder. The pandemic gave us the opportunity to reconsider so much: where we live, how we work, whom we date, and what kinds of families, chosen and biological, we want to cultivate. Amid the anxiety of Covid, and the dating drought that it precipitated, many of those who could afford it—or who still worked for employers that pay for it—invested in egg freezing.

There were practical reasons for why many women felt that the pandemic offered them more of a window to pursue egg freezing. Thousands of them suddenly found themselves with more time, working remotely and traveling less. Many had more funds available since they were spending less money. Others, who combated isolation by moving back in with their families, had more emotional support as well. Existential reasons played a role, too. Sharon Covington, director of psychological support services at Shady Grove Fertility, told me that as many women sat at home, unable to date, considering what they most valued in life, "they realize that time is ticking. They feel extremely alone and isolated and think, 'Well, I don't know if I'm going to find a partner, but I know I want to have a family and I want to keep that option open.' And so they decide to pursue egg freezing."

This was true for Fatima,* who told me the pandemic prompted her to freeze her eggs in September 2020, when she was thirty-six. Originally from Pakistan and now living in Los Angeles, Fatima told me about the pressure she'd felt from cultural norms to get married and start a family in her twenties. She'd wanted to be a mother for a long time, but in her thirties she began to make peace with not having biological children when she realized she was one of the last of her siblings and cousins to not have kids. But then the pandemic brought on an overwhelming sense of grief that she might be out of options if she did decide to one day have children. Then her employer—she works in the education sector—started offering fertility treatment coverage through Carrot, a fertility benefits company. "The pandemic made me feel such a lack of control over everything in my life," said Fatima. "There's so much uncertainty and ambiguity. Freezing my eggs was something I could have control over. And that felt really empowering."

You would think, perhaps, that in this context—when life is on hold but eggs continue aging, as they are wont to do—I, too, might have decided to do it. It was, on paper, an extremely appropriate moment. I was thirty now. I wasn't dating; no one was, really, and our social lives were on hold for the foreseeable future. I sometimes caught myself mulling over the prospect of children with more urgency than I

---

* Name has been changed.

ever had before. You'd think it would be easier for me to rationalize egg freezing in the absence of the "right" partner. And so you might think that, more than at any other point in my journey, this was the opportune time to freeze my eggs. You'd probably be right on all counts. But as logical as it very well might be, I couldn't seem to make the logic work. I'd done the research, thoroughly examined all the angles. And yet I still didn't arrive at the conclusion I'd thought I would, the one that would allow me to freeze my eggs and sleep at night, confident in my decision.

I am not alone in not knowing how to navigate this moment, I thought what felt like a thousand times during the pandemic. Control was on my mind in a different way now, my brain ablaze with the frustrated urge to "take control" that had come to dominate my and so many others' lives during this unprecedented event. How do we navigate the loss of control? My answer, at least in part, was to throw myself into learning about what the future might hold for egg freezing—the final puzzle piece of my quest.

One aspect of egg freezing that had not changed during the pandemic, despite the droves of women doing it, was the fear that the technology would ultimately not deliver on its promises. Perhaps it was naïve of me to think the data on success rates would have materialized by now, but for the most part, they hadn't.

"I really believe that the generation of women now who are freezing their eggs are trailblazers," said Dr. Shahine, the reproductive endocrinologist in Seattle, on a video call in April 2020. "And these are the people who, in five or ten years, will help us find out really how well it works for people. Because, right now, we just don't have the data." Through my computer screen, I noticed her face showed real concern. I wasn't used to seeing her brow furrowed; on Dr. Shahine's educational TikTok and Instagram videos, which are famous in the fertility world, she's usually lighthearted and sarcastic, in a funny way. "I worry that there's going to be a huge backlash against my industry and the doctors," she went on. "That when people come back to use their eggs and they don't work, they're going to be really angry because they'll feel like they weren't counseled well."*

Deborah Anderson-Bialis, of FertilityIQ, had mentioned this potential backlash to me a while back. "I think it's inevitable that a large number of people will be disappointed when their eggs don't work," she said. "There will be a reckoning. And I believe that will make the places that are marketing this as a very easy quick fix and a guarantee look bad—and I don't think that's a bad thing." In a 2021 *New Yorker* article, Peter Klatsky, a San Francisco–based reproductive endocrinologist and co-founder of Spring Fertility, put it more strongly: "When women come back for their eggs, it's going to be a nightmare," he said. "It's going to be really bad for our whole field. It could make people say, 'Well, egg-freezing doesn't work,' because there's massive variability" in outcomes between clinics. The experts I spoke with agreed that it was a matter not of *if* an egg freezing backlash would occur but *when*. One way to mitigate it: more honest and educational conversations *now* about the likelihood of using frozen eggs successfully.

In the several years I'd been researching and reporting on egg freezing, two major changes had transpired: one, the decreased stigma surrounding egg freezing, and two, the massive jump in employers paying for it—although accessibility and affordability remained major issues. Soon, hopefully, we'll be able to add increased transparency and realistic expectation-setting to that list, as potential egg freezers become better informed.†

---

* Now, however, Dr. Shahine is more optimistic. She feels people *are* more aware about egg freezing's lack of guarantee these days, as well as about the procedure's pros and cons. She's less worried today than she was when egg freezing cocktail parties were all the rage years ago. And she's heartened by the increasing number of people who share their egg freezing stories—not just successes, but failures, too. "People are much better prepared for egg freezing's [various] potential outcomes," she said. I can't say I fully agree with her, but her changed stance made me feel more hopeful.

† Researchers are working on tools to help people considering egg freezing make the right decision for them. I'm hopeful that this represents a move toward more openness about the real costs and benefits of egg freezing.

As I continued to think about the technology's flaws, I also kept dwelling on how the dawn of egg freezing coincided with a relatively novel sentiment: For many women, being able to have children when they want them is the ultimate sign of independence. This symbol of autonomy is more central to a modern woman's sense of self than perhaps anything else. We may look back and be able to say egg freezing was the next revolution for women's reproductive lives. But even if it's not—even if it doesn't end up affording women the chance to recalibrate their baby-making timelines the way they hope it will—we will almost certainly acknowledge egg freezing's powerful role in changing how we think about fertility, family, and feminism over the past decade.

Then, while sitting at home during the pandemic thinking about the many women rushing to freeze their eggs and wondering why I wasn't, I learned about a fertility technology company that had the potential to, at long last, solve one of the industry's biggest problems: the protection and well-being of eggs and embryos on ice. As soon as it was safe to do so, I got on a plane to see for myself.

Fertile Ground

In April 2022, I flew to New York City to visit TMRW Life Sciences, a biotech start-up whose technology automates reproductive tissue's storage and management. All the buzz I'd heard about the company— backed by Peter Thiel, Google Ventures, even Amy Schumer—had me thinking that this cryostorage venture was the future of fertility in the way that mattered most.

Walking up to the company's U.S. headquarters in Lower Manhattan, I passed kids playing dodgeball in the sun next to a school, the sort of normal scene that now, two years into the pandemic, struck me as precious. I rode an elevator up to TMRW's main floor and was escorted to a small room where I took off my mask and took a rapid test, per the company's Covid protocols. Several minutes later, Cynthia Hudson greeted me. With her pearl studs, gray loafers, and collared shirt under a blue half-zip pullover, Hudson gave off both scientist and corporate vibes, which was fitting, since she's TMRW's vice president of clinical strategy and an embryologist with more than two decades of experience. She led the way to a massive room on the street level, where TMRW's white, sleek cryogenic freezers—the company's CryoRobots—are kept. The company's latest model, the CryoRobot Select, looked as if Apple had made a super-sophisticated extra-large ATM machine that stored and dispensed frozen eggs and embryos.

Of the many advancements ART has seen since the beginning of human IVF nearly fifty years ago, one major facet has remained mostly unchanged: the shockingly analog method of storing frozen repro-ductive tissue. Founded in 2018, TMRW is changing that with what it calls "the world's first automated platform" of integrated software and hardware that digitally tracks frozen embryos, eggs, and sperm. The software developed by the company uses radio frequency identi-fication, or RFID, an identity management coding system. RFID, which works similar to the way a car's VIN number or a book's ISBN number does but also uses tags and readers, replaces the handwritten labels that most fertility clinics use to identify patients' gametes and embryos. The wireless system also records an audit trail, which auto-matically captures the data of who did what and when and constantly monitors tanks' levels and temperatures. The company's hardware is the CryoRobots, which are similar to the storage tanks, or dewars, that most clinics use to store frozen reproductive cells. Traditional dewars, though, resemble old-fashioned metal milk cans that you might find on a farm; TMRW's tanks reminded me of a refrigerator-sized R2-D2, the *Star Wars* droid, for their technology-powered ca-pabilities.

With the TMRW's FDA-cleared system, when a patient is ready to use their eggs or embryos, a robotic mechanism picks the specimen and delivers it to the embryologist, as a vending machine might. Sen-sors within the CryoRobots conduct thousands of automated checks daily to monitor the safety and well-being of the tissues inside. (The company's motto: "TMRW never sleeps so you can.") This is espe-cially impressive considering that the only way to check on a person's eggs or embryos with the current method of frozen tissue storage is to manually open the tank and lift them out of the liquid nitrogen, which disturbs other patients' specimens unnecessarily.*

As we stood talking next to one of the massive freezers, Hudson alternated between standing with her hands tucked in the pockets of her dark jeans and excitedly demonstrating to me how the Cryo-Robot Select's iris-scan security feature worked. As a seasoned embryologist, Hudson knew firsthand how unsustainable the current low-tech and human-error-prone systems used by most of the country's fertility labs were. "These are incredible professionals," she said, referring to embryologists, "but we've got to arm them with better tools. And I think patients are very quickly going to start insisting on that, as soon as they know that they're an option." Maybe Hudson's passion was contagious, or maybe it was remembering what it felt like interviewing patients at the cemetery in Ohio after the tank failures and seeing dewars lined up wall-to-wall and shoved under desks in the back offices of fertility clinics I'd visited, but as I peered inside a CryoRobot, I felt a rush of excitement, convinced I was looking at one of the fertility industry's biggest advances in decades.

If Kindbody is the SoulCycle of fertility, TMRW's monitoring system is the industry's Google Nest Cam meets ADT Home Security, providing real-time information about frozen specimens and identifying issues *before* something happens. The command center manages data from every TMRW CryoRobot in the country, remotely monitoring clinics' systems through its predictive analytics. Eventually, patients will be able to check in virtually on their eggs or embryos, too, via TMRW's app (which is still in development). A pre-baby baby monitor, one might say.

TMRW works with more than fifty clinics across the country, some of which operate networks of multiple centers, who have or are

---

* One dewar—the type typically used at fertility clinics—can usually hold the specimens of about two hundred patients. TMRW's machine can hold about twenty times more.

in the process of ditching their dewars for TMRW's CryoRobots and automated system. The company is expanding overseas, too. It's also developing several regional bio-repositories that it plans to use, in addition to its New York facility, to store gametes and embryos from patients around the country. Patients can store with TMRW through their fertility clinic or individually; the company charges individual consumers about $600 a year, as of this writing, to store with TMRW directly, which is on the lower end of average annual storage costs.*

TMRW begins its pitch by predicting that between two hundred million and three hundred million IVF babies will have been born by the end of this century. Some fertility experts find that number too conservative, actually, but TMRW's point is that most of these IVF births will rely on tens of millions of frozen eggs and embryos— a mind-boggling amount that would quickly overwhelm the current IVF infrastructure. TMRW sees itself as the solution for the hundreds of thousands of fertility patients requiring frozen gamete storage in coming years. And we do need a solution. In the wake of the 2018 tank failures and as embryo mix-ups make headlines with more frequency, patients have every reason to be scrutinous about how their frozen reproductive tissue is handled. Joshua Abram, TMRW's founder, likened the catastrophes to the sinking of the *Titanic*. "When we think about the *Titanic* on its inevitable path to the iceberg, it's clear now that the failure was in not having enough lifeboats—and in not having the foresight to see issues before they become problems," said Abram when we first spoke. "That's a fairly apt metaphor for what's happening in fertility clinics today. The risks are hidden most of the time." Hidden though they may be, risks should be planned for, before they lead to devastating consequences—as indeed they have. TMRW hopes to preempt the extreme headlines as well as the day-to-day fertility clinic lab errors that go unseen, making the loss or mixing up of eggs and embryos never-events.

* TMRW offers discounts if a patient prepays for multiple years of storage. ReproTech, a large network of cryobanks, offers patients similar prepay discounts, and also has lower-than-average storage prices. Generally speaking, a patient can often bring down their egg storage costs—sometimes by half—if they arrange to have them moved from the clinic she froze at to an offsite storage facility.

Tara Comonte, who served as TMRW's CEO until June 2023, came to the femtech start-up from Shake Shack, where she was president and chief financial officer. Like many women in the fertility technology space, Comonte is also an IVF mom; she had her daughter when she was in her early forties. The five frozen embryos left over from her IVF cycles are housed at TMRW's cryobank at its Manhattan headquarters, to which, in early 2023, Comonte moved them from the clinic where she'd undergone fertility treatment. "We're in a whole new generation of patient transparency and I think it is overdue," said Comonte, who is fifty, when we spoke a few weeks after my visit. "[Most] patients have no idea how outdated the processes are for storing their precious eggs and embryos. And I think there will be shock and reality checks when it's realized how many decades the storage process has sat unchanged."

A few months later, I spoke with a woman whose story was one of several I'd heard that made the need for more reliable storage options for reproductive cells painfully clear. In June 2022, Danielle was eight months pregnant and scrambling to figure out how to move her and her husband's remaining frozen embryos out of Texas. *Roe v. Wade* had just been overturned, and Danielle, like many people across the country living in more restrictive states who have eggs and embryos left over from fertility treatment on ice, was afraid of how the ruling would impact her embryos. She and her husband decided to move them to a different state; they'd travel there to use them if they chose to have another child.

When Danielle called her fertility clinic to ask about moving her embryos, she was told the clinic didn't know where they were. The clinic eventually located them, but Danielle was shaken. "It was something I never questioned until now: where my embryos are, who's watching them, and how safe they are," she told me. I was reminded of how most fertility patients have no good alternative with regard to storing their genetic material once they choose a clinic and are locked into their facility's storage methods and prices. Then, on social media, Danielle learned about TMRW and reached out right away. She was the first individual patient whose embryos TMRW arranged to transport to its New York facility.

Of course, there are risks to replacing humans with digital machines as custodians, but the likelihood of human error surpasses that of a CryoRobot confusing barcodes on petri dishes. The more I considered TMRW's revolutionary technology, the worse the fertility industry's status-quo method of storing and monitoring reproductive tissue seemed. What kind of investment—which frozen eggs and embryos certainly are—can you never see, check up on, verify? When do you ever spend thousands of dollars and not receive reassurance that what you paid for and entrusted the safekeeping to has gone unharmed? It seemed so obvious, the fertility industry's need for a long-overdue redo of a faulty system. But even obvious deficiencies take time to fix.

Groundbreaking reproductive technology lingered in my mind in the weeks after my TMRW trip. A crucial component of cryopreservation's future, it was clear, is automation. Scientists will continue to shape the future of fertility, of course, because they're the ones who've brought us the techniques we have today. But egg freezing isn't the only innovation changing ART's landscape. "The ability to fertilize an egg outside of a woman's body, without sexual congress between two human beings, has led to a host of other advances and reproductive improvisations that can extend and expand the scope of possibility for when and with whom (if anyone) we can have children," writes Rebecca Traister in her book *All the Single Ladies*. Entire texts have been written about what's on reproductive medicine's horizon, but a few of the discoveries and technologies in development are too wild for me not to mention.

Ovarian tissue freezing could be the next egg freezing. The procedure's experimental label was removed in 2019, and as the technique has continued to advance, hundreds of live births have resulted. Doctors surgically remove a woman's ovary, or part of it, then freeze the egg-producing portion of the ovary—the outer layer of ovarian tissue that contains the follicles. When the woman is ready to try to get pregnant, the strips of ovarian tissue are thawed and transplanted back into

her body to restore fertility and endocrine function.* The procedure
has mostly been performed on prepubescent girls about to undergo
chemotherapy to treat cancer who want to preserve their fertility (egg
freezing isn't an option for them). But it can also be—and is being—
used by adult women who don't have time to freeze eggs before cancer
treatment, transgender men hoping to retain the chance to have biological children, and women wanting to delay menopause. In this case,
a woman has slices of her ovary taken out (as with egg freezing, the
younger she is, the better) and, once she enters menopause years later,
doctors graft the tissue back into her body, thereby restoring her sex
hormones, which pauses menopause and its unpleasant side effects.

Uterine transplants. In December 2017, in Dallas, Texas, a woman
who was born without a uterus gave birth. That landmark event, part
of an ongoing uterus transplant clinical trial at Baylor University Medical Center, was the first of its kind in the United States. "When I
started my career, we didn't even have sonograms," said Dr. Robert T.
Gunby Jr., the OB/GYN who delivered the baby, in an interview
with *Time.* "Now we are putting in uteruses from someone else and
getting a baby." While uterine transplants likely won't become
mainstream—there's no need for them to—it's a revolutionary procedure for the right type of patient, and a big breakthrough for reproductive science.†

Drugs that could prolong female fertility. Ovarian aging has long been
an understudied field, but that's starting to change, as experts studying

---

* Where the ovarian tissue is reimplanted depends on the patient's circumstances.
If her entire ovary wasn't removed, the tissue can be placed near it, where it re-
gains blood supply, and ovarian activity—including egg production—resumes
after a few months. Doctors have also transplanted ovarian tissue to the forearm,
the abdominal wall, and the area just above the pubic bone—places that have
several blood vessels, which help the ovarian tissue grow and produce eggs. (If
ovarian tissue is transplanted someplace other than the pelvis, the patient would
only be able to get pregnant via IVF.)

† Perhaps even more remarkable than the science is the fact that more than seventy women contacted Baylor expressing interest in donating their uterus. These
women—many of whom have no relationship with a potential recipient—
volunteered to have their uterus removed and transplanted not to prolong the life
of the recipient (as is the case with most organ transplants) but to offer a stranger
a shot at motherhood.

reproductive longevity attract more funding and attention for their efforts to figure out how to make ovaries work for longer. Their research could lead to learning how to extend a person's reproductive years, and potentially life span, by delaying menopause. Scientists have also identified a drug that prolongs egg viability in microscopic roundworms—their unfertilized eggs show an age-related decline in quality similar to that of human eggs—which could theoretically extend women's fertility by three to six years. Drugs that slow down menopause and prolong the ovaries' natural functioning are already in development.

Artificial intelligence is helping embryologists better select embryos most likely to result in a healthy birth. On a larger scale, the ability to more precisely pick viable embryos to implant could improve success rates, reduce the risk of pregnancy loss, and bring IVF costs down. Also in the works: editing eggs and sperm to rid them of diseases.

Artificial wombs. Researchers have developed rudimentary artificial uteruses, proving that it's possible to separate natural gestation from the process of having biological children. And human embryos have been grown in ectogenesis, the process of human or animal gestation in an artificial environment, for several years now. Although years away from being a reality, complete human ectogenesis and the potential for "motherless births" will have myriad moral and legal implications, particularly with regard to abortion rights.

Ovaries grown in a lab. In 2021, five years after successfully converting skin cells from a mouse into fertile eggs, two Japanese reproductive biologists constructed an ovary organoid—a mini organ-like structure—made entirely from stem cells in mice. The pair of scientists are now trying to repeat the construction of mini-ovaries with human stem cells, also with the goal of using them to grow an egg. New ovarian stem cell discoveries have researchers working on building an artificial ovary that could produce eggs and jump-start hormonal function for cancer survivors, as well as potentially delay menopause.

Egg-making technology. IVG, or in vitro gametogenesis, refers to converting nonreproductive adult human cells into artificial gametes. The emerging technology involves custom-making human eggs and sperm in the laboratory from any cell in a person's body. For fertility patients, IVG would solve the problem of not having enough eggs, because there'd be no need to harvest them. And if lab-made eggs and sperm could be derived from a person's stem cells to create embryos, solo parents could create a child on their own and same-sex couples could have biological children that share the genes of both partners. Finally, this technology could remove, or at least dramatically reduce, the concerns about exposing young, generally healthy women to the high doses of hormones that are currently necessary to stimulate egg production. IVG "is on the precipice of materialization," a reproductive biology specialist told NPR in 2023. "And IVF will probably never be the same."

Researchers have also spent years exploring how to mature eggs that have been extracted from the body. This process, called in vitro maturation, or IVM, is when a woman's immature oocytes are extracted and then "ripened" outside the body. The ASRM recently declared the technology to be nonexperimental. IVM, which eradicates the need for most of the self-injected, ovary-stimulating drugs and thus requires less medication, money, and time than conventional IVF and egg freezing, is the primary focus of Gameto, a biotech start-up founded in 2020.* The company, which hopes to make fertility treatment safer and more widely accessible, was co-founded by Martin Varsavsky—who, you'll recall, founded Prelude, the nationwide fertility clinic mega-network.

Fertility treatment for women has been focused on making the best possible use of whatever women have left. That will change when we discover a way to regenerate human eggs via stem cell technology, perhaps the most consequential of the on-the-cusp technologies mentioned above. Part of the future of fertility will lie in developing new procedures and techniques—but part of it lies in better understanding the technologies we already employ. When the Italian doctors who

---

* Dina Radenkovic, a physician turned entrepreneur and Gameto's CEO, said in a 2023 *New Yorker* article: "We're really hopeful of allowing women to go through I.V.F. with much fewer side effects, less clinical time, and a lower cost—something that you could do in, like, egg freezing kiosks. I see it almost like an extension of the beauty studio, where being proactive about your reproduction and longevity just seems like an act of self-care."

developed egg freezing technology started working together in the 1980s, they never envisioned egg freezing as a way to fulfill women's desires to "have it all." Except that's precisely how we've come to view it—and we're rapidly embracing egg freezing without pausing to consider, for one thing, how society is changing as more and more people postpone childbearing. Or what it means—what it says about our modern culture, about *us*—that so many women, myself included, do not feel free to be pregnant when we are fertile and young.*

Revolutionary technology is by nature bound up with contentious benefits and repercussions, as well as terribly exciting implications. And the fact that it is now possible for almost anyone with adequate resources to become a parent *is* terribly exciting. When you stop to think about it, it's wild that humans are reproducing in ways that would have been unimaginable just several decades ago. As social ideas about coupling, mating, and parenting continue to change, the pioneering technological developments in the works mark the beginning of a new era of reproductive medicine, with major implications for fertility research and beyond.

Medicine, Morality, and the Pursuit of Parenthood

Around this time, I caught up with my cousin Bridget. Needing to start cancer treatment immediately meant she couldn't freeze her eggs beforehand. Instead, she received monthly Zoladex shots—a type of hormone therapy that stops the release of LH, so that her body stopped producing estrogen—which effectively shut down her ovaries during chemotherapy, the aim being to help preserve her fertility.

---

* I remain torn by the popular view that egg freezing, and ART in general, equals reproductive freedom. I think about this often, most recently while listening to the podcast *The Retrievals,* a chilling five-part narrative series from Serial Productions and *The New York Times.* "One of the central tensions of fertility treatment, basically since its inception, has been: Is this a patriarchal system or a feminist one?" said reporter and host Susan Burton. "On the one hand, you have a top-down system that, frankly, was designed by men, and there's tons of drugs and doctors telling you what to do with your body. On the other hand, being able to decide when and how to have a baby—and the possibilities that fertility medicine opens up for patients in all kinds of situations—this is also reproductive freedom. If you have access to it."

When Bridget woke up after her mastectomy in more pain than she has ever experienced before or since, her first thought was: *I never want my daughter or granddaughter to go through this.* She and Chris knew it would be a while before she was cleared to try to become pregnant, but they started to delve into family planning options, aware of the 50 percent chance that their children would inherit the gene mutation. They decided that if her fertility held up and if they could afford it—two very big ifs—they would genetically test their embryos and select the healthiest one to get pregnant with via IVF. They'd use PGT-M, a test performed on embryos that looks for the presence of a specific, disease-causing gene, making it possible to identify which embryos do not have a BRCA gene mutation.* By now, Bridget was confident she was going to survive cancer, but she was consumed with worry that it was going to prevent her from having a healthy family. *Of course I'll beat cancer,* she wrote in her journal the week she was diagnosed. *But to think that this may rob us of the ability to have a family is something that I can't get over.* At Chris's graduation from business school, Bridget sat in the audience crying, thinking about how in a different version of life she'd be sitting there with their toddler, instead of wondering if she'd ever have one.

When Bridget's period came back a few months after she finished chemotherapy, her oncologist told her she had "very strong ovaries." She was elated. While she waited for the okay from her doctors to begin freezing embryos, she did what she normally does in stressful situations: making to-do lists. She researched insurance options, joined online support groups, and stared at her and Chris's savings account balance.† Roughly two years after she was diagnosed and six months after completing cancer treatment, Bridget underwent her

---

* PGT-A, a more generic form of preimplantation genetic testing, screens for common chromosomal abnormalities. Selective embryo transfer—the process of identifying and using an embryo with a high chance of successful pregnancy—is an option for many couples who are at risk for transmitting an inherited condition.

† She also spent many hours on the phone with insurance companies and doctors jumping through hoops to get approval to access ART benefits without an infertility diagnosis.

first egg retrieval, fertilizing the eggs with Chris's sperm and genetically testing the resulting embryos. Over the next three years, she
raced the clock, undergoing six egg retrievals in an effort to get as
many BRCA1-negative embryos on ice before needing to have her
fallopian tubes and ovaries surgically removed.* Because of IVF and
the ability to genetically test and select embryos, Bridget was freed
from the worry and guilt of potentially passing on BRCA1 via a
spontaneous pregnancy.† Using her and Chris's chromosomally normal frozen embryos, she gave birth to a son when she was thirty-three
and, later, a daughter. Neither child has the BRCA1 mutation.

"I feel overwhelmingly grateful that science allows us to make this
choice to give the rest of our family a little bit of a safer life, and that
we have had the insurance coverage to do it," Bridget told me.‡ People
with fertility-threatening medical conditions often struggle to cobble
together funding from various sources to preserve their fertility, which
adds significant financial pressure to an already stressful situation. The
current political climate surrounding reproductive rights has made her
gratitude swell, too. "When I needed an abortion, I almost immediately got a safe and legal appointment at a clinic less than three miles
from my house," she said. "I could afford it. I think about this a lot:
how many women and couples, especially now, who have to make the
same heartbreaking decision we did, don't have the access or means to
give themselves the best possible chance to treat cancer. How infuriating that is. How that's the opposite of 'pro-life.'"

Genetically testing embryos is complicated, and there are certainly
drawbacks in addition to the many positives. But Bridget's story is a

---

* To reduce the risk of ovarian cancer mortality, surgeons generally remove the
ovaries as well as the fallopian tubes in women with a BRCA1 genetic mutation,
typically between the ages of thirty-five and forty. Ideally, the women will have
completed childbearing by then.

† Nineteen of their resulting embryos were tested for BRCA1 using PGT-M; five
were non-BRCA1-affected and chromosomally normal.

‡ Four rounds of IVF were covered through Chris's employer at the time; the last
two rounds were covered by Bridget's employer. Later, Bridget reflected: "I cannot overstate that if we hadn't had insurance coverage, IVF with PGT-M would
likely not have been an option for us, and a lot of my feelings on my fertility and
this situation would probably be very different."

clear-cut example of the power of both IVF and genetic testing. As I reflected on all she'd gone through, I was once again struck by remarkable science and technologies that enabled her to have biological children—why such technologies were invented and what they make possible, as well as all they were leading to. ART has already changed millions of lives for the better. It will continue to do so. But I also understood another, more dispassionate, perspective: Just because we can make a baby using certain tools does not mean we should. Biological boundaries and ethical guidelines demand that we consider the question that's on the tip of our tongues: Just how far can science push the boundaries of human fertility? Just how far *should* it?

Our field, more than ANY field in medicine, has the ability to literally change society as we know it, the text on my phone screen read. It was from Dr. Anate Brauer, director of IVF at Shady Grove Fertility New York. I'd been pinging her with questions about the implications of the latest biomedical technologies I'd been learning about. Fertility doctors like Dr. Brauer, I knew, had long been weighing the potential ramifications of these newer ART developments, and my recent conversations with her and other experts had helped me to clarify some of their moral and ethical implications.

As genetic testing becomes more sophisticated and commonplace, decisions about screening embryos and making disposition choices about them will become more difficult. It's a slippery slope. IVG could supercharge the path to designer children. DNA editing in human embryos raises ethical questions about the prospect of controversial gene-editing techniques being used clinically to correct defects in, or even enhance, embryos. Such a laboratory process would also permit unfettered genetic editing with DNA engineering tools such as CRISPR,* which is already sharpening some of the old tensions that came with IVF: the specter of selective abortion and eugenic selection of offspring. Before this happens, though, advances in human

---

* CRISPR stands for "clustered regularly interspaced short palindromic repeats." (Quite the mouthful.)

genetic engineering are likely to play out through preimplantation genetic testing. As geneticists become more proficient in mapping out DNA sequences that correspond to specific human attributes, PGT—which already allows sex selection, used by IVF patients in the United States all the time—may be increasingly used to screen embryos with far more detail, including for intelligence and even cosmetic traits. For people like Bridget, PGT is life-changing, making it possible to have children without passing on certain debilitating gene mutations, but it's not difficult to imagine the procedure becoming another form of ART adopted for elective, widespread use by the public.

And so the ethical and philosophical debate about the reproductive revolution rages on, bringing us back to the lack of regulation in ART and how that lack has contributed to the fertility industry growing rapidly, without many legal or ethical constraints. To that end, the authors of the book *Babies of Technology* have outlined what it would look like to create a federal administrative agency that would be responsible for maintaining a database of all ART cycles and use of eggs and sperm in the United States. Advantages of having such an agency, the authors say, include monitoring advertisements for fertility clinics to ensure accuracy and—arguably most important—assuring equal access to fertility treatments for people of all socioeconomic levels. This regulatory body could also establish detailed rules governing how clinics operate and provide consequences for those that do not comply. It's a compelling vision—and a shame nothing like this is in the works yet.

More broadly, these scientific developments point to a future in which reproduction is moved entirely outside the body. In *The End of Sex,* the Stanford bioethicist Henry Greely writes about the coming obsolescence of sex for the purpose of conceiving children. He contends that the technological developments within genetics and stem cell research mean that, in the near future, "humans will begin, very broadly, to select consciously and knowingly the genetic variations and thus at least some of the traits and characteristics of our children." So we're dealing with a real beast here, a fact I did not fully grasp or appreciate until well into this journey. The more I learned about how technology is fundamentally altering reproduction, the more enthralled I've become with the inefficient, complex, impossibly random act that is creating human life. I have also grown quite fond of my single ovary and would like for it to someday produce an egg that meets a nice sperm to grow in a welcoming nest of a uterus inside me. Most women are still having babies the old-fashioned way. But if Greely's prediction is accurate and the act of sex to make a baby is going by the wayside, well, I look forward to a ride at the carnival before it closes.

A few years ago, on the day after Christmas, my brother and sister-in-law pushed a holiday card across the dinner table for my mother to open. Inside was a sonogram, the expected due date handwritten on the back. My parents beamed—their wish to be grandparents was coming true—and I burst into tears that were partly from shock and partly from joy, completely overwhelmed with emotion. My brother and sister-in-law's first child, a healthy baby girl, was born several months later, in the middle of the pandemic. It was a humbling reminder that, for all we try to anticipate and control, choices around some of life's biggest moments unfold differently for all of us.

Throughout the pandemic, I found myself thinking about how I felt after Ben and I broke up: unsure of so much, except for knowing that something fundamental was missing from our relationship—a mutual deep level of trust and respect, I realized only in hindsight—and how, without it, I couldn't move forward, couldn't make it work in my head or my heart. I now felt a similar way about egg freezing. For a while, I couldn't trust whatever decision I made or unmade about egg freezing unless I was sure I'd done my due diligence to understand every aspect of it. And so as my journey progressed, I went farther and deeper to find the answers I sought, trusting the world—science, stories, stone-cold facts—more than I trusted myself. But the farther afield I went, the more I realized that the answers to this particular search lay closer to hand. It was an inkling I'd first had on a trip to Italy, not so long ago—a moment when everything shifted.

A Journalist and Her Ovary

~~~~~~

Walking into the Past

It was September, a few years ago, and I was flying to Italy for the wedding of a family friend. Before I left, I emailed Dr. Raffaella Fabbri and Dr. Eleonora Porcu—the biologist and fertility doctor who had forever altered egg freezing's trajectory with their discoveries at the University of Bologna three decades earlier—asking to meet. I wanted to know what they thought about the technology now, decades after they'd developed it and a few years since it had become mainstream. Where were we headed?

On the train from Milan to Bologna, I reviewed my notes. When I arrived, I walked from the train station to the university, marveling at the impressive porticoes—column-lined sheltered walkways—that the city is famous for. I passed boutique clothing stores and alleys lined with parked mopeds. Statues of the Virgin Mary were scattered everywhere, the city's Catholic roots in evidence on every corner. The University of Bologna was exactly as I had envisioned it, regal and old-looking. I walked inside the university's hospital building and called Dr. Fabbri, the biologist, to let her know I'd arrived. (The doctors no longer work together, so I met them in their separate offices.) A few minutes later, she greeted me.

Dr. Fabbri wore a white lab coat, pens sticking out of the breast pocket, and pink glasses on a chain around her neck. Her hair was white-blond and straight, and her skin pale; her eyelashes were coated in blue mascara, and her fingernails were unpolished. I followed her through the bowels of the building to her basement office, near the laboratory she worked in. The drab-colored hallways reminded me of a 1970s locker room. It couldn't have looked or felt more different from the bright, modern egg freezing clinics I'd visited back home, although this probably shouldn't have come as a surprise, considering this was a research hospital.

"Sit, sit," Dr. Fabbri said when we entered her small office. I sat in the chair across from her desk and looked around. Piles of paperwork, lanyards from several conferences, a small wall mirror. Behind her, plastic file organizers were stacked tall. Pops of personality stood out amid the clutter—there was a greeting card with an egg and sperm talking to each other, and her computer's screensaver was a photo of a bowl of risotto.

We spoke about the worldwide patent she received in 2001 for her novel (pre-vitrification) method for successfully cryopreserving human eggs, and how she started flying to laboratories and symposiums around the world to talk about it. When we got to discussing where the industry was headed, I asked Dr. Fabbri if she thought ovary—as opposed to egg—freezing was the future of fertility preservation. "It's not the future—it's now," she corrected me, then gushed excitedly about a twenty-year clinical study their department had recently published detailing more than one thousand patients who had undergone ovarian tissue cryopreservation and transfer. Ovarian tissue freezing, Dr. Fabbri explained, is the only fertility preservation technique currently available for prepubescent girls and for adult patients for whom freezing eggs isn't possible. In her opinion, women freezing for non-medical reasons might be better off freezing ovarian tissue than eggs, in part because this isn't just about eggs and babies, as we've seen; it's also connected to restarting hormone production and postponing menopause. The logic makes sense: Why preserve a dozen cars when you could preserve the entire factory and the ability to make new cars? "If Google decided to cryopreserve the ovary," she said, meaning if Google paid for its female employees to freeze ovarian tissue the way they do eggs, "everyone, every clinic in the world, would start doing this."

Later that day, I sat on a stone wall in front of the university hospital and waited for Dr. Porcu. It began to rain lightly, a late summer drizzle. Several minutes after the time when we'd arranged to meet, a dark car sped up to the entrance, brushing against a tall stone pillar. I stood up, alarmed. *Did that car just hit that pillar? And why is it on the walkway and not the road?* I watched as a tall woman dressed all in black emerged from the driver's side. She stepped around the pillar, which the car was still touching. *No way is that Dr. Por—*

"Natalia?" the woman half-yelled in my direction, peering over at me.

I slung my bag over my shoulder and began walking toward her. "Dr. Porcu," I said, extending my hand. She grasped it briefly.

"The rain," she said, motioning at her car by way of explanation. "Come," she said, heading for the glass doors. We walked briskly and silently down the first floor's main hallway. I wondered about her leaving the car on the walkway and touching the pillar.

Dr. Porcu's office was spacious, with big windows, and when we walked in I was blasted with air-conditioning. "Would you like a chocolate egg?" she asked, offering me a candy wrapped in pink foil. My first thought when I saw Dr. Porcu was how much her looks contrasted with Dr. Fabbri's. Roughly the same age as her former colleague, in her mid-sixties, Dr. Porcu was tan, with dark curly hair, and wore a long black dress and black shoes. A complete dark vision compared to Dr. Fabbri's light and bright.

Dr. Porcu sat at her desk while we spoke. Behind her, pinned to a bulletin board, was a picture of herself on a page of a newspaper from October 1999. "It seemed like a miracle because nobody trusted the capacity of human eggs to be fertilized and give rise to a pregnancy," she said, reflecting on her and Dr. Fabbri's first frozen-egg birth in 1997. Dr. Fabbri was responsible for the game-changing cryoprotectant solution, and Dr. Porcu had figured out that using ICSI, the method by which doctors inject sperm directly into eggs to fertilize them, was crucial. Dr. Porcu told me about the several interviews she'd given to journalists at the annual ASRM conference shortly after their paper was published and how proud she'd been when fertility doctors from the United States came to Italy to learn the technique. When I asked about her commitment to egg freezing research, she explained it was largely due to the thousands of embryos that were being frozen and abandoned. "I believe that you can make progress in medicine without destroying and involving the root of life in this bad manner," she said.

I had decided I'd take advantage of sitting down with two of the world's leading egg freezing specialists and ask them both about my particular ovary-and-eggs conundrum. When I told Dr. Fabbri I'd gone back and forth about whether or not to freeze my eggs, she made a face—without trying to hide it—and when I asked why the concerned look, she told me I was young but warned against waiting until my mid- to late thirties to do it. "That's closer to the dangerous period," she said, referring to follicles decreasing month by month, "when the decline is more steep." Dr. Porcu was more blunt. "In your case, you should freeze," she said matter-of-factly. "Every day, every month, you risk ovarian torsion again. If you got pregnant now, that would be a good thing. But even then, if you are prone to having ovarian torsion, it can happen during pregnancy."

I didn't know what I wanted Dr. Porcu to say, but this wasn't it. Before I could respond, she went on: "Do it here," she said, in a persuasive tone that struck me as pushy but warm, very Italian. "Save your money and do the procedure in the first and still best place where you can do this." In Italy, Dr. Porcu explained, a woman can undergo egg freezing for free if she has a medical reason to do so. The government foots the bill. When I reminded her I was not an Italian citizen, she brushed off the concern, telling me it might cost me 5,000 euros or so—a fraction of what egg freezing would cost me in the United States. "In the United States, the prices are crazy," she said. "Where the money is the main goal, the medicine is bad. Bad for patients and bad for medicine." She paused, craning her neck to look through the window. "Oh, good, my car is still there." Sometimes, she explained, university staff removed it when she parked on the walkway in front of the building's entrance, but today she'd gotten lucky.

I was relieved we'd moved on from the risk of something happening to my ovary during pregnancy—one more item to add to my growing list of ovary-related worries—until Dr. Porcu said, almost as an afterthought: "One ovary left is a risk condition. If you were my daughter, I would do it for you." I raised my eyebrows in surprise. Without prompting, Dr. Porcu had said more or less the same thing Dr. Noyes had told me when I last saw her—at the last appointment I'd have with her, though I didn't know it then: *If you were my daughter, I'd tell you to freeze.* When I mentioned this to Dr. Porcu, she said, "You know that Nicole Noyes learned the technique here."

By this point, I probably shouldn't have been so surprised at the way my egg freezing journey had come full circle.

The sun was starting to set when I stepped out of the hospital building. I ran to make the train back to Milan, my black flats slippery on the uneven cobblestones. I made it just in time, collapsing into a seat, sweaty and out of breath. I turned to the scenery flying by and pressed my nose against the window. The horizon was a bleeding line of color. It would be months before I connected the dots: that exactly four years earlier, on a similarly warm September day an ocean away, I'd walked into a buzzing room inside a Manhattan hotel and into the future of egg freezing. That was where this journey had begun. Today I had stepped into egg freezing's beginnings—and, I'd realize a while later, a part of this journey's end.

A few days later, I flew home. As the plane approached the Rocky Mountains and began to descend, I looked out the window and into a much larger story. I had had a front-row seat to egg freezing's transformation, both as a young woman pursuing the procedure and as a young reporter writing about the changing landscape of fertility and revolutionary reproductive technologies. I considered the plot twists in my journey, moments that hinged on uncertainty, and the versions of me grappling with this decision. Twenty years old, in the hospital, ovary miraculously saved. Twenty-five, chuckling at the egg freezing ad on the subway, feeling smug with how ahead of the game I was from the moment I stepped into the first egg freezing cocktail party. On the cusp of thirty, single and unsure, the lens now turned inward, as I found myself shining a light on a conviction I'd held my entire life: that I am destined to be a mother.

Most journeys have stages, and this one, it dawned on me now, was no different. First there was confusion, then apprehension and fear, and now a fuzzy sort of acceptance and resolve. It wasn't time I needed to make the decision about freezing my eggs, I realized. It wasn't years of reporting or scrutinizing my medical records in my attempt to piece together painful surgeries and the story of what happened to my reproductive system and why. It was this: allowing myself to let the decision go, to know that I could make and unmake this choice countless times and neither answer would be fully right.

Changed Narratives

Back in Colorado, I started dating a man a few years older than I was. He was a filmmaker, clever and complex and a bit contrarian. Deeply sensitive and patient, with a wild mind and a silly irreverent side I adored. A bit self-absorbed, in the way artists can be. He taught me how to rock-climb, surf, and smoke a cigarette. He challenged me, in ways that were a mix of annoyance and frustration leading to growth. We'd talk fervently for hours, about dreams and ambitions, books and music we loved, narrative films we'd make together. The sex was so good that it left us stunned, nearly every time.

Falling in love with the filmmaker felt like traveling together to somewhere that didn't exist yet. It was a dizzying thrill, like when we were surfing and we'd straddle our boards side by side and watch for the big waves, the ones that made us feel terribly small but the op-posite of alone. Sometimes I would look at the filmmaker and know, simply and clearly, that we had something others spent their lives searching for. On a black-sand beach we stumbled upon in Hawaii, in the kitchen of my parents' mountain house on Thanksgiving, hand in hand on a cobblestone street in Soho, from my surfboard to his out in the deep blue in Baja—a small but powerful swell would make my heart skip a beat, some cosmic force playing the strings of our connection.

Our relationship did not have a clean through line, a sensible narrative arc. He would come and go, leaving Boulder for long stretches in other places, which I didn't mind until I did. We broke up; we got back together. He waffled about commitment while I swallowed my needs and struggled to be honest about what I wanted. The truth was, I had never felt with anyone the way I did with him. Never felt *for* anyone what I did for him. But I was afraid to admit that to myself—much less to him, especially when he always had one foot out the door—which made it easy for us both to go all-in with our white-hot chemistry and intellectual kinship but balk in the face of emotional intimacy and doing the real work required to make a relationship last. Despite how much I wanted it to be, feeling complicated and incredibly alive together wasn't enough. And then there were our differing desires when it came to kids. The filmmaker would make an incredible father, I knew, but he vacillated between saying he didn't want children and saying he wasn't sure. A familiar story to many, but new for me, and after some time I reluctantly extricated myself from our exquisite, intense tangle. This time, each of us bolstered by our own sad but real reasons to be walking away, it felt like it was for good.

Love can make you feel both held and free; it does not have to be clamored for and clutched tight to be real. The filmmaker helped me learn that. He also taught me—showed me, rather—that questioning even the things that seem surest can be healthy and helpful. When he and I discussed a future in which we might have kids together, he would sometimes gently challenge my impenetrable "I want children and always have" stance—not because he wanted me to change my mind but because he was genuinely curious about the roots of my conviction. It was, frankly, a great question: How *did* my lifelong desire to have biological children become the one, and maybe only, thing I have ever known for certain? I didn't have a thorough, cogent answer; I still don't. But while examining this in-my-heart certainty hasn't diminished its potency, it has helped me cling less tightly to my carefully constructed vision of babies and parenthood—and embrace the possibility that, for me, as it has for so many others, motherhood may unfold in any number of unexpected ways.

This story could have been written very differently. Here is what could have happened on that breezy summer day several years ago: I could have lost my remaining ovary. It would have been the first day of the rest of my life, a twenty-year-old who couldn't have biological children. Instead, it was the day of surgery number two, and my rescued ovary prompted the beginning of a complicated journey of questions that otherwise I never would've needed to or thought to ask—about eggs and ovaries, and so much more: the degree to which I'd staked my identity on my fertility and ability to become pregnant on my terms and timeline; the power and ramifications of reproductive technologies; my habit of craving guarantees and being in control.

Changed narratives on my mind, I caught up with Mandy, Remy, and Lauren.

Mandy, now in her mid-thirties, and Quincy were still in Oakland, in the same house I'd visited before. We'd been on the phone for less than a minute when she shared the big news: She was three months pregnant. Her and Quincy's embryos remained on ice, untouched. "When I was trying to get pregnant, I was so relieved I'd frozen embryos," Mandy said when I asked if conceiving naturally had changed how she thought about egg freezing. "Even though I knew we couldn't 100 percent bank on them, they still brought comfort." For a while, motherhood remained a never-ending list of pros and cons, but sometime after freezing embryos she'd begun to feel attached to the idea of having biological children. "I've always been afraid of uncertainty, and here I am, having a kid, which is the most uncertain thing," she said, chuckling. "It was only once I accepted that uncertainty that I started to feel excited about it. Now I'm embracing whatever is to come. There's no more ambivalence on my end. Be-

cause I went all in." I was used to hearing anxiety in her voice, but
tonight on the phone, she sounded calm. There was a strength, wisdom, even, underlying all she was telling me, and it made me tear up.

While Mandy had felt good about her decision to freeze embryos
for a long time after she did so, she felt differently now about all the
money, time, and stress that had gone into it. She and Quincy were
thrilled, and surprised, when they conceived so quickly. But now,
she told me, "I felt like I was tricked. I've been scared for the last ten
years, ever since I found these cysts on my ovaries. And then I got
pregnant so fast and I was like, 'So what was all of that *for*?'" Looking
back, she wishes she hadn't felt so steered by her anxiety. She got
sucked into what she now describes as an industry trying to instill
fear. "Egg freezing is seen as a solution, but it's not, really—and
often, like in my case, I didn't even truly know if there was a problem," she said. "I spent thousands of dollars, did all those extreme
injections, went through a lot of emotional suffering. I did all that to
feel more secure, to try and control my future. But I've learned that
you can't control life. You just can't." As for where she stands now
with egg freezing, she told me, "I wish I hadn't done it. Of course
that's easy to say now, because I'm pregnant. But I don't think we'll
ever use those backup frozen embryos. If I do want more kids in the
future and I can't conceive naturally, I really believe I'll be okay with
that."

She paused. "Not only are my ovaries more resilient than I thought
they were, but I was, too," she said, her voice soft and steady. "And I
still am."

Before we hung up, Mandy told me when the baby was due, and
I gasped: her due date was my birthday. We laughed at how full-circle
it felt. A few weeks before she gave birth, Mandy texted to tell me
that her pregnancy app had told her, *If you're having a girl, she will already have all the eggs she'll have in her lifetime.* Mandy had groaned,
with a laugh, and when I read her message, I laughed, too.

For Remy, nearing her late thirties, life had changed quite a bit. Days
after we last spoke, she met a fella on a dating app and sent me a

photo of the two of them on a hike, looking smitten. *Meet Thomas,*★ her message read. *99.9% this is THE ONE.* A few months later, she texted me a picture of a positive pregnancy test. They'd stopped using protection only the month before, thinking it might take them up to a year to conceive because of Remy's age, but were happily surprised when she'd gotten pregnant almost right away. They married at a courthouse in North Carolina, and then moved back to California, where Remy's from. When we caught up over video, Remy, now an attending physician, was on maternity leave. She was glowing, her hair fixed high on her head, breastfeeding her one-month-old daughter. In the background, the mantel was decorated with Christmas stockings and several of Remy's crystals, lovingly arranged by Thomas.

She and Thomas had talked about her frozen eggs soon after they began dating. "Having them in the background makes me feel very at ease," Remy said. "We'd love a second baby, but not too soon." She once joked to Thomas that he had all the characteristics she would've chosen if she'd gone the route of using a sperm donor to fertilize her frozen eggs, telling him, "You're exactly the kind of phenotype that I wanted to mate with! You're my million-dollar sperm." Remy was often upbeat, even when she was tired, but as we talked I noticed how grounded and happy she seemed. And she was. "I couldn't have in a million years dreamed up the reality I'm living now," she said as her daughter nuzzled away.

Then, when their daughter was four months old, Remy discovered she was pregnant again. Baby number two was very much not planned. Once she and Thomas recovered from the shock, they were thrilled. During her first pregnancy Remy had told me it was very likely they'd use her frozen eggs for future babies. Now she said, "So much for freezing those eggs!"

On a warm autumn morning, I met Lauren, now in her mid-forties, at a coffee shop near my apartment. The last time I'd seen her was in

★ Name has been changed.

Houston, after she'd unexpectedly gotten pregnant—after her terrible egg freezing experience, but not with her frozen eggs. Now she was parenting mostly solo; her son, Ethan, sat between us licking sour cream off of his breakfast burrito while he played with toy cars scattered across the table. They were in town visiting a friend; Lauren had gone to college in Boulder and was excited to show Ethan her old stomping grounds. She wore jeans, a red flowy top, and oversized sunglasses, her dark brown hair pulled back in a bun. I had wondered about her frozen eggs, whatever happened to them, and was shocked when Lauren told me she doesn't know where they are. She's received storage bills from different vendors—the clinic where she froze her eggs has changed its billing system multiple times over the years—and assumes her eggs remain at the clinic but isn't sure.★ "I have zero faith that my eggs are safe and sound," she told me. She ultimately abandoned pursuing legal action related to the Lupron error and first botched egg freezing cycle; it would've ended up costing her a fortune, and even more distress. "I was so stressed out and upset at the time, I couldn't afford the added stress of a lawsuit," she told me.

While she remains somewhat bitter, thanks to her unexpected happy ending, Lauren doesn't lose sleep over the fate of her frozen eggs. They represent a backup plan she never ended up needing. "I never would have had Ethan if I hadn't frozen my eggs," she told me as she handed the four-year-old a dollar bill to give to the musician playing the cello nearby. A few minutes later, he scampered back to the table with a happy grin. Lauren hadn't been sure how she would have a child until she began considering egg freezing when she was almost forty, and, she told me, doubts she would have had the guts to become a solo parent. Then, the night of her trigger shot and in the months after, her life changed in a way she never could have predicted. If she could do it all over again, she would, though she would've frozen her eggs at a younger age. She had Ethan despite her awful egg freezing ordeal, or maybe because of it—she'll never know.

★ Lauren's made several phone calls attempting to confirm her eggs' location and gotten nowhere. She has not paid the storage bills, unwilling to give any more money to the clinic, or associated vendor, where her egg freezing cycles were such a nightmare.

But she wouldn't change a single thing that happened if it changed where she'd ended up.

Eleven Beautiful Follicles

So, what did I decide to do about my ovary?

Part of me wants this to be a wise recounting, not a wishy-washy one. But I have lost track of how many times I sat down with this question that I desperately wanted to answer and then put to rest. It took me years to make my egg freezing decision. It took me this entire book.

One day in the heart of winter, I lay on my bed staring at the icy branches outside my window. In my hands: the ultrasound image of my ovary from years ago, the photo now grayed and fading, and my most recent image, shiny and crisp, from my annual OB/GYN visit days earlier. At the appointment, I asked for a transvaginal ultrasound to check up on my ovary. "Yes, I remember, you've got the one ovary," the technician said, remembering me from two years earlier, when I'd last requested an ultrasound. "You know the drill," she said on her way out of the room. I undressed from the waist down and lay back on the table, stirrups holding my feet. The technician returned and dimmed the lights. Several minutes later: "You have eleven beautiful follicles," she remarked, swiveling the monitor around to show me. There was my ovary, and there were the follicles inside, squishy black ovals on the screen that almost seemed to pulse as she counted them out to me. "Yay!" I said, grinning. *Little, lovely ovary,* I thought, flushing with a strange mix of pride and relief. *Look at you, still doing your thing. Eleven potential eggs. And we're not even trying; we don't even need them yet.* "You've got time," my doctor told me after she completed my checkup and we discussed my follicle count. She was talking about my eggs, but she might as well have been speaking of a paradigm shift in my life. My age meant the odds were in my favor, even with just one ovary—for now, at least, and for several more years, best-case. I left the gynecologist's office feeling deeply comforted, even though I hadn't thought anything was wrong, and hopeful, even though I wasn't trying to get pregnant.

Time. I've got it, so I'm told. Many don't.

If you were my daughter, I'd absolutely tell you to freeze your eggs. The doctors' words echoed in my thoughts. It seemed foolish to disregard the advice of the many doctors whose advice I sought. Still does.

But that's exactly what I did.

After my eleven-beautiful-follicles appointment, I made a new decision about egg freezing: I stopped trying to decide. Deciding to stop trying to decide was a simpler way of deciding no. Clarity comes when we pivot, change course, leave, let go. Clarity comes when we surrender. Not always, maybe, but often. The act of deciding helps us get where we're going. Put a stake in the ground and continue on. I realized, finally, it's not about the eggs. It's about what the deciding, or the ceasing to decide, yields. So I let go of the notion of a "right" decision and the pressure to make it. After trusting the world more than trusting myself for so long, after years of looking for evidence and answers only *out there* and almost never *in here*—I arrived at some in-between state. It's hazy, uncomfortable, and undeniably real.

Egg freezing is a powerful, if imperfect, technology. It is a worthwhile option for many, many women. But not, I've determined at long last, for me.

If money were not an issue and if we knew more about the potential risks of fertility drugs and if I was certain I would use my frozen eggs within five years and if reliable data proved more eggs survived being thawed, I would probably freeze my eggs tomorrow. For now, I've determined that—barring some sort of emergency or urgent medical necessity in which I would almost certainly decide to freeze my eggs—the best thing I can do for my ovary and desire to have biological children is to take care of my body, and my heart, as best I can. To stay on the Pill, per my doctors' instructions, in order to protect my ovary and keep it hibernating. If, when I am ready to become pregnant, I find myself confronting infertility, I may decide to pursue IVF. I will cross that river if and when I come to it. And if I do undergo IVF and I'm not able to have biological children, I can only hope it won't be the end-all scenario I once imagined it would be. My mother's words from all those years ago come back to me now: *You still would have had kids,* she'd said softly, squeezing my hand as I woke up from the surgery that saved my ovary. *Even if they'd had to take it out, you would still someday be a mother.*

Outside, dark shadows danced against the late afternoon twilight. I cocooned myself in a blanket and gazed out my bedroom window, the ultrasound images next to my pillow. I thought about all I had learned and all I couldn't yet know—and how I would look back at all this someday, and especially this moment, when I finally accepted that not knowing is okay. How I would remember feeling, as I settled into my early thirties: An entire decade is knocking and I am revising my questions.

For a while, I'd sometimes catch myself thinking I still might freeze my eggs. So let me put this journey I have taken to good use in a practical sense. I offer the following thoughts in this spirit.

If I were to freeze my eggs now, here is what I would do: I'd take a few of FertilityIQ's comprehensive online courses and use its verified reviews to help me decide on a reputable doctor and clinic, one that offers a low-interest finance option and a discount for multiple cycles. I'd strongly consider freezing outside the United States, probably in Europe, for a fraction of the cost. I'd inquire about the clinic's embryology staff, lab protocols, and pregnancy rates from frozen eggs. I'd research specialty pharmacies before ordering the pricey meds. I'd store my frozen eggs at a clinic that uses TMRW's storage technology or at a TMRW biorepository, and certainly in a state that was friendly to reproductive choice. I'd go off the Pill—this time, after a lengthy discussion with my OB/GYN—then test my hormone levels with Modern Fertility's at-home kit before following up with a reproductive endocrinologist. I'd use an online egg freezing predictive calculator, inputting my specific numbers, to gauge how many eggs I might get. If I was in a committed relationship with a person I could see myself having kids with, I'd likely freeze embryos instead of eggs.

Finally—and if you take away anything from this list of recommendations, let it be this—I would not mistake freezing eggs for freezing time. I would do my best to not let my frozen eggs be a sort of Band-Aid, a thinly veiled rationale to postpone confronting the difficult questions that arise in my relationships, in my desire to have children, in my life. Because while egg freezing can spark a positive, powerful psychological shift, it does not guarantee a woman more control over her life. She may believe that it does—Remy, Mandy, and Lauren all felt that way—but while the feeling of assurance is very real indeed, the actual control piece is an illusion. Accepting this makes all the difference.

I get that you're concerned. I understand that you may feel swept up in the glitz and glamour, the potential and the power, the sleek reassurances. I got swept up, too. The perfect storm of ignorance, money, and fear makes this an incredibly alluring world to get lost in. I, too, craved the answers and was worried about not knowing enough, not being prepared for whatever might come next, all of the uncertainties we cannot plan for that alter our trajectory.

I know you want someone or something else to tell you what to do. Unfortunately, there are so many someones and somethings who can and will do just that. Your body says, *Tick-tock.* Your gynecologist says, *Don't be silly, you're young. Come back to see me after trying for a year.* Your parents say, *Haven't you figured out your career and love life yet? By the time I was your age . . .* Your ex-boyfriend says, *Maybe you should've just stayed with me.* Your social media feeds say, *Everyone you know is getting married and having babies and so here is an ad for egg freezing that you will see a thousand times.* Your employer says, *We'll pay for it; we've got you covered. So go freeze your eggs, keep working, and don't have kids yet.* (Or maybe your work says, *Egg freezing? We don't even cover flu shots.*) I know all this is true for you because I lived it, too. I had my own way of weighing the risks and benefits, and so do you. The best we can do is make an informed decision with the facts and knowledge we have, inside of ourselves and out there, available to us to learn about.

Only you can make these determinations about your eggs, your ovaries, and your fertility, both present and future. But it's not really about the yes/no of egg freezing, is it? It's about not buying into the notion that your fertility is something to be conquered. It's about not handing over the power to all the someones and somethings asking you to yield it. It's about recognizing that weighing the pros and cons is hard, *really* hard. It's about saying, *For now, no.* So that you can be better at saying, *Yes, oh yes.*

When I set out to write this book, I was determined to arrive at clear answers. My quest turned into something else. For Remy, Mandy, and Lauren, freezing their eggs invited what came next. It helped them be more open, willing, and accepting. Deciding not to did the same for me. Now, I'm giving up on certainty. I've stopped trying to crystal-ball my fertility and figure out my possible future of pregnancy, motherhood, and building a family with a partner. I've stopped trying to picture the ending.

And yet. I had wanted to report from the other side of a decision many people make and say, yes, you should freeze your eggs, or no, you shouldn't. Reader, I cannot offer you that. What I can give you instead are signposts for your journey. Murmurings about the side roads I took or almost took. Gentle reminders to loosen your grip on the steering wheel. Use this information to navigate the decisions you are or soon will be facing. Allow this technology and its possibilities to challenge you. Embrace the questions, even when they are anxiety-inducing and uncomfortable. Unseen forces will continue to buffer you, as they did me. See your life as the series of choices that it is. Do not postpone whatever reckoning you are invited into. And, above all else: Give yourself permission to not have all the answers.

I offer up my experience, as a woman and a journalist, navigating this fertile soil.

The science and the story are still unfolding.

Acknowledgments

In many ways, I had to grow up fast to write this book. Now that I've written it, what I most want to say is: YAY.

We are who we are, we do what we do, because of the team around us. And while writing a book can be a lonely task, it is not one that can be done alone. This book would not have been possible without the incredible people—family, friends, mentors, teachers, editors—who supported and encouraged me these past several years. I am forever grateful.

I know there's no way to write these acknowledgments without leaving someone out. If I've forgotten a mention, please understand it's a failure of my cluttered mind, not my heart.

I am immensely thankful to all those I interviewed for their openness and generosity of spirit, especially the women who graciously shared their personal journeys. My deep gratitude to Remy, Mandy, and Lauren, who let me into their lives and their egg freezing experiences, and whom I hope will find that I was fair and true to them in my writing. And to Ben, aka Ponman: I'm so glad you didn't run away from the table when I told you on our first date about this book and the possibility of you being in it. Thank you for your unwavering belief in journalism and in my work, for your grace, and for introducing me to cheese curds.

I owe more than I can say to my literary agent, Elias Altman, who enthusiastically took on this book and championed it from the beginning. Not every writer is fortunate enough to have an agent who is also a talented editor; I could not ask for a better reader and advocate. Thank you for the reassuring notes of encouragement—still taped to the wall above my desk—and for being a steadfast guide throughout this process. Onward.

My sincerest gratitude to Susanna Porter, a dream editor, for her incisive comments and tireless work helping me wrestle this narrative into shape. Being a first-time author is nerve-racking, and when I stumbled along the way, she met me with boundless patience and compassion. Thank you for the many hours you poured into helping make this book the best it could be.

Many other good people at Ballantine and Penguin Random House worked hard on behalf of this book, especially Cindy Berman, Kim Hovey, Pam Alders, Sue Warga, Carolyn Foley, Brianna Kusilek, Allison Schuster, Robin Schiff, Barbara Bachman, and Anusha Khan. Thank you for all you did to usher this book into the world.

I am so fortunate to have extraordinary teachers and mentors who have guided me along the way. The wonderful professors at New York University's Arthur L. Carter Journalism Institute helped mold me as a young journalist and offered vast wisdom. Profound thanks to Robert Boynton, for his mentorship and continued support; Brooke Kroeger, who encouraged me to pitch what became my first published story about egg freezing; Ted Conover, for his inspiring teachings in immersive reporting; and Perri Klass, who helped me shape this material from graduate school thesis to book proposal. Thank you to Lauren Sandler for her advice and from whom I learned important lessons about both journalism and life. I am deeply grateful to Bud and Beth Warner, Cassie Kircher, Crista Arangala, and Drew Perry at Elon University for shaping me as a writer, a thinker, and a human learning how to make her way in the world. And to Heather Gatley, a powerful early influence.

A great debt is owed to Katherine Zoepf, who saw this book in me before I had the confidence to write it—and without whom it would not exist. Thank you for your invaluable guidance, your friendship, and for making me feel like I had something to say.

I am indebted to Kelsey Lannin, who shouldered the challenging task of fact-checking this book and left no stone unturned, and to Kelsey Kudak, who provided significant fact-checking support and did so with sensitivity. Endless thanks to you both for making these pages incalculably better. Thank you also to Sarah Stodder, researcher extraordinaire, who tumbled down many-a-rabbit-hole with me early on.

This book was supported by a grant from the Alfred P. Sloan Foundation Program for Public Understanding of Science and Technology, and I am eternally beholden to them for making it possible for me to do fact-checking and additional research. Sincere thanks to FASPE and the lessons and professional connections the illuminative fellowship provided. For the gift of space and time to figure out what this book could be, I am enormously grateful to the Logan Nonfiction Program and the Carey Institute for Global Good. Thank you also to the talented writers and creatives of my Logan cohort for seeing what was needed, and to Adrian Nicole LeBlanc, Rafil Kroll-Zaidi, and Mark Kramer, who helped me untangle the threads.

My sincere gratitude to the reproductive endocrinologists, embryologists, founders, and other experts, many of whom are mentioned in the book or cited in the Notes, who shared their knowledge and time with me and played crucial roles in the reporting. I am grateful to the journalists, authors, and scholars whose writing on reproduction and fertility I've referenced, and whose work in this space have been both helpful and inspiring, especially that of Marcia C. Inhorn, Anna Louie Sussman, and Rachel E. Gross. Enormous thanks also to the following people for their expertise and fact-checking assistance, often with little or no advance warning, and for helping me identify some of my own blind spots and omissions: Temeka Zore, Lora Shahine, Leslie Ramirez, Natalie Crawford, Julie Lamb, and Anate Brauer. For providing and helping me interpret egg freezing statistics, thank you to Amy Sparks, Timothy Hickman, and especially Ethan and Pat with the Society for Assisted Reproductive Technology.

A heartfelt thank-you to Bridget Jameson and Jenn Brown for reading an early draft and offering valuable contributions; to Alex Brokaw, for the tough love; and to my mother, who is the first person to read anything I write and was this book's first reader as well. Many thanks also to Susan Knoppow for her support and gracious feedback when this book was merely a smattering of Google docs, and to Shannon Offerman for her helpful comments.

Several friends and family members very kindly provided editorial service, and I am grateful for their help. Michael Pearl, Hannah Stadlober, Katrina Lampert, and Molly Varoga transcribed interviews; Rachel Wood fielded numerous reproductive health–related medical questions; and Sean O'Connor helped generate ideas for the cover and offered shrewd insights along the way. Thank you to Elena Horn, Michael Orleans, and Peter Cooper for accompanying me on reporting trips in Italy and Ghana, and to DeeDee Montgomery for facilitating an important discussion.

A special thanks to all those who gave me a table to write at and a bed to crash on in various cities while I was reporting and writing portions of this book, especially the Brokaw, Montgomery, and Corrao families. Thank you to my former therapists in Colorado and New York who helped me maintain my sanity along the way: Nancy, Evan, Rich, Marjorie, and Emily. Thank you also to the publications that gave portions of this book's reporting early homes and the talented editors I've had the privilege of working with, especially Jessica Reed at *The Guardian,* Erik Vance at *The New York Times,* and Bijan Stephen, then at *The New Republic.*

Many incredible humans, too numerous to name here, buoyed me up with their friendship during this arduous endeavor, especially in the home stretch. A few must be singled out: Rachel Wood, Alex Brokaw, Jenn Brown, and Sam Kern, who keep me going on a daily basis. Endless thanks to Andrew Hyde for your out-of-this-world generosity, and for providing a haven, patronage, and Dram when I needed it the most. To Sarah Maslin, Lindsey Smith, Laura Orland, Christine Cassaro, Hannah Stadlober, Lauren Lambert, and Emily Montgomery—amazing women I'm lucky to have in my life—who gave me a steady stream of support. To Kyle for the puddles-on-the-floor moments and for being a cheerleader when I needed it the most. To Julie for the ways in which you always lifted me up, and to Maggie for nourishing me with words and popcorn for years.

Hugs one, two, and five hundred to the Brumbaugh/Hiller clan, whom I am so grateful to call family. Thank you for the laughs, the warmth, and for accepting and loving me in all the ways that you do.

My grandparents are in the spaces between these words. My mother's mother, Patricia Jameson, passed away while I was writing this book; I miss your laugh and wit, Grandma. I am eternally thankful to my father's parents, Lauren and Sidney Ann Lampert, who helped put me through college and graduate school and made it possible for me to pursue a career as a writer. Granddaddy: How I wish I could place a copy of this book in your hands.

It is very hard to write this part, because I don't know that my dear grandpa, George "Bud" Jameson, will still be with us when this book comes out. But Grandpa, if you're reading this, know that there is no one I am more excited to see hold this book than you. Thank you for long being one of my biggest fans. You, and the life you've lived, will forever be an inspiration to me.

A last deep bow and eternal gratitude to my family: Peter Lampert, Alison Jameson, Katrina Lampert, Ben Lampert, Ali Lampert, Pete Groves. (Also, Indy, Bear, and Teddy. And Piper: We miss you, sweet girl.) Your love and support are the foundation of everything good and true in my life.

I am profoundly fortunate to have parents who raised me to pursue my passions and who taught me that a spirit of adventure will usually suffice. Their unwavering faith and encouragement mean more than I'll ever be able to say. Mom, you are the wind beneath my wings. Dad, my rock; you'll always be my first call. Hugs and pats forever.

And, finally, to Jonathan, aka the Filmmaker: Our story has been the most unexpected and wonderful part of this journey. When I told you about this book on our first hike six years ago, I couldn't have imagined that we'd be getting married three weeks before it published. You've lived with this book almost as long as I have and believed in me in times when I forgot to. Thank you for everything, but especially for braving with grace and patience the long days I had to "be in the book cave" and for seeing me through the hardest bits. More today, now more than ever—I love you.

Notes

INTRODUCTION

xvi **a third of American adults say:** Pew Research Center, "A Third of U.S. Adults Say They Have Used Fertility Treatments or Know Someone Who Has," July 17, 2018, pewresearch.org/short-reads/2018/07/17/a-third-of-u-s-adults-say-they-have-used-fertility-treatments-or-know-someone-who-has/.

xvi **Sperm freezing is on the rise:** Gururaj M. Borate and Ajay Meshram, "Cryopreservation of Sperm: A Review," *Cureus* 14, no. 11 (2022), doi.org/10.7759/cureus.31402.

CHAPTER 1

4 **"We will be like Uber":** Danielle Paquette, "How Fear Fuels the Business of Egg Freezing," *Washington Post,* March 6, 2015, washingtonpost.com/business/economy/how-fear-fuels-the-business-of-egg-freezing/2015/03/06/87fd068c-c294-11e4-9271-610273846239_story.html.

10 **the impact of mining industries:** Aboka Yaw Emmanuel, Cobbina Samuel Jerry, and Doke Adzo Dzigbodi, "Review of Environmental and Health Impacts of Mining in Ghana," *Journal of Health and Pollution* 8, no. 17 (2018): 43–52, doi.org/10.5696/2156-9614-8.17.43.

14 **By all accounts:** A 2023 study published in the *Journal of Clinical Medicine* summarized egg freezing's growth plainly: "It has been indisputably evident from the current data that the demand for social egg freezing has been growing exponentially over the last decade." See Pragati Kakkar, Joanna Geary, Tania Stockburger, Aida Kaffel, Julia Kopeika, and Tarek El-Toukhy,

"Outcomes of Social Egg Freezing: A Cohort Study and a Comprehensive Literature Review," *Journal of Clinical Medicine* 12, no. 13 (2023), doi.org/10 .3390/jcm12134182.

14 **a mere 482:** A note on reporting the number of distinct egg freezing patients versus the number of egg freezing cycles: It's easy to misinterpret the published data, and many people—including journalists—have. The Society for Assisted Reproductive Technology collects and publishes online the number of egg freezing cycles each year, but neither SART nor the CDC publicly reports the number of women freezing their eggs, i.e., distinct egg freezing patients. Also, many women do multiple cycles, which is one reason that the cycle numbers in the official annual egg freezing reports are higher. I obtained the numbers of patients who froze eggs for non-medical reasons from 2009 to 2022 from SART directly.

14n **the latest year:** Preliminary 2022 egg freezing data came out in early 2024. There's typically a two-year lag when it comes to compiling ART statistics. It takes a while to wait for live-birth outcomes, and then there's the collection of the data by the fertility clinics, which SART audits before submitting it to the CDC for analysis and official publication.

14 **22,967 did:** I obtained the numbers of patients who froze eggs for non-medical reasons from 2009 to 2022 from SART directly.

14n **The United Kingdom has also seen:** Human Fertilisation and Embryology Authority (HFEA), "Fertility Treatment 2021: Preliminary Trends and Figures," 2023, hfea.gov.uk/about-us/publications/research-and-data/fertility -treatment-2021-preliminary-trends-and-figures/.

14 **"one of the most significant":** Sonia Allan et al., "International Federation of Fertility Societies' Surveillance (IFFS) 2019: Global Trends in Reproductive Policy and Practice, 8th Edition," *Global Reproductive Health* 4, no. 1 (2019): 51, doi.org/10.1097/grh.0000000000000029.

15 **young users extol:** Naomi May, "Gen Z Are Freezing Their Eggs. Why?," *Vice,* July 20, 2023, vice.com/en/article/bvj7nz/why-gen-z-are-freezing -eggs.

15 **"I would've given anything":** Danielle Pergament, "Jennifer Aniston Has Nothing to Hide," *Allure,* December 2022, allure.com/story/jennifer -aniston-december-2022-cover-interview.

16 **in the next twenty to forty years:** Henry T. Greely, *The End of Sex and the Future of Human Reproduction* (Cambridge, MA: Harvard University Press, 2016).

16n **Remy:** She asked for her name to be changed to protect the privacy of her family.

17 **"geriatric pregnancy" and "advanced maternal age":** Historically, "advanced maternal age" has been defined as women who are thirty-five years of age or older at estimated date of delivery. This—rudely—used to be called a "geriatric pregnancy." The age cutoff was based on evidence of declining fertility and concern surrounding increasing risks for genetic

abnormalities identified in the offspring of pregnant women older than thirty-five. As of 2022, "pregnancy at age 35" is the term preferred by the American College of Obstetricians and Gynecologists. To simplify things, ACOG recommends that doctors and researchers indicate patients' age in five-year increments (35–39 years, 40–44 years, etc.), which better stratifies the possible pregnancy risks associated with advancing age. See "Pregnancy at Age 35 Years or Older," *American College of Obstetricians and Gynecologists* 140, no. 2 (2022): 348–366, doi.org/10.1097/aog.0000000000004873.

CHAPTER 2

20   **bacterial vaginosis:** Bacterial vaginosis, or BV, is the most common vaginal condition in women ages fifteen to forty-four. Douching, not using condoms, and having new or multiple sex partners can upset the normal balance of vaginal bacteria and increase a woman's risk of getting BV.

21   **since sex ed was introduced:** Jonathan Zimmerman, *Too Hot to Handle: A Global History of Education* (Princeton, NJ: Princeton University Press, 2015).

21   **The vast majority:** "The SIECUS State Profiles 2022," Sexuality Information and Education Council of the United States (SIECUS), accessed January 3, 2023, siecus.org/the-siecus-state-profiles-2022/.

21   **school districts aren't required:** Guttmacher Institute, "Sex and HIV Education," last modified September 1, 2023, guttmacher.org/state-policy /explore/sex-and-hiv-education.

21   **little evidence that providing:** Kathrin Stanger-Hall and David Hall, "Abstinence-Only Education and Teen Pregnancy Rates: Why We Need Comprehensive Sex Education in the U.S.," *PLOS One* 6, no. 10 (2011), doi.org/10.1371/journal.pone.0024658.

21   **teen births and risky sexual behaviors:** American College of Obstetricians and Gynecologists, "Committee Opinion No. 678: Comprehensive Sexuality Education," *Obstetrics and Gynecology* 128, no. 5 (2016; reaffirmed 2020): 9–10, doi.org/10.1097/AOG.0000000000001769.

22   **risk of being sexually abused:** Eva S. Goldfarb and Lisa D. Lieberman, "Three Decades of Research: The Case for Comprehensive Sex Education," *Journal of Adolescent Health* 68, no. 1 (2021): 13–27, doi.org/10.1016/j .jadohealth.2020.07.036.

22   **twenty-five states:** Guttmacher Institute, "Sex and HIV Education."

22   **seventeen states:** Guttmacher Institute, "Sex and HIV Education."

23   **young people are less likely:** Laura D. Lindberg and Leslie M. Kantor, "Adolescents' Receipt of Sex Education in a Nationally Representative Sample, 2011–2019," *Journal of Adolescent Health* 70, no. 2 (2022): 290–297, doi.org/10.1016/j.jadohealth.2021.08.027.

23   **"It was as if":** Katie Wheeler, "We Teach Girls to Be Ashamed in Sex Ed. This Has to Change," *The Lily,* November 5, 2017, thelily.com/we-teach -girls-to-be-ashamed-in-sex-ed-this-has-to-change-2/.

23 **Fewer than half:** Laura D. Lindberg and Leslie M. Kantor, "Adolescents' Receipt of Sex Education in a Nationally Representative Sample, 2011–2019," *Journal of Adolescent Health* 70, no. 2 (2022): 290–297, doi.org/10.1016/j.jadohealth.2021.08.027.

23 **barred from demonstrating:** Mississippi Legislature, 2023 Regular Session, House Bill 1390, Section 37-13-171, billstatus.ls.state.ms.us/documents/2023/html/HB/1300-1399/HB1390IN.htm.

23 **"homosexual conduct":** Bills have been introduced to remove the requirement that Texas sex education curricula include that "homosexual conduct is not an acceptable lifestyle and is a criminal offense," but they have failed. Technically, the ban isn't enforceable because of a 2003 U.S. Supreme Court ruling that declared state laws criminalizing homosexual behavior to be unconstitutional. But the Texas ban remains in the state's penal code. Texas Health and Safety Code Sec. 85.007, "Educational Materials for Minors," statutes.capitol.texas.gov/docs/HS/htm/HS.85.htm.

23 **In Tennessee:** "Tennessee State Profile," SIECUS, accessed January 25, 2023, siecus.org/state_profile/tennessee-state-profile.

23 **"Kissing and hugging":** Stephen Colbert, *The Colbert Report,* Comedy Central, April 18, 2012, cc.com/video/er0kn7/the-colbert-report-the-word-gateway-hug.

24 **Only ten states:** Guttmacher Institute, "Sex and HIV Education."

24 **instruction that discriminates** *against:* SIECUS, "The SIECUS State Profiles 2022."

24 **people ages fifteen to twenty-four:** NCHHSTP, "Incidence, Prevalence, and Cost of Sexually Transmitted Infections in the United States," last modified March 16, 2022, cdc.gov/nchhstp/newsroom/fact-sheets/std/STI-Incidence-Prevalence-Cost-Factsheet.html.

24 **one in five people:** NCHHSTP, "Incidence, Prevalence, and Cost of Sexually Transmitted Infections in the United States."

25 **"There still seems to be":** Jenna Wortham, "We're More Honest with Our Phones than with Our Doctors," *New York Times Magazine,* March 23, 2016, nytimes.com/2016/03/27/magazine/were-more-honest-with-our-phones-than-with-our-doctors.html.

25 **religious underpinnings:** Planned Parenthood Federation of America, "History of Sex Education in the U.S.," 2016, cdn.plannedparenthood.org/uploads/filer_public/da/67/da67fd5d-631d-438a-85e8-a446d90fd1e3/20170209_sexed_d04_1.pdf.

25 **difficult to pass legislation:** Rachel Janfaza, "The Nuanced Push for American Sex Education," *Harvard Political Review,* January 24, 2020, harvardpolitics.com/american-sex-education/.

27 **knew that the ovaries:** Department of Health and Human Services, "Fertility Knowledge Survey, 2020: Findings Report," 2020, opa.hhs.gov/sites/default/files/2021-01/fertility-knowledge-survey-findings-exec-summary-2020.pdf.

27   **"may have grave implications":** Department of Health and Human Services, "Fertility Knowledge Survey, 2020."

27   **Other research focused on fertility awareness:** Juliana Pedro, Tânia Brandão, Lone Schmidt, Maria E. Costa, and Mariana V. Martins, "Families Formed through Assisted Reproductive Technology: Causes, Experiences, and Consequences in an International Context," *Upsala Journal of Medical Sciences* 123, no. 2 (2018): 71–81, doi.org/10.1080/03009734.2018.1480186.

28   **"If you have never":** Natalie Angier, *Woman: An Intimate Geography* (New York: Anchor, 2000), 4–5.

29   **three and five hundred thousand oocytes:** American College of Obstetricians and Gynecologists and American Society for Reproductive Medicine, "Committee Opinion No. 589: Female Age-Related Fertility Decline," *Fertility and Sterility* 101, no. 3 (2014; reaffirmed 2022): 633–634, doi.org/10.1016/j.fertnstert.2013.12.032.

29   **"The eggs do not":** Angier, *Woman,* 3.

30   **the ovary is the first organ:** Jiachen Wu, Yang Liu, Yinhua Song, Lingjuan Wang, Jihui Ai, and Kezhen Li, "Aging Conundrum: A Perspective for Ovarian Aging," *Frontiers in Endocrinology* 13 (2022), doi.org/10.3389/fendo.2022.952471.

30n **While it's a biological reality:** Emily Witt, "The Future of Fertility," *New Yorker,* April 17, 2023, newyorker.com/magazine/2023/04/24/the-future-of-fertility.

31   **"There's no one age":** Christina Caron, "Raising Concerns About a Widely Used Test to Measure Fertility," *New York Times,* October 16, 2017, nytimes.com/2017/10/16/health/fertility-test-ovarian-reserve.html.

CHAPTER 3

37   **the country's first birth control clinic:** "Seventy-Fifth Anniversary of the Brownsville Clinic," Margaret Sanger Papers Project, 1991, sanger.hosting.nyu.edu/articles/seventieth_anniversary_of_brownsville/.

37n **Before I tell you more:** "Our History," Planned Parenthood Federation of America, accessed August 2, 2022, plannedparenthood.org/about-us/who-we-are/our-history.

37   **For the next several days:** William Clifford Roberts, "Facts and Ideas from Anywhere," *Baylor University Medical Center Proceedings* 28, no. 3 (2015): 421–432, doi.org/10.1080/08998280.2015.11929297.

38   **Sanger was arrested:** Sam Roberts, "Trotsky's Bronx Headquarters and Other New York Arcana," *New York Times,* September 10, 1995, nytimes.com/1995/09/10/nyregion/trotsky-s-bronx-headquarters-and-other-new-york-arcana.html.

38   **"Woman can never":** Margaret Sanger, "Morality and Birth Control," February 1918, Margaret Sanger Papers Project, sanger.hosting.nyu.edu/documents/speech_morality_and_bc/.

38   **"the key word was 'control' ":** Jonathan Eig, *The Birth of the Pill: How Four Crusaders Reinvented Sex and Launched a Revolution* (New York: W. W. Norton, 2014), 46.

39   **bestselling method:** Libby Copeland, "From Medical Pariah to Feminist Icon: The Story of the IUD," *Smithsonian Magazine,* June 15, 2017, smithsonianmag.com/science-nature/medical-pariah-feminist-icon-story -iud-180963699/.

39n   **Prior to FDA approval:** Megan Gibson, "One Factor That Kept the Women of 1960 Away from Birth Control Pills: Cost," *Time,* June 23, 2015, time.com/3929971/enovid-the-pill/.

39n   **Enovid clinical trials:** "The Puerto Rico Pill Trials," Public Broadcasting Service (PBS) and WGBH Educational Foundation, 2023, pbs.org/wgbh /americanexperience/features/pill-puerto-rico-pill-trials/.

39   **nearly 10 percent of women:** Copeland, "From Medical Pariah to Feminist Icon."

40   **Thousands of patients suffered:** "The story of the Dalkon Shield is a story of loss and suffering and bitterness and pain," began a 1987 *New York Times* article about the early IUD. "It is a story of individual heartbreak and corporate defeat. And it is a story that points up the difference between science and law." Gina Kolata, "The Sad Legacy of the Dalkon Shield," *New York Times Magazine,* December 6, 1987, nytimes.com/1987/12/06 /magazine/the-sad-legacy-of-the-dalkon-shield.html.

40   **After paying billions:** "Guide to the Dalkon Shield Claimants Trust Collection," 1970–1988, MSS 00-4, Special Collections, University of Virginia Law Library, archives.law.virginia.edu/resources/guide-dalkon -shield-claimants-trust-collection.

40   **dented the legitimacy and popularity:** "Pharmaceutical companies witnessed how one IUD caused billions of dollars in liabilities and the bankruptcy of a major pharmaceutical company. They also realized that IUDs were not as profitable as their less controversial oral contraceptive product lines." Because of this, between 1983 and 1988 there were no IUDs on the market in the United States. See Clare L. Roepke and Eric A. Schaff, "Long Tail Strings: Impact of the Dalkon Shield 40 Years Later," *Open Journal of Obstetrics and Gynecology* 4, no. 16 (2014): 996–1005, doi.org/10 .4236/ojog.2014.416140.

41   **Across the globe:** M. Laopaiboon, P. Lumbiganon, N. Intarut, R. Mori, T. Ganchimeg, J. P. Vogel, J. P. Souza, and A. M. Gülmezoglu, "Advanced Maternal Age and Pregnancy Outcomes: A Multicountry Assessment," *British Journal of Obstetrics and Gynaecology* 121, no. S1 (2014): 49–56, doi .org/10.1111/1471-0528.12659.

41   **Now it's twenty-eight:** U.S. Census Bureau, "Estimated Median Age at First Marriage, by Sex: 1890 to Present," Historical Marital Status Tables, last modified November 2022, census.gov/data/tables/time-series/demo /families/marital.html.

41 **Women with college degrees:** National Center for Health Statistics, Centers for Disease Control and Prevention, "Fertility of Men and Women Aged 15–49 in the United States: National Survey of Family Growth, 2015–2019," 2023, cdc.gov/nchs/data/nhsr/nhsr179.pdf.

41 **roughly seven years later:** Quoctrung Bui and Claire Cain Miller, "The Age That Women Have Babies: How a Gap Divides America," *New York Times,* August 4, 2018, nytimes.com/interactive/2018/08/04/upshot/up-birth-age-gap.html.

41 **The median age:** U.S. Census Bureau, "Stable Fertility Rates 1990–2019 Mask Distinct Variations by Age," April 6, 2022, census.gov/library/stories/2022/04/fertility-rates-declined-for-younger-women-increased-for-older-women.html.

41 **Now it's twenty-seven:** National Center for Health Statistics, Centers for Disease Control and Prevention, "Births: Final Data for 2021," 2023, cdc.gov/nchs/data/nvsr/nvsr72/nvsr72-01.pdf.

41 **fewer children overall:** Pew Research Center, "Key Facts About Moms in the U.S.," May 9, 2023, pewresearch.org/short-reads/2023/05/09/facts-about-u-s-mothers/.

41 **15 percent to 30 percent:** U.S. Census Bureau, "More Women in Early 30s Are Childless," November 30, 2017, census.gov/library/stories/2017/11/women-early-thirties.html.

41 **86 percent of American women:** Pew Research Center, "They're Waiting Longer, but U.S. Women Today More Likely to Have Children than a Decade Ago," January 18, 2018, pewresearch.org/social-trends/2018/01/18/theyre-waiting-longer-but-u-s-women-today-more-likely-to-have-children-than-a-decade-ago.

41n **"refers to any woman":** Pew Research Center, "They're Waiting Longer."

41 **birth rates have declined:** U.S. Census Bureau, "Stable Fertility Rates 1990–2019."

42 **earnings take a significant hit:** Center for Economic Studies, "The Parental Gender Earnings Gap in the United States," November 2017, www2.census.gov/ces/wp/2017/CES-WP-17-68.pdf.

42 **only 83 percent:** U.S. Department of Labor, "5 Fast Facts: The Gender Wage Gap," March 14, 2023, blog.dol.gov/2023/03/14/5-fast-facts-the-gender-wage-gap.

42 **"motherhood penalty":** American Association of University Women, "The Motherhood Penalty," accessed April 20, 2023, aauw.org/issues/equity/motherhood.

42n **"Having a first child":** National Center for Health Statistics, "Fertility of Men and Women Aged 15–49 in the United States."

43 **about one in five babies:** National Center for Health Statistics, "Births: Final Data for 2021."

43 **nearly 20 percent:** National Center for Health Statistics, "Births: Final Data for 2021."

43n **"subsided in 2020":** Sabrina Tavernise, "The U.S. Birthrate Has Dropped Again. The Pandemic May Be Accelerating the Decline," *The New York Times,* May 5, 2021, nytimes.com/2021/05/05/us/us-birthrate-falls-covid .html.

43   **nine million babies:** Anne-Kristin Kuhnt and Jasmin Passet-Wittig, "Families Formed through Assisted Reproductive Technology: Causes, Experiences, and Consequences in an International Context," *Reproductive Biomedicine and Society Online* 14 (2022): 289–296, ncbi.nlm.nih.gov/pmc /articles/PMC8907601/.

44   **nearly 80 percent:** Centers for Disease Control and Prevention, "ART Success Rates: 2021 Preliminary Data," last modified May 31, 2023, cdc.gov /art/artdata/index.html.

44   **has been heralded:** Julia Calderone, "10 Years of Fertility Advances," *New York Times,* April 19, 2020, nytimes.com/2020/04/19/parenting/fertility /fertility-advances.html.

44   **"If women had the power":** Eig, *The Birth of the Pill,* 6.

45   **mid- to late thirties:** E. Chronopoulou, C. Raperport, A. Sfakianakis, G. Srivastava, and R. Homburg, "Elective Oocyte Cryopreservation for Age-Related Fertility Decline," *Journal of Assisted Reproduction and Genetics* 38, no. 5 (2021): 1177–1186, doi.org/10.1007/s10815-021-02072-w.

45n **"The average age":** Naomi May, "Gen Z Are Freezing Their Eggs. Why?," *Vice,* July 20, 2023, vice.com/en/article/bvj7nz/why-gen-z-are-freezing -eggs.

45   **In 1965, after seeing promising results:** James L. Burks, M. Edward Davis, Aimee H. Bakken, and Jerry J. Tomasovic, "Morphologic Evaluation of Frozen Rabbit and Human Ova," *Fertility and Sterility* 16, no. 5 (1965): 638–641, doi.org/10.1016/S0015-0282(16)35710-7.

46   **In 1986, in Australia:** Christopher Chen, "Pregnancy After Human Oocyte Cryopreservation," *The Lancet* 327, no. 8486 (1986): 884–886, doi.org/10 .1016/S0140-6736(86)90989-X.

46   **the Church's denunciation of embryo freezing:** A 1987 document known as *Donum Vitae* (The Gift of Life), an authoritarian proclamation on reproductive science, addressed the morality of many at-the-time-modern fertility procedures, and specifically IVF. The Vatican's declarations guide Catholic doctors and hospitals around the world, and the *Donum Vitae* governed the Church's stance on embryo freezing while Dr. Fabbri and Dr. Porcu were doing their research in the 1980s and 1990s. In 2008, the Vatican issued a new document, *Dignitas Personae,* which gives doctrinal directives on certain embryonic ethical controversies that had emerged since 1987, after *Donum Vitae* was released. The thirty-five-page document denounces most forms of fertility treatment, including egg freezing, which it deems immoral when used for artificial procreation. (The Vatican hadn't commented on egg freezing in its 1987 document.) In addition to being

against egg freezing, the Catholic Church still condemns IVF and other forms of assisted reproductive technology (as well as contraception and abortion).

47 **Dr. Fabbri tried adjusting:** R. Fabbri, E. Porcu, T. Marsella, G. Rocchetta, S. Venturoli, and C. Flamigni, "Human Oocyte Cryopreservation: New Perspectives Regarding Oocyte Survival," *Human Reproduction* 16, no. 3 (2001): 411–416, doi.org/10.1093/humrep/16.3.411.

47 **a new method, called intracytoplasmic sperm injection:** ICSI was the first truly successful treatment for male infertility and today is often used when prior IVF cycles have failed or a couple is confronting unexplained infertility.

48 **a baby born from a frozen egg using ICSI:** The child was born February 17, 1997, from an egg that had been frozen for four months. Later that year, the first successful pregnancy in the United States from frozen eggs resulted in the birth of twins, in Georgia. Eleonora Porcu, Patrizia M. Ciotti, Raffaella Fabbri, Otello Magrini, Renato Seracchioli, and Carlo Flamigni, "Birth of a Healthy Female After Intracytoplasmic Sperm Injection of Cryopreserved Human Oocytes," *Fertility and Sterility* 68, no. 4 (1997): 724–726, doi.org/10.1016/s0015-0282(97)00268-9.

48 **Until 2003, when it was proven:** Tae Ki Yoon, Thomas J. Kim, Sung Eun Park, Seung Wook Hong, Jung Jae Ko, Hyung Min Chung, and Kwang Yul Cha, "Live Births After Vitrification of Oocytes in a Stimulated In Vitro Fertilization–Embryo Transfer Program," *Fertility and Sterility* 79, no. 6 (2003): 1323–1326, doi.org/10.1016/S0015-0282(03)00258-9.

48 **Vitrification significantly improved egg survival:** "A Review of Best Practices of Rapid-Cooling Vitrification for Oocytes and Embryos: A Committee Opinion," *Fertility and Sterility* 115, no. 2 (2021): 305–310, doi.org/10.1016/j.fertnstert.2020.11.017.

49 **lifted the "experimental" label on egg freezing:** American Society for Reproductive Medicine (ASRM) and Society for Assisted Reproductive Technology (SART) Committee Report, "Mature Oocyte Cryopreservation: A Guideline," *Fertility and Sterility* 99, no. 1 (2013): 37–43, doi.org/10.1016/j.fertnstert.2012.09.028.

50 **More than nine hundred babies:** Charlotte Schubert, "Egg Freezing Enters Clinical Mainstream," *Nature,* October 23, 2012, scientificamerican.com/article/egg-freezing-enters-clinical-mainstream/.

50 **With that designation:** ASRM and SART Committee Report, "Ovarian Tissue and Oocyte Cryopreservation," *Fertility and Sterility* 90, no. 5 (2008): 241–246, doi.org/10.1016/j.fertnstert.2008.08.039.

50 **Despite the society's recommendation:** Briana Rudick, Neisha Opper, Richard Paulson, Kristin Bendikson, and Karine Chung, "The Status of Oocyte Cryopreservation in the United States," *Fertility and Sterility* 94, no. 7 (2010): 2642–2646, doi.org/10.1016/j.fertnstert.2010.04.079.

50   **after reviewing nearly:** Josephine Johnston and Miriam Zoll, "Is Freezing Your Eggs Dangerous? A Primer," *New Republic,* November 1, 2014, newrepublic.com/article/120077/dangers-and-realities-egg-freezing.

50   **"There are not yet sufficient data":** ASRM and SART Committee Report, "Mature Oocyte Cryopreservation," 42.

50   **simply to delay childbearing:** It could be argued that there wasn't enough quality research to go on even when it came to removing the experimental label from the procedure. At the time, only four randomized clinical egg freezing trials had been conducted. And of the 981 fairly small egg freezing studies ASRM reviewed, only 112 addressed safety and efficacy concerns.

51   **"While a careful review of the literature":** "Highlights from the 68th Annual Meeting of the American Society for Reproductive Medicine," *Texas Fertility Center,* October 22, 2012, ASRM, txfertility.com/wp-content/uploads/2014/01/ASRMeggfreezerelease.pdf.

51   **in its 2008 report:** ASRM and SART Committee Report, "Essential Elements of Informed Consent for Elective Oocyte Cryopreservation," *Fertility and Sterility* 88, no. 6 (2008): 134, doi.org/10.1016/j.fertnstert.2007.10.009.

51   **"while this technology may appear to be":** ASRM and SART Committee Report, "Mature Oocyte Cryopreservation," 41.

51   **"Marketing this technology":** ASRM and SART Committee Report, "Mature Oocyte Cryopreservation," 41.

51   **Apple and Facebook announced:** Danielle Friedman, "Perk Up: Facebook and Apple Now Pay for Women to Freeze Eggs," NBC News, October 14, 2014, nbcnews.com/news/us-news/perk-facebook-apple-now-pay-women-freeze-eggs-n225011.

51   **debate ensued:** Miriam Zoll, "Freezing Eggs Puts Women and Infants' Health at Stake," *New York Times,* October 16, 2014, nytimes.com/roomfordebate/2014/10/15/freezing-plans-for-motherhood-and-staying-on-the-job/freezing-eggs-puts-women-and-infants-health-at-stake.

52   **nearly 115,000 women:** I obtained the numbers of patients who froze eggs for non-medical reasons from 2009 to 2022 from SART directly.

57   **"Not since the birth control pill":** Emma Rosenblum, "Later, Baby: Will Freezing Your Eggs Free Your Career?," Bloomberg, April 17, 2014, bloomberg.com/news/articles/2014-04-17/new-egg-freezing-technology-eases-womens-career-family-angst.

CHAPTER 4

63   **Dr. Ruth Lewis:** At one of her first egg freezing appointments, Remy introduced me to her doctor as a friend and someone writing about egg freezing. I agreed not to use her doctor's real name.

70n **"a crackling network":** Rachel E. Gross, *Vagina Obscura: An Anatomical Voyage* (New York: W. W. Norton & Company, 2022), 161.

74n **conceived at the same rates:** Alexandra Farrow, M.G.R. Hull, K. Northstone, H. Taylor, W.C.L. Ford, and Jean Golding, "Prolonged Use of Oral Contraception Before a Planned Pregnancy Is Associated with a Decreased Risk of Delayed Conception," *Human Reproduction* 17, no. 10 (2002): 2754–2761, doi.org/10.1093/humrep/17.10.2754.

74 **roughly 20 percent:** Guttmacher Institute, "Contraceptive Use in the United States by Method," May 2021, guttmacher.org/fact-sheet/contraceptive -method-use-united-states.

79n **female sterilization:** United Nations, "Contraceptive Use by Method 2019," 2019, digitallibrary.un.org/record/3849735.

80n **which proved 99 percent effective:** Dani Blum, "Despite Encouraging Research, a Male Birth Control Pill Remains Elusive," *New York Times,* March 25, 2022, nytimes.com/2022/03/25/well/male-birth-control-pills .html.

80n **An injectable hydrogel:** Paul Anderson, Damien Bolton, and Nathan Lawrentschuk, "Preliminary Results of a First in Human Dose-Ranging Clinical Trial of ADAM, a Nonhormonal Hydrogel-Based Male Contraceptive," *Journal of Urology* 209, no. 4 (2023), doi.org/10.1097/JU .0000000000003352.08.

80 **About 65 percent of reproductive-age women:** National Center for Health Statistics, Centers for Disease Control and Prevention, "Current Contraceptive Status Among Women Aged 15–49: United States, 2017– 2019," 2020, cdc.gov/nchs/products/databriefs/db388.htm.

80 **four in ten women:** Kaiser Family Foundation, "Contraception in the United States: A Closer Look at Experiences, Preferences, and Coverage," 2022, kff.org/womens-health-policy/report/contraception-in-the-united -states-a-closer-look-at-experiences-preferences-and-coverage.

81 **more than six million:** Guttmacher Institute, "Contraceptive Use in the United States by Method."

81 **hundreds of millions:** United Nations, "Contraceptive Use by Method 2019."

81n **many women struggle:** Lauren N. Lessard, Deborah Karasek, Sandi Ma, Philip Darney, Julianna Deardorff, Maureen Lahiff, Dan Grossman, and Diana Greene Foster, "Contraceptive Features Preferred by Women at High Risk of Unintended Pregnancy," *Perspectives on Sexual and Reproductive Health* 44, no. 3 (2012): 194–200, doi.org/10.1363/4419412.

81 **mood disorders:** Eveline Mu and Jayashri Kulkarni, "Hormonal Contra-ception and Mood Disorders," *Australian Prescriber* 45, no. 3 (2022): 75–79, doi.org/10.18773/austprescr.2022.025.

81 **serious health risks:** "Hormonal Methods of Contraception," Merck Manual Consumer Version, last modified August 2023, merckmanuals.com /home/women-s-health-issues/family-planning/hormonal-methods-of -contraception.

CHAPTER 5

Portions of this chapter were previously published in The New York Times *on May 1, 2020, under the title "Fertility Clinics Stay Open Despite Unclear Guidelines."*

93 **more than 50 percent:** According to the (meager) research available. The World Health Organization says the statistic is even higher, up to a worrying 70 percent. Wendy Wolf, Rachel Wattick, Olivia Kinkade, and Melissa Olfert, "Geographical Prevalence of Polycystic Ovary Syndrome as Determined by Region and Race/Ethnicity," *International Journal of Environmental Research and Public Health* 12, no. 11 (2018), doi.org/10.3390/ijerph15112589.

96 **demographics are beginning to shift:** Dayna Evans, "'I've Just Spent $14,000 on One Egg': Five People on Their Egg Freezing Experience," *Buzzfeed News,* January 26, 2023, buzzfeednews.com/article/daynaevans/egg-freezing-stories-what-to-expect.

96 **roughly 35 percent:** Alisha Haridasani Gupta and Dani Blum, "Hope, Regret, Uncertainty: 7 Women on Freezing Their Eggs," *New York Times,* December 28, 2022, nytimes.com/2022/12/23/well/family/egg-freezing-fertility.html.

96 **more than 80 percent:** Marcia Inhorn, Daphna Birenbaum-Carmeli, Ruoxi Yu, and Pasquale Patrizio, "Egg Freezing at the End of Romance: A Technology of Hope, Despair, and Repair," *Science, Technology, & Human Values* 47, no. 1 (2021), doi.org/10.1177/0162243921995892.

97 **Inhorn identified:** Matilda Hay, "What the Egg-Freezing Process Feels Like: One Woman's Fertility Journey," *Washington Post,* September 25, 2023, washingtonpost.com/wellness/2023/09/25/egg-freezing-fertility-motherhood-emotions/.

97 **"a reproductive backstop":** Marcia C. Inhorn, *Motherhood on Ice: The Mating Gap and Why Women Freeze Their Eggs* (New York: New York University Press, 2023).

98 **largest egg freezing ethnographic study to date:** The two-year study comprised 150 women who had completed at least one cycle of non-medical egg freezing and volunteered to participate in the study. At the time of egg freezing, 85 percent of the women were single, and of these single women, 35 percent had experienced a breakup. Additionally, 26 percent of the married and partnered women in the study were in the midst of separations.

98 **"For women whose":** Inhorn, *Motherhood on Ice,* 57.

99n **one in six adults:** World Health Organization, "Infertility Prevalence Estimates," 2023, who.int/publications/i/item/978920068315. For a full discussion on male infertility and the plummeting sperm levels among men in Western countries, see *Count Down: How Our Modern World Is Threatening Sperm Counts, Altering Male and Female Reproductive Development, and*

Imperiling the Future of the Human Race by Shanna H. Swan, in which she writes, ". . . it's that the chemicals in our environment and unhealthy lifestyle practices in our modern world are disrupting our hormonal balance, causing varying degrees of reproductive havoc that can foil fertility and lead to long-term health problems even after one has left the reproductive years."

CHAPTER 6

106 **the fun really begins:** Once past the obstacle of the cervix's muscular contractions, sperm must then "choose" and swim up one of two fallopian tubes, while the egg only travels down one. Then, the egg can affect which sperm wins the race—the audition, really—with the chemicals it releases in the follicular fluid that surrounds the egg. The sperm that gets there first and is able to penetrate the egg shell—via the very complex biological process that has to occur—gets the starring role in conceiving a baby.

109 **"Your menstrual cycle is not something":** Toni Weschler, *Taking Charge of Your Fertility*, 20th Anniversary Edition (New York: William Morrow, 2015).

111 **Fertilization happens when:** The establishment of a pregnancy is a process: first fertilization, then implantation. Between one-third and one-half of all fertilized eggs never fully implant in a woman's uterine lining. Also worth noting: The term "conception" isn't actually a medical term, and it's often mistakenly used synonymously with "fertilization," when technically it's equated with implantation.

111 **they'd use a condom:** Although, Will noted, there was something to be said for having to wait. As Weschler writes: "By choosing to postpone sex rather than using a barrier method during the fertile phase, people often feel they're living in harmony with their fertility, rather than fighting it." Weschler, *Taking Charge of Your Fertility*, 164.

117 **$100 billion by 2030:** According to a 2023 report by Precedence Research, a worldwide research and consulting organization. Precedence Research, "Femtech Market Size to Surpass US $108.78 Billion by 2032," 2023, precedenceresearch.com/femtech-market.

117 **the only:** The app Natural Cycles, when combined with the wearable Oura ring, is also FDA-approved for fertility tracking.

117 **with 90 percent accuracy:** Brianna Goodale, Mohaned Shilaih, Lisa Falco, Franziska Dammeier, Györgyi Hamvas, and Brigitte Leeners, "Wearable Sensors Reveal Menses-Driven Changes in Physiology and Enable Prediction of the Fertile Window: Observational Study," *Journal of Medical Internet Research* 21, no. 4 (2019): e13404, doi.org/10.2196/13404.

121 **users were dissatisfied:** Daniel A. Epstein, Nicole B. Lee, Jennifer H. Kang, Elena Agapie, Jessica Schroeder, Laura R. Pina, James Fogarty, Julie A. Kientz, and Sean Munson, "Examining Menstrual Tracking to Inform the Design of Personal Informatics Tools," *CHI '17: Proceedings of the 2017 CHI*

Conference on Human Factors in Computing Systems (New York: ACM, 2017), 6876–6888, doi.org/10.1145/3025453.3025635.

121 **an unintended pregnancy:** One of the more alarming studies illustrating the unreliability of fertility-tracker apps was a case study in 2018, when thirty-seven women who relied on the European fertility app Natural Cycles as their contraception method reported unwanted pregnancies. Authorities in Sweden investigated the app, which is certified in Europe for birth control and approved for marketing as a contraceptive in the United States by the FDA. Natural Cycles has since further clarified the risk for users.

122 **"share some user data":** Catherine Roberts, "These Period Tracker Apps Say They Put Privacy First. Here's What We Found," *Consumer Reports,* May 25, 2022, consumerreports.org/health/health-privacy/period-tracker -apps-privacy-a2278134145/.

122 **federal safeguards for patient privacy:** It's better in Europe, though. One reason I decided to use Clue's app is that the company that developed it is based in Germany, where it's subject to stricter regulations. The company follows the same EU restrictions for every person using the app, including those in the United States. Clue also makes it easy for users to understand how it shares users' information—its privacy policy is light on jargon and broken down into readable chunks—and lets people opt out of having their data shared.

122 **just 1 percent:** McKinsey & Company, "Unlocking Opportunities in Women's Healthcare," 2022, mckinsey.com/industries/healthcare/our -insights/unlocking-opportunities-in-womens-healthcare.

123 **"And here lies the":** Alisha Haridasani Gupta and Natasha Singer, "Your App Knows You Got Your Period. Guess Who It Told?," *New York Times,* January 28, 2021, nytimes.com/2021/01/28/us/period-apps-health -technology-women-privacy.html.

123 **"I thought how simple":** Bonhams, "Voices of the 20th Century," auction in New York, June 16, 2015, bonhams.com/auction/22407/lot/37/crane -margaret-inventorthe-first-home-pregnancy-test-original-predictor-home -pregnancy-test-prototype-1968/.

124 **"Unlike medical tests that reveal":** Cari Romm, "Before There Were Home Pregnancy Tests," *The Atlantic,* June 17, 2015, theatlantic.com/health /archive/2015/06/history-home-pregnancy-test/396077/.

124 **"Regardless of who":** Romm, "Before There Were Home Pregnancy Tests."

124 **"a private little revolution":** "The Thin Blue Line: The History of the Pregnancy Test," National Institutes of Health, accessed August 8, 2022, history.nih.gov/display/history/Pregnancy+Test+-+A+Thin+Blue+Line +The+History+of+the+Pregnancy+Test.

125 **"I feel that the reputations":** P. A. Entwistle, "Do-It-Yourself Pregnancy Tests: The Tip of the Iceberg," *American Journal of Public Health* 66, no. 11

(1976): 1108–1109, ncbi.nlm.nih.gov/pmc/articles/PMC1653504/pdf/amjph00498-0064c.pdf.

129n **can impact AMH and suppress follicle count:** Scott M. Nelson, Benjamin J. Ewing, Piotr S. Gromski, and Sharon F. Briggs, "Contraceptive-Specific Antimüllerian Hormone Values in Reproductive-Age Women: A Population Study of 42,684 Women," *Fertility and Sterility* 119, no. 6 (2023): 1069–1077, doi.org/10.1016/j.fertnstert.2023.02.019.

129 **AMH testing:** "What Low AMH Means and How It Affects Fertility," Ro, last modified April 27, 2021, ro.co/health-guide/how-does-low-amh-affect-fertility.

130 **AMH does not reveal:** Anne Z. Steiner, David Pritchard, Frank Z. Stanczyk, James S. Kesner, Juliana W. Meadows, Amy H. Herring, and Donna D. Baird, "Association Between Biomarkers of Ovarian Reserve and Infertility Among Older Women of Reproductive Age," *Journal of the American Medical Association* 318, no. 14 (2017): 1367–1376, doi.org/doi:10.1001/jama.2017.14588.

130 **"These tests are":** Julia Belluz, "The Fertility Testing Racket Just Got Debunked by Science," *Vox,* October 11, 2017, vox.com/science-and-health/2017/10/11/16453714/ovarian-reserve-test-science-results-fertility.

131 **"fertile as hell":** "I Tested My Fertility Hormones and Discovered I Had Low AMH at Age 29. It Changed My Life," Ro, last modified April 21, 2021, ro.co/fertility/caroline-lunny-fertility-story.

135n **but several studies have concluded:** Yao Lu, Yuan Wang, Ting Zhang, Guiquan Wang, Yaqiong He, Steven R. Lindheim, Zhangsheng Yu, and Yun Sun, "Effect of Pretreatment Oral Contraceptives on Fresh and Cumulative Live Birth In Vitro Fertilization Outcomes in Ovulatory Women," *Fertility and Sterility* 114, no. 4 (2020): 779–786, doi.org/10.1016/j.fertnstert.2020.05.021.

CHAPTER 7

137 **"We all knew that":** Grace Paley, *Just As I Thought* (New York: Macmillan, 1999), 13.

138 **twenty-four states restrict:** Brooke Whitfield, Elsa Vizcarra, Asha Dane'el, Lina Palomares, Graci D'Amore, Julie Maslowsky, and Kari White, "Minors' Experiences Accessing Confidential Contraception in Texas," *Journal of Adolescent Health* 72, no. 4 (2023): 591–598, doi.org/10.1016/j.jadohealth.2022.11.230.

138 **a stark difference:** "Parental Consent and Notice for Contraceptives Threatens Teen Health and Constitutional Rights," Center for Reproductive Rights, November 1, 2006, reproductiverights.org/parental-consent-and-notice-for-contraceptives-threatens-teen-health-and-constitutional-rights/.

140n **about one in ten:** National Center for Health Statistics, Centers for Disease

Control and Prevention, "Current Contraceptive Status Among Women Aged 15–49: United States, 2017–2019," 2020, cdc.gov/nchs/products /databriefs/db388.htm.

140 **"Taught that their anatomy":** Janice P. Nimura, "Why 'Unwell Women' Have Gone Misdiagnosed for Centuries," *New York Times,* June 8, 2021, nytimes.com/2021/06/08/books/review/unwell-women-elinor-cleghorn .html.

141 **50 percent of reproductive-age women:** Lisbet S. Lundsberg, Lubna Pal, Aileen M. Gariepy, Xiao Xu, Micheline C. Chu, and Jessica L. Illuzzi, "Knowledge, Attitudes, and Practices Regarding Conception and Fertility: A Population-Based Survey Among Reproductive-Age United States Women," *Fertility and Sterility* 101, no. 3 (2014): 767–774.E2, doi.org/10.1016/j .fertnstert.2013.12.006.

141n **"We found that 40 percent":** "The Science of Baby-Making Still a Mystery for Many Women," *YaleNews,* January 27, 2014, Yale Office of Public Affairs and Communications, news.yale.edu/2014/01/27/science-baby-making -still-mystery-many-women.

141 **less than one-third:** The survey concluded that the OB/GYNs' limited consultation time and their limited knowledge were among the most frequently reported barriers when counseling patients about reproductive aging. Rani Fritz, Susan Klugman, Harry Lieman, Jay Schulkin, Laura Taouk, Neko Castleberry, and Erkan Buyuk, "Counseling Patients on Reproductive Aging and Elective Fertility Preservation—A Survey of Obstetricians and Gynecologists' Experience, Approach, and Knowledge," *Journal of Assisted Reproduction and Genetics* 35, no. 9 (2018): 1613–1621, doi .org/10.1007/s10815-018-1273-7.

141 **Nearly half of U.S. counties:** Michael Ollove, "A Shortage in the Nation's Maternal Health Care," *Stateline,* August 15, 2016, stateline.org/2016/08 /15/a-shortage-in-the-nations-maternal-health-care/.

142 **not that TV, music, and movies:** Books such as the revolutionary feminist health book *Our Bodies, Ourselves* I mentioned earlier have helped, but after being consistently revised over the decades, it stopped printing new editions in 2018.

142 **"There's nowhere else":** Maggie Jones, "What Teenagers Are Learning from Online Porn," *New York Times Magazine,* February 7, 2018, nytimes .com/2018/02/07/magazine/teenagers-learning-online-porn-literacy-sex -education.html.

142 **one hundred most-frequented:** Jones, "What Teenagers Are Learning from Online Porn."

142 **shaping their early ideas about sex:** Amaze.org is an excellent resource for reliable sex ed information for both kids and parents. Scarleteen.com offers "sex ed for the real world," with inclusive, comprehensive info for teens and emerging adults. For parents with younger kids, *It's Not the Stork* by Robie H. Harris is a great place to start.

145n **abortion very rarely affects:** National Academies of Sciences, Engineering, and Medicine, *The Safety and Quality of Abortion Care in the United States* (Washington, D.C.: National Academies Press, 2018), doi.org/10.17226 /24950; Jen Gunter, "Can an Abortion Affect Your Fertility?," *New York Times,* May 30, 2019, nytimes.com/2019/05/30/well/can-an-abortion -affect-your-fertility.html.

149　**"Older female age":** American Society for Reproductive Medicine, "Planned Oocyte Cryopreservation for Women Seeking to Preserve Future Reproductive Potential: An Ethics Committee Opinion," *Fertility and Sterility* 110, no. 6 (2018): 1022–1028, doi.org/10.1016/j.fertnstert.2018 .08.027.

150　**"Fertility meant nothing":** Ariel Levy, *The Rules Do Not Apply* (New York: Random House, 2018), 85.

150　**"We lived in a world":** Levy, *The Rules Do Not Apply,* 10.

CHAPTER 8

168　**nearly 115,000 healthy women:** I obtained the numbers of patients who froze eggs for non-medical reasons from 2009 to 2022 from SART directly. The actual number for this 2009–2022 timeframe is higher, though. There are women electively freezing eggs and embryos in the United States who aren't part of SART's data set, which relies on data reporting from SART-member clinics. About 85 percent of U.S. fertility clinics are members of SART and report their ART data to SART each year. So, egg freezers from at least 15 percent of additional fertility clinics aren't included in this figure, but there's no way of knowing exactly how many are left out.

168　**the latest year:** As mentioned in chapter 1, preliminary 2022 egg freezing data came out in 2024. There's typically a two-year lag when it comes to compiling ART statistics. It takes a while to wait for live-birth outcomes, and then there's the collection of the data by the fertility clinics, which SART audits before submitting it to the CDC for analysis and official publication.

168n **data do differentiate:** SART began collecting the reason for fertility preservation from clinics in 2016. Prior to 2016, when clinics submitted their annual data to SART, they did not specify whether the egg freezing cycles they'd conducted that year were for women undergoing gonadotoxic treatments (chemotherapy or radiation) or for women freezing for non-gonadotoxic reasons (healthy women seeking fertility preservation). Now clinics do, although the field is not mandatory.

168n **the vast majority:** In 2022, for example, fewer than 4 percent of women who froze their eggs did so because they had to get chemotherapy or other potentially debilitating treatments.

168　**73 percent increase:** From 16,786 egg freezing cycles in 2020 to 29,083 cycles in 2022. Society for Assisted Reproductive Technology, "Preliminary

National Summary Report for 2022," 2022, sartcorsonline.com/rptCSR
_PublicMultYear.aspx?reportingYear=2022.

168 **40 percent:** Centers for Disease Control and Prevention, "ART Success
Rates: 2021 Preliminary Data," last modified May 31, 2023, cdc.gov/art
/artdata/index.html.

169 **the low thousands:** In 2022, nearly 92,000 babies were born in the United
States using ART. (That includes IVF using donor eggs, fresh eggs, and
frozen eggs; the data only partially differentiates among the three.) Out of
those ninety thousand or so babies, around 250 were born from frozen non-
donor eggs, based on data from SART. (This data isn't publicly available;
SART provided me with a year-by-year breakdown of live births from
frozen eggs in the United States from 2009 to 2022.)

169 **only 6 percent:** Karin Hammarberg, Maggie Kirkman, Natasha Pritchard,
Martha Hickey, Michelle Peate, John McBain, Franca Agresta, Chris Bayly,
and Jane Fisher, "Reproductive Experiences of Women Who Cryopreserved
Oocytes for Non-Medical Reasons," *Human Reproduction* 32, no. 3 (2017):
575–581, doi.org/10.1093/humrep/dew342.

170 **"the average return rate":** Pragati Kakkar, Joanna Geary, Tania Stockburger, Aida Kaffel, Julia Kopeika, and Tarek El-Toukhy, "Outcomes of
Social Egg Freezing: A Cohort Study and a Comprehensive Literature
Review," *Journal of Clinical Medicine* 12, no. 13 (2023): 4182, doi.org/10
.3390/jcm12134182.

170 **oft-discussed scary statistic:** The original ASRM report seems to have
been wiped from the internet, but in 2014, major outlets, from *The New
York Times* to *The New Republic* to PBS—and, more recently, in 2017 (*The
Washington Post*)—repeated this misleading statistic, again and again.

171 **"While anecdotal evidence suggests":** Charlotte Alter, "The Truth About
Freezing Your Eggs," *Time,* July 16, 2015, time.com/3960528/the-truth
-about-freezing-your-eggs/.

171 **74 percent of eggs:** All frozen egg cycles performed after July 2011, which
was about 70 percent of the cycles in the study, involved vitrification. The
study's first egg freezing-and-thaw cycle was performed in 2006; a sharp
increase in thaws occurred after, with 70 percent occurring from 2016 to
2020. Sarah Druckenmiller Cascante, Jennifer K. Blakemore, Shannon
DeVore, Brooke Hodes-Wertz, M. Elizabeth Fino, Alan S. Berkeley, Carlos
M. Parra, Caroline McCaffrey, and James A. Grifo, "Fifteen Years of
Autologous Oocyte Thaw Outcomes from a Large University-Based
Fertility Center," *Fertility and Sterility* 118, no. 1 (2022): 158–166, doi.org
/10.1016/j.fertnstert.2022.04.013.

172 **The younger a woman was:** Eighty percent of patients were between thirty-
five and forty, and 12 percent were over the age of forty-one. Just 8 percent
of patients were under the age of thirty-five when they underwent their first
egg freezing cycle; the youngest patient was twenty-seven years old.

173n **transfer a single embryo:** Embryos are graded at each point in their development to determine which ones are most likely to grow successfully when implanted. Thanks to scientific advances, doctors are now better able to select the best embryos to implant, which in turn allows them to transfer just one, rather than multiple, embryos into the womb at a time. Almost 95 percent of ART babies born in 2021 were singletons, compared to 80 percent in 2015.

174 **twenty eggs are recommended:** E. Chronopoulou, C. Raperport, A. Sfakianakis, G. Srivastava, and R. Homburg, "Elective Oocyte Cryo-preservation for Age-Related Fertility Decline," *Journal of Assisted Reproduction and Genetics* 38, no. 5 (2021): 1177–1186, doi.org/10.1007/s10815-021-02072-w.

174 **"irrespective of age at freezing":** Kakkar et al., "Outcomes of Social Egg Freezing," 4182.

174n **"clearly suggest that":** Chronopoulou et al., "Elective Oocyte Cryopreservation for Age-Related Fertility Decline," 1177–1186.

174 **assign probabilities to egg freezing:** R. H. Goldman, C. Racowsky, L. V. Farland, S. Munné, L. Ribustello, and J. H. Fox, "Predicting the Likelihood of Live Birth for Elective Oocyte Cryopreservation: A Counseling Tool for Physicians and Patients," *Human Reproduction* 32, no. 4 (2017): 853–859, doi.org/10.1093/humrep/dex008.

175 **That's pretty good:** It's worth noting, however, that in the paper's conclusion the authoring physicians conceded that the numbers may be too optimistic, given "the paucity of validation data" available from women who have actually used frozen eggs to try to become pregnant.

175 **publicly available calculators:** The one I like best is Spring Fertility's, found at springfertility.com/eggcalc/.

182 **"when it comes to":** Jessica Hamzelou, "How Do I Know if Egg Freezing Is for Me?," *MIT Technology Review,* January 27, 2023, technologyreview.com/2023/01/27/1067333/how-do-i-know-if-egg-freezing-is-for-me/.

CHAPTER 9

Additional resources for topics mentioned in this chapter:

Comprehensive breakdown of egg freezing's costs, including average costs by region:

• fertilityiq.com/egg-freezing/the-costs-of-egg-freezing

Navigating specialty pharmacies:

• resolve.org/learn/what-are-my-options/medications/specialty-pharmacies/

If you're a self-pay fertility patient, be sure to ask the clinic(s) if they have discounted self-pay options for patients not using insurance. Speak with the specialty pharmacy where you're buying fertility meds from about discounts, too.

State-by-state information about fertility insurance coverage laws (updated regularly):

- resolve.org/learn/financial-resources-for-family-building/insurance
  -coverage/insurance-coverage-by-state/

Financial resources and financial assistance programs for fertility treatment:

- resolve.org/learn/financial-resources-for-family-building/
- allianceforfertilitypreservation.org/financial-assistance-programs/

Grants and charities:

- fertilityiq.com/topics/fertilityiq-data-and-notes/free-ivf-grants-and
  -charities

Refund and "freeze-and-share" programs:

- fertilityiq.com/topics/cost/ivf-refund-and-package-programs
- cofertility.com/freeze-learn/the-ultimate-guide-to-the-split-program

185 **"How do you build":** Kaitlyn Tiffany, "The SoulCycle of Fertility Sells Egg-Freezing and 'Empowerment' to 25-Year-Olds," *The Verge,* September 11, 2018, theverge.com/2018/9/11/17823810/kindbody-startup-fertility-clinic -egg-freezing-millennials-location.

187 **"Just like Uber":** Angelina Chapin, "Egg Freezing for Millennials: The Latest Start-up Trend," *The Cut,* February 28, 2017, thecut.com/2017/05 /egg-freezing-clinics-for-millennials-a-new-start-up-trend.html.

189 **roughly $16,000 per cycle:** As egg freezing has exploded in popularity over the last several years, I've seen cost estimates ballparked as low as $7,000 and as high as $20,000. One reason it's hard to get a handle on the costs is that many clinics are not transparent about their pricing. Another is that the cost of egg freezing varies due to several factors: where in the country a woman is doing it; the amount of hormone medications required for her particular cycle; how long she pays to keep them stored on ice; what the clinic charges for ultrasound monitoring, anesthesia, and lab processing; and more. Also, fertility treatment prices across the board have gone up in recent years as materials and operating costs have increased. Finally, women often end up paying more for egg freezing than the sticker price they've seen advertised. The current cost estimates I explain here take all this into account.

189n **And they're going up:** Yeganeh Torbati, "With Egg Freezing Increasingly Common, Fertility Clinics Hike Storage Fees," *Washington Post,* April 14, 2023, washingtonpost.com/business/2023/04/12/egg-freezing -storage-prices/.

189 **on average, 2.1 cycles:** FertilityIQ, "Egg Freezing: The Costs of Egg

Freezing," accessed January 8, 2023, fertilityiq.com/egg-freezing/the-costs -of-egg-freezing.

189   **"Welcome to the fertility casino":** Ron Lieber, "A Baby or Your Money Back: All About Fertility Clinic Package Deals," *New York Times,* April 14, 2017, nytimes.com/2017/04/14/your-money/baby-fertility-clinic-package -deals.html.

190   **"Meet Prelude Fertility":** Miguel Helft, "Meet Prelude Fertility, The $200 Million Startup That Wants to Stop the Biological Clock," *Forbes,* October 17, 2016, forbes.com/sites/miguelhelft/2016/10/17/prelude-fertility-200 -million-startup-stop-biological-clock/?sh=7c175af87260.

190   **"envisioned a new norm":** Anna Louie Sussman, "The Promise and Perils of the New Fertility Entrepreneurs," *New Yorker,* May 19, 2021, newyorker .com/tech/annals-of-technology/the-promise-and-perils-of-the-new -fertility-entrepreneurs.

190   **Bundl also promises:** Bundl, "Peace of Mind with Shared Risk IVF," accessed August 27, 2022, bundlfertility.com/peace-of-mind-with-shared -risk-ivf/.

191   **"We are now targeting":** Ruth La Ferla, "These Companies Really, Really, Really Want to Freeze Your Eggs," *New York Times,* August 29, 2018, nytimes.com/2018/08/29/style/egg-freezing-fertility-millennials.html.

192   **"The more friends":** OVA, "OVA Programs," accessed November 18, 2022, ovaeggfreezing.com/programs/.

192   **"freeze and share":** Kristine Thomason, "New Programs Allow Women to Freeze Their Eggs for Free—As Long as They Donate Half of Them," *Women's Health,* womenshealthmag.com/health/a43621157/egg-freezing -donation-programs-national-infertility-awareness-week-2023/.

192   **package or "shared risk" programs:** When patients do multiple IVF cycles, the costs climb fast. To offset this, roughly half of U.S. fertility clinics offer the chance to pay up front to buy a package of treatments at a discount, sometimes with a refund if the patient doesn't "succeed," i.e., go home with a baby. This is a gamble on the patient's part. If you need to use these extra treatments, you purchased them at a discount. But if you have a baby or get pregnant before using all these cycles, you don't get your money back.

192n **SART found that:** Society for Assisted Reproductive Technology, "Preliminary National Summary Report for 2022," 2022, sartcorsonline .com/rptCSR_PublicMultYear.aspx?reportingYear=2022.

192   **Shady Grove Fertility:** Shady Grove Fertility, "Shared Risk 100% Refund Program," accessed August 6, 2023, shadygrovefertility.com/refund-programs -for-infertility-treatment/.

192   **Spring Fertility:** When I emailed Spring Fertility to clarify their money-back policy, a company spokesperson explained that, for a patient who meets their refund program criteria, Spring refunds all money the patient paid to Spring, which constitutes all treatment costs. This doesn't include medication costs, which the patient paid to the pharmacy, or anesthesia

costs, which were paid to Spring's anesthesiologists. Spring Fertility, "Live Your Life. Own Your Options," accessed August 6, 2023, springfertility.com /knowyouroptions/.

193 **twenty-one states:** RESOLVE: The National Infertility Association, "Insurance Coverage by State," last modified September 2023, resolve.org /learn/financial-resources-for-family-building/insurance-coverage /insurance-coverage-by-state/.

193 **to cover or offer:** The distinction is important. A "mandate to cover" is when state law requires health insurance plans to include coverage for a specific benefit (in this case, fertility treatments). A "mandate to offer" requires health insurers to offer coverage, but the person or group buying the policy doesn't necessarily have to elect coverage for that benefit.

193 **state-specific examples:** RESOLVE, "Insurance Coverage by State."

194n **Infertility, a disease:** The World Health Organization (WHO), American Medical Association, and ASRM are part of the growing worldwide trend of recognizing infertility as a disease. These entities (and several others) view reproduction as a fundamental interest and human right and maintain that the access, treatment, and outcome disparities associated with infertility care and ART warrant correction. WHO, "Infertility," April 3, 2023, who.int /news-room/fact-sheets/detail/infertility.

194n **defined by physicians:** Centers for Disease Control and Prevention, "Infertility FAQs," last modified April 26, 2023, cdc.gov/reproductivehealth /infertility/index.htm.

194 **at least partial coverage:** Sometimes, for example, initial diagnostic testing and screening procedures are covered, but the actual fertility treatment isn't; many insurance plans that *do* pay for fertility testing say that once an infertility diagnosis has been established, they'll no longer pay for fertility-related services. That's absurd, but it comes back to the price tag: Covering diagnostic testing doesn't cost them very much. Treatment, in the form of IVF or egg freezing, does.

195 **less limited reasons:** Some private sector companies include surrogacy and adoption in their coverage, but most don't. According to FertilityIQ, only one in five companies that offered fertility coverage also offered coverage for adoption or foster assistance—although average levels of coverage for the latter amounted to around $8,000 per employee versus the $36,000 level allocated for fertility.

195 **hot new perk:** Avery Stone, "More and More Companies Are Covering the Cost of Egg Freezing. But Who Is It Really For?," *Vice,* May 26, 2020, vice .com/en/article/ep448j/more-companies-are-covering-the-cost-of-egg -freezing-who-is-it-really-for-v27n2.

195 **19 percent:** Mercer, "New Survey Finds Employers Adding Fertility Benefits to Promote DEI," May 6, 2021, mercer.com/en-us/insights/us -health-news/new-survey-finds-employers-adding-fertility-benefits-to -promote-dei/.

195 **become a staple:** Mercer, "New Survey Finds Employers Adding Fertility Benefits to Promote DEI."

195 **Each member receives:** Progyny, *Member Guide: Understanding Your Progyny Benefit,* 2020.

196 **in their mid-thirties:** E. Chronopoulou, C. Raperport, A. Sfakianakis, G. Srivastava, and R. Homburg, "Elective Oocyte Cryopreservation for Age-Related Fertility Decline," *Journal of Assisted Reproduction and Genetics* 38, no. 5 (2021): 1177–1186, doi.org/10.1007/s10815-021-02072-w.

197 **travel abroad for a better deal:** Alyson Krueger, "Have Eggs, Will Travel. To Freeze Them," *New York Times,* April 8, 2023, nytimes.com/2023/04/08/style/egg-freezing-procedure-travel.html.

197 **alimony can finance:** Marcia C. Inhorn, *Motherhood on Ice: The Mating Gap and Why Women Freeze Their Eggs* (New York: New York University Press, 2023), 74–75.

197 **"We pay too much":** Jia Tolentino, *Trick Mirror: Reflections on Self-Delusion* (New York: Random House, 2020), 87.

199 **twenty-one states:** "Tracking Abortion Bans Across the Country," *New York Times,* last modified December 8, 2023, nytimes.com/interactive/2022/us/abortion-laws-roe-v-wade.html.

200 **"The United States has":** Emily Witt, "The Future of Fertility," *New Yorker,* April 17, 2023, newyorker.com/magazine/2023/04/24/the-future-of-fertility.

200 **could mean impaired access:** Gerard Letterie and Dov Fox, "Legal Personhood and Frozen Embryos: Implications for Fertility Patients and Providers in Post-Roe America," *Journal of Law and the Biosciences* 10, no. 1 (2023), doi.org10.1093/jlb/lsad006.

200 **"personhood laws":** Wendy Davis, "The Next Big Battle in America's Abortion Fight Will Be over Fetal Personhood," NBC News, October 23, 2022, nbcnews.com/think/opinion/americas-abortion-law-fight-will-fetal-personhood-rcna53477.

200 **raises all sorts of questions:** Chabeli Carranza and Jennifer Gerson, "IVF May Be in Jeopardy in States Where Embryos Are Granted Personhood," *The Guardian,* July 16, 2022, theguardian.com/society/2022/jul/16/ivf-anti-abortion-states-embryos-personhood.

200 **could become illegal:** Krys Mroczkowski, Colleen Ammerman, and Rembrand Koning, "How Abortion Bans Will Stifle Health Care Innovation," *Harvard Business Review,* August 8, 2022, hbr.org/2022/08/how-abortion-bans-will-stifle-health-care-innovation.

201n **public universities in Idaho:** Rebecca Boone, "Idaho Universities Disallow Abortion, Contraception Referral," Associated Press, September 27, 2022, apnews.com/article/abortion-health-legislature-idaho-birth-control-bd238c572da10d812ef5ba93f1860fc5.

201 **Time will tell:** Ariana Eunjung Cha and Emily Wax-Thibodeaux, "Overturn of Roe Could Make IVF More Complicated, Costly," *Washington*

Post, May 11, 2022, washingtonpost.com/health/2022/05/11/roe-overturn -ivf/.

202   **about 12 percent:** National Center for Health Statistics, Centers for Disease Control and Prevention, "Key Statistics from the National Survey of Family Growth," last modified June 20, 2017, cdc.gov/nchs/nsfg/key_statistics/i .htm.

203   **twice as likely:** Jamila Perritt and Natalia Eugene, "Inequity and Injustice: Recognizing Infertility as a Reproductive Justice Issue," *F&S Reports* 3, no. 2 (2022): 2–4, fertstertreports.org/article/S2666-3341(21)00103-3/.

203   **twice as long:** Helen B. Chin, Penelope P. Howards, Michael R. Kramer, Ann C. Mertens, and Jessica B. Spencer, "Racial Disparities in Seeking Care for Help Getting Pregnant," *Paediatric and Perinatal Epidemiology* 29, no. 5 (2015): 416–425, doi.org/10.1111/ppe.12210.

203n   **lack of ethnic diversity:** Angela Hatem, "Sperm Donors Are Almost Always White, and It's Pushing Black Parents Using IVF to Start Families That Don't Look Like Them," *Insider,* September 17, 2020, insider.com/egg -sperm-donor-diversity-lacking-race-2020-9.

203   **have reported that:** American Society for Reproductive Medicine, "Disparities in Access to Effective Treatment for Infertility in the United States: An Ethics Committee Opinion," *Fertility and Sterility* 116, no. 1 (2021): 54–63, doi.org/10.1016/j.fertnstert.2021.02.019.

203   **wouldn't feel comfortable:** Jihan Thompson, "Why Are So Many Black Women Suffering Through Infertility in Silence?," *Women's Health,* October 29, 2018, womenshealthmag.com/health/a23320626/infertility -race-survey/.

203   **raises deeper questions:** Avery Stone, "More and More Companies Are Covering the Cost of Egg Freezing. But Who Is It Really For?," *Vice,* May 26, 2020, vice.com/en/article/ep448j/more-companies-are-covering -the-cost-of-egg-freezing-who-is-it-really-for-v27n2.

204   **7 percent are Black:** Genevieve Glass, "America Expected a Pandemic Baby Boom. It Got an Egg-Freezing One Instead," *The Lily,* June 7, 2021, thelily.com/america-expected-a-pandemic-baby-boom-it-got-an-egg -freezing-one-instead/.

205   **understudied and underreported:** Leena Nahata, Amy C. Tishelman, Nicole M. Caltabellotta, and Gwendolyn P. Quinn, "Low Fertility Preservation Utilization Among Transgender Youth," *Journal of Adolescent Health* 61, no. 1 (2017): 40–44, sciencedirect.com/science/article/abs/pii /S1054139X16309582.

206   **"There's no question that":** Shira Stein, "Fertility Practices, Coverage Lacking for Transgender People," Bloomberg Law, May 17, 2019, news .bloomberglaw.com/health-law-and-business/fertility-practices-coverage -lacking-for-transgender-people.

CHAPTER 10

209 **most ethnically diverse place:** Brittny Mejia, "How Houston Has Become the Most Diverse Place in America," *Los Angeles Times,* May 9, 2017, latimes .com/nation/la-na-houston-diversity-2017-htmlstory.html.

215 **most widely prescribed:** Brown University, "50 Years Ago, Clomid Gave Birth to the Era of Assisted Reproduction," September 13, 2017, brown.edu /news/2017-09-13/clomiphene.

215 **"involving the Pope's blessing":** Oliver Staley, "The Strange Story of a Fertility Drug Made with the Pope's Blessing and Gallons of Nun Urine," *Quartz,* June 26, 2016, qz.com/710516/the-strange-story-of-a-fertility-drug -made-with-the-popes-blessing-and-gallons-of-nun-urine.

215 **"Donini called":** Staley, "The Strange Story of a Fertility Drug."

216 **"Within two years":** Staley, "The Strange Story of a Fertility Drug."

216 **from Chinese hamsters:** Nadezhda A. Orlova, Sergey V. Kovnir, Yulia A. Khodak, Mikhail A. Polzikov, Victoria A. Nikitina, Konstantin G. Skryabin, and Ivan I. Vorobiev, "High-Level Expression of Biologically Active Human Follicle Stimulating Hormone in the Chinese Hamster Ovary Cell Line by a Pair of Tricistronic and Monocistronic Vectors," *PLOS One* 14, no. 7 (2019): e0219434, doi.org/10.1371/journal.pone.0219434.

217 **quite low:** Paolo Emanuele Levi-Setti, Federico Cirillo, Valeria Scolaro, Emanuela Morenghi, Francesca Heilbron, Donatella Girardello, Elena Zannoni, and Pasquale Patrizio, "Appraisal of Clinical Complications After 23,827 Oocyte Retrievals in a Large Assisted Reproductive Technology Program," *Fertility and Sterility* 109, no. 6 (2018): 1038–1043e1, doi.org/10 .1016/j.fertnstert.2018.02.002.

218 **experience mild OHSS:** "Ovarian Hyperstimulation Syndrome (OHSS) Caused by Fertility Treatment," Embryo Project Encyclopedia, last modified October 20, 2020, hdl.handle.net/10776/13175.

218 **severe case:** It's rare to die from OHSS, but the condition can lead to other immediate and serious health issues. In one case I read, a twenty-four-year-old Florida woman who had forty-five eggs retrieved had a stroke the next day, likely due to the blood clots caused by severe OHSS.

219n **Lupron label warns of:** "Lupron Injection," Food and Drug Administration, accessed June 19, 2023, accessdata.fda.gov/drugsatfda_docs/label/2014 /019010s037lbl.pdf.

219 **off-label:** Rebecca S. Usadi and Kathryn S. Merriam, "On-Label and Off-Label Drug Use in the Treatment of Female Infertility," *Fertility and Sterility* 103, no. 3 (2015): 583–594, doi.org/10.1016/j.fertnstert.2015.01 .011.

219 **has been linked with:** "Women Fear Drug They Used to Halt Puberty Led to Health Problems," Christina Jewett, *Kaiser Health News* and *Reveal,* February 2, 2017, kffhealthnews.org/news/women-fear-drug-they-used-to

-halt-puberty-led-to-health-problems/; Jenny Sadler Gallagher, Stacey A. Missmer, Mark D. Hornstein, Marc R. Laufer, Catherine M. Gordon, and Amy D. DiVasta, "Long-Term Effects of Gonadotropin-Releasing Hormone Agonists and Add-Back in Adolescent Endometriosis," *Journal of Pediatric and Adolescent Gynecology* 31, no. 4 (2018): 376–381, doi.org/10.1016/j.jpag .2018.03.004.

219n **"evaluating the need":** "Potential Signals of Serious Risks/New Safety Information Identified by the FDA Adverse Event Reporting System (FAERS)," Food and Drug Administration, last modified January 6, 2023, fda.gov/drugs/questions-and-answers-fdas-adverse-event-reporting-system -faers/january-march-2017-potential-signals-serious-risksnew-safety -information-identified-fda-adverse.

219 **petitioned Congress:** "Investigation into Lupron Side Effects (Leuprolide Acetate)," Petition2Congress.com petition, accessed July 2, 2023, petition2congress.com/ctas/investigation-lupron-side-effects-leuprolide -acetate.

220 **don't appear to increase:** American Society for Reproductive Medicine, "Fertility Drugs and Cancer: A Guideline," *Fertility and Sterility* 106, no. 7 (2016): 1617–1626, doi.org/10.1016/j.fertnstert.2016.08.035.

221 **may increase a woman's risk of cancer:** Aus Tariq Ali, "Fertility Drugs and Ovarian Cancer," *Current Cancer Drug Targets* 18, no. 6 (2018): 567–576, doi.org/10.2174/1568009617666170620102049.

221 **an episode on *Reveal*:** Emily Harger and Olivia Merrion, "Is Egg Donation Safe?," *Reveal*, June 1, 2017, revealnews.org/article/is-egg-donation-safe/.

221 **Jessica said:** Jane E. Brody, "Do Egg Donors Face Long-Term Risks?," *New York Times*, July 10, 2017, nytimes.com/2017/07/10/well/live/are-there -long-term-risks-to-egg-donors.html.

221 **no history of:** Center for Bioethics and Culture Network, "Egg Donor Registry Needed," November 3, 2008, cbc-network.org/2008/11/egg -donor-registry-needed/.

221 **a multimillion-dollar and poorly regulated industry:** Paris Martineau, "Inside the Quietly Lucrative Business of Donating Human Eggs," *Wired*, April 23, 2019, wired.com/story/inside-lucrative-business-donating-human -eggs/.

222n **closest statistic I could find:** Centers for Disease Control and Prevention, "2020 Assisted Reproductive Technology Fertility Clinic and National Summary Report," 2022, cdc.gov/art/reports/2020/pdf/Report-ART -Fertility-Clinic-National-Summary-H.pdf.

223 **it's impossible to:** Jennifer Schneider, Jennifer Lahl, and Wendy Kramer, "Long-Term Breast Cancer Risk Following Ovarian Stimulation in Young Egg Donors: A Call for Follow-Up, Research and Informed Consent," *Reproductive Biomedicine Online* 34, no. 5 (2017): 480–485, doi.org/10.1016 /j.rbmo.2017.02.003.

223 **"Better understanding":** Harger and Merrion, "Is Egg Donation Safe?"

224 **informed consent:** Schneider et al., "Long-Term Breast Cancer Risk Following Ovarian Stimulation in Young Egg Donors."

224n **"I specifically remember":** Reema Khrais and Alice Wilder, "The Price of Eggs," *This Is Uncomfortable* (podcast), produced by Marketplace, May 18, 2023, marketplace.org/shows/this-is-uncomfortable-reema-khrais/the-price -of-eggs/.

225 **"We have no idea":** Maya Dusenbery, "What We Don't Know About I.V.F.," *New York Times,* April 16, 2020, nytimes.com/2020/04/16/parenting /fertility/ivf-long-term-effects.html.

CHAPTER 11

233 **rose nearly 60 percent:** This figure is for frozen embryos created using a patient's own frozen eggs (either they previously froze embryos or they created embryos using their previously frozen eggs), not frozen embryos using donor eggs. The point being, women are increasingly choosing to freeze embryos (using their own eggs with either donor sperm or their partner's sperm) over just freezing eggs. See Society for Assisted Reproductive Technology, "Final National Summary Report for 2020," 2020, sartcorsonline.com/CSR/PublicSnapshotReport?ClinicPKID=0& reportingYear=2020.

249 **"Freezing my eggs":** Sarah Elizabeth Richards, *Motherhood, Rescheduled: The New Frontier of Egg Freezing and the Women Who Tried It* (New York: Simon & Schuster, 2015), 59.

249 **spent $50,000:** Sarah Elizabeth Richards, "Why I Froze My Eggs (And You Should, Too)," *Wall Street Journal,* May 3, 2013, wsj.com/articles /SB10001424127887323628004578458882165244260.

CHAPTER 12

252 **six more years:** Sarah Zhang, "A Woman Gave Birth from an Embryo Frozen for 24 Years," *The Atlantic,* November 25, 2017, theatlantic.com /science/archive/2017/12/frozen-embryo-ivf-24-years/548876/.

252 **longest-frozen embryos:** Frozen in 1992, the embryos were in the care of the National Embryo Donation Center and had been created for an anonymous married couple using IVF. Elise Solé, "Oregon Parents Welcome Twins from Donated Embryos Frozen 30 Years Ago," NBC News, November 22, 2022, nbcnews.com/news/us-news/oregon-parents-welcome-twins-donated -embryos-frozen-30-years-ago-rcna58442.

255 **"These investments materialize":** Lucy van de Wiel, *Freezing Fertility: Oocyte Cryopreservation and the Gender Politics of Aging* (New York: New York University Press, 2020), 96.

256n **"We've had ten oocyte thaw cycles":** Margaret Ryan, vice president of Communications at Kindbody, email messages to the author, April 18, 2022, and October 10, 2023.

256 **"credits private equity":** Anna Louie Sussman, "The Promise and Perils of the New Fertility Entrepreneurs," *New Yorker,* May 19, 2021, newyorker .com/tech/annals-of-technology/the-promise-and-perils-of-the-new -fertility-entrepreneurs.

256 **"volume-driven":** Sussman, "The Promise and Perils of the New Fertility Entrepreneurs."

256 **Studies in:** Kiri Beilby, Ingrid Dudink, Deanna Kablar, Megan Kaynak, Sanduni Rodrigo, and Karin Hammarberg, "The Quality of Information About Elective Oocyte Cryopreservation (EOC) on Australian Fertility Clinic Websites," *Australian and New Zealand Journal of Obstetrics and Gynaecology* 60, no. 4 (2020): 605–609, doi.org/10.1111/ajo.13174; Zeynep B. Gürtin and Emily Tiemann, "The Marketing of Elective Egg Freezing: A Content, Cost and Quality Analysis of UK Fertility Clinic Websites," *Reproductive Biomedicine and Society Online* 12 (2020): 56–68, doi.org/10 .1016/j.rbms.2020.10.004.

256 **more persuasive:** Christopher Barbey, "Evidence of Biased Advertising in the Case of Social Egg Freezing," *New Bioethics* 23, no. 3 (2017): 195–209, doi.org/10.1080/20502877.2017.1396033.

256 **fudge the numbers:** Jessica Hamzelou, "Fertility Clinics Are Fudging IVF Stats to Look More Successful," *New Scientist,* November 29, 2017, newscientist.com/article/mg23631542-700-fertility-clinics-are-fudging-ivf -stats-to-look-more-successful/.

257 **a form of self-care:** Rebecca Grant, "How Egg Freezing Got Rebranded as the Ultimate Act of Self-Care," *The Guardian,* September 30, 2020, theguardian.com/us-news/2020/sep/30/egg-freezing-self-care-pregnancy -fertility.

258 **"Beneath the firm's Instagrammable aesthetic":** Jackie Davalos, "Embryo Errors, Flooded Clinics: Kindbody and IVF's Risky Business," *Bloomberg,* October 13, 2023, bloomberg.com/news/articles/2023-10-13/kindbody -fertility-clinic-embryo-mix-ups-spotlight-ivf-business-risks.

259 **"Kindbody's challenges":** Davalos, "Embryo Errors, Flooded Clinics."

259 **"Data suggest that":** Michelle J. Bayefsky, Alan H. DeCherney, and Louise P. King, "Respecting Autonomy—A Call for Truth in Commercial Advertising for Planned Oocyte Cryopreservation," *Fertility and Sterility* 113, no. 4 (2020): 743–744, doi.org/10.1016/j.fertnstert.2019.12.039.

259 **"If a woman younger":** Bayefsky et al.," Respecting Autonomy."

260 **aggressive form of:** Specifically, triple-negative invasive ductal carcinoma. The "triple-negative" meant her cancer wasn't driven by estrogen, pro-gesterone, or HER2 (human epidermal growth factor receptor 2, a gene that makes a protein found on the surface of all breast cells).

CHAPTER 13

Portions of this chapter, including data from the survey conducted by FertilityIQ, were previously published in The New York Times Magazine *on December 11, 2019, under the title "The Unexpected Freedom That Comes with Freezing Your Eggs."*

269 **60 percent reported:** B. Hodes-Wertz, S. Druckenmiller, M. Smith, Y. G. Kramer, and N. Noyes, "Beating Biology and Buying Time: An Update Survey of Womens' Experiences After Oocyte Cryopreservation (OC) for Deferred Reproduction," *Fertility and Sterility* 106, no. 3 (2016): e61–e62, doi.org/10.1016/j.fertnstert.2016.07.1079.

270 **91 percent:** Benjamin P. Jones, Lorraine Kasaven, Ariadne L'Heveder, Maria Jalmbrant, Joy Green, Mahmoud Makki, Rabi Odia, et al., "Perceptions, Outcomes, and Regret Following Social Egg Freezing in the UK; A Cross-Sectional Survey," *Acta Obstetricia et Gynecologica Scandinavica* 99, no. 3 (2020): 324–332, doi.org/10.1111/aogs.13763.

270n **Twenty percent:** Jones et al., "Perceptions, Outcomes, and Regret Following Social Egg Freezing in the UK."

270 **egg freezing helps women:** Eliza Brown and Mary Patrick, "Time, Anticipation, and the Life Course: Egg Freezing as Temporarily Disentangling Romance and Reproduction," *American Sociological Review* 83, no. 5 (2018): 959–982, doi.org/10.1177/0003122418796807.

270 **"hoped to bracket":** Brown and Patrick, "Time, Anticipation, and the Life Course."

272 **"has created a new drive":** Peggy Orenstein, *Don't Call Me Princess: Essays on Girls, Women, Sex, and Life* (New York: HarperCollins, 2018), 188.

275n **"Two recessions before":** Hillary Hoffower and Andy Kiersz, "Millennials Make More Money than Any Other Generation Did at Their Age, but Are Way Less Wealthy. The Affordability Crisis Is to Blame," *Insider,* September 22, 2021, businessinsider.com/millennials-highest-earning-generation-less-wealthy-boomers-2021-9.

276 **unlikely to ever have children:** Pew Research Center, "Growing Share of Childless Adults in U.S. Don't Expect to Ever Have Children," 2021, pewresearch.org/short-reads/2021/11/19/growing-share-of-childless-adults-in-u-s-dont-expect-to-ever-have-children/.

276 **Why are young adults:** Claire Cain Miller, "Americans Are Having Fewer Babies. They Told Us Why," *New York Times,* July 5, 2018, nytimes.com/2018/07/05/upshot/americans-are-having-fewer-babies-they-told-us-why.html.

276n **Their reasons:** Miller, "Americans Are Having Fewer Babies."

276 **climate change affects their decision:** Catherine Clifford, "53% of Parents Say Climate Change Affects Their Decision to Have More Kids," CNBC, cnbc.com/2023/06/20/climate-change-affects-53percent-of-parents-decision-to-have-more-kids.html.

276 **adjusted their family planning:** Danielle McNally, "Women Are Deciding
     to Have Fewer Children, and Global Warming Is to Blame," *Marie Claire,*
     February 7, 2022, marieclaire.com/politics/climate-change-fertility-modern
     -fertility-survey/.

276 **"Around the world":** Anna Louie Sussman, "The End of Babies," *New York
     Times,* November 16, 2019, nytimes.com/interactive/2019/11/16/opinion
     /sunday/capitalism-children.html.

276 **"our workweeks":** Sussman, "The End of Babies."

276 **brutal:** See, for example, Claire Cain Miller, "The Relentlessness of Modern
     Parenting," *New York Times,* December 25, 2018, nytimes.com/2018/12/25
     /upshot/the-relentlessness-of-modern-parenting.html.

276 **most educated generations:** Pew Research Center, "Millennial Life: How
     Young Adulthood Today Compares with Prior Generations," 2019,
     pewresearch.org/social-trends/2019/02/14/millennial-life-how-young
     -adulthood-today-compares-with-prior-generations-2/.

277 **don't have biological children:** National Center for Health Statistics,
     Centers for Disease Control and Prevention, "Fertility of Men and Women
     Aged 15–49 in the United States: National Survey of Family Growth,
     2015–2019," 2023, cdc.gov/nchs/data/nhsr/nhsr179.pdf.

277 **decades-long trend:** National Center for Health Statistics, Centers for
     Disease Control and Prevention, "Fertility of Men and Women Aged 15–49
     in the United States." Delayed childbearing, the report also notes, increased
     ninefold between 1972 and 2012.

278 **"When I was much younger":** Jan Moir, "The Rules Every Woman Should
     Live By: She's One of the World's Most Celebrated (and Colorful) Feminists.
     At 81, Gloria Steinem Reveals What She's Learned," *Daily Mail,* March 16,
     2016, dailymail.co.uk/debate/article-3468553/The-rules-women-live-s-one
     -world-s-celebrated-colourful-feminists-81-Gloria-Steinem-reveals-s
     -learned.html.

CHAPTER 14

Portions of this chapter were previously published in The Guardian *on May 13, 2018,
under the title "Their Embryos Were Destroyed. Now They Mourn the Children They'll
Never Have."*

*Facts about the Ohio and California tank failures were gathered from the author's own
reporting, legal documents, news reports, state health department findings, and documentation
that affected patients received from University Hospitals Cleveland Medical Center and
Pacific Fertility.*

292n **"After the March 2018 mishap":** Nicholas Iovino, "Tank Manufacturer
     Accuses Fertility Clinic of Falsifying Data in Frozen Eggs Trial," Courthouse
     News Service, May 27, 2021, courthousenews.com/tank-manufacturer
     -accuses-fertility-clinic-of-falsifying-data-in-frozen-eggs-trial/.

292n **One recent example:** Neil Vigdor, "'We Had Their Baby, and They Had Our Baby': Couple Sues over Embryo 'Mix-Up,'" *New York Times,* November 9, 2021, nytimes.com/2021/11/09/us/fertility-clinic-embryo-mixup.html.

293 **at least nine:** Anar Murphy, Sindhu Gollapudi, and Michael G. Collins, "Legal Case Study of Severe IVF Incidents Worldwide: Causes, Consequences, and High Emotional, Financial, and Reputational Costs to Patients and Providers," *North American Proceedings in Gynecology & Obstetrics* 2, no.1 (2022): 22, doi.org/10.54053/001c.37563.

293 **nearly 30 percent:** "FertilityIQ Protocol: How to Pick a Fertility Doctor," FertilityIQ, accessed February 3, 2023, fertilityiq.com/topics/ivf/fertilityiq-protocol-how-to-pick-a-fertility-doctor.

293 **misdiagnosed, mislabeled, or mishandled:** Dov Fox, "What Happens When Reproductive Tech Like IVF Goes Awry?" *Wired,* July 17, 2019, wired.com/story/when-ivf-goes-awry.

294 **restrict federal funding:** National Academies of Sciences, Engineering, and Medicine, *Fetal Research and Applications: A Conference Summary* (Washington, D.C.: National Academies Press, 1994), doi.org/10.17226/4797.

294 **states are left to:** Kirstin R. W. Matthews and Daniel Morali, "Can We Do That Here? An Analysis of US Federal and State Policies Guiding Human Embryo and Embryoid Research," *Journal of Law and the Biosciences* 9, no. 1 (2022): 124, doi.org/10.1093/jlb/lsac014.

294 **complex patchwork:** I. Glenn Cohen, "The Right(s) to Procreate and Assisted Reproductive Technologies in the United States" in *The Oxford Handbook of Comparative Health Law,* ed. Tamara K. Hervey and David Orentlicher (Oxford, United Kingdom: Oxford University Press, 2021), 1009.

294n **In contrast:** Vishan Dev Singh Jamwal and Arun Kumar Yadav, "The Assisted Reproductive Technology (Regulation) Act, 2021: A Step in the Right Direction," *Indian Journal of Community Medicine* 48, no. 1 (2023): 4–6, doi.org/10.4103/ijcm.ijcm_169_22.

295n **CLIA doesn't extend:** American Society for Reproductive Medicine (ASRM) and the Society for Reproductive Biologists and Technologists (SRBT), "Comprehensive Guidance for Human Embryology, Andrology, and Endocrinology Laboratories: Management and Operations: A Committee Opinion," *Fertility and Sterility* 117, no. 6 (2022): 1183–1202, doi.org/10.1016/j.fertnstert.2022.02.016.

295 **required to report:** In 1992, Congress passed the Fertility Clinic Success Rate and Certification Act—the only federal legislation that specifically pertains to assisted reproductive technology—which requires all U.S. clinics performing ART to report data annually to the CDC. In addition to providing pregnancy success rates, clinics must provide details of treatment cycles, including infertility diagnosis, number of embryos transferred, and use of fresh or frozen embryos and donor or non-donor eggs. The CDC

works in consultation with SART and ASRM to report ART success rates each year.

295 **donor tissue:** This includes the screening and testing of reproductive tissue, such as donor eggs and sperm, to ensure it's free from disease.

295 **disclosure of medical errors:** ASRM and SRBT Committee Report, "Comprehensive Guidance."

295n **"might improve the uniformity":** ASRM, "Oversight of Assisted Reproductive Technology," updated 2021, asrm.org/globalassets/_asrm /advocacy-and-policy/oversiteofart.pdf.

298 **Arizona passed:** Arizona Revised Statutes, 2018, Section 25-318.03, "Marital and Domestic Relations," law.justia.com/codes/arizona/2018/title -25/section-25-318.03.

298n **"Just like a judge":** Kathy Ritchie, "Arizona Governor Signs Bill to Change Laws Concerning Frozen Embryos," *KJZZ,* April 5, 2018, kjzz.org/content /633242/arizona-governor-signs-bill-change-laws-concerning-frozen -embryos.

299 **a Virginia judge:** Matthew Barakat, "Judge Uses a Slavery Law to Rule Frozen Embryos Are Property," Associated Press, March 9, 2023, apnews .com/article/embryos-slavery-chattel-custody-virginia-82e1f36ecbcf35ec4 659e8e2c3443c4f.

299 **embryos as "juridical persons":** Hannah C. Catchings, "A 'Modern Family' Issue: Recategorizing Embryos in the 21st Century," *Louisiana Law Review* 80, no. 4 (2020): 1521–1556, digitalcommons.law.lsu.edu/lalrev /vol80/iss4/12/.

299 **foreshadows:** Gerard Letterie and Dov Fox, "Legal Personhood and Frozen Embryos: Implications for Fertility Patients and Providers in Post-*Roe* America," *Journal of Law and the Biosciences* 10, no. 1 (2023): 1–13, doi.org /10.1093/jlb/lsad006.

299 **legal gray area:** Julianna Goldman, "Why Many IVF Patients Worry About the Antiabortion Movement," *Washington Post,* July 29, 2023, washingtonpost .com/wellness/2023/07/29/dobbs-abortion-ivf-embryos-impact/.

299 **courts struggled:** American Bar Association, "In Case of Divorce, Destroy the Eggs," December 9, 2015, americanbar.org/groups/litigation/committees /minority-trial-lawyer/practice/2015/in-case-of-divorce-destroy-the-eggs/.

299 **1.5 million frozen embryos:** Gerard Letterie, "In Re: The Disposition of Frozen Embryos: 2022," *Fertility and Sterility* 117, no. 3 (2022): 477–480, doi.org/10.1016/j.fertnstert.2022.01.001.

299 **"I live in a freezer now":** Susanna Fogel, "Your Frozen Egg Has a Question," *New Yorker,* May 15, 2017, newyorker.com/magazine/2017/05 /22/your-frozen-egg-has-a-question.

300 **nine hundred babies:** N. Noyes, E. Porcu, and A. Borini, "Over 900 Oocyte Cryopreservation Babies Born with No Apparent Increase in Congenital Anomalies," *Reproductive BioMedicine Online* 18, no. 6 (2009): 769–776, doi.org/10.1016/s1472-6483(10)60025-9.

300 **A 2013 study:** Paolo Emanuele Levi Setti, Elena Albani, Emanuela Morenghi, Giovanna Morreale, Luisa Delle Piane, Giulia Scaravelli, and Pasquale Patrizio, "Comparative Analysis of Fetal and Neonatal Outcomes of Pregnancies from Fresh and Cryopreserved/Thawed Oocytes in the Same Group of Patients," *Fertility and Sterility* 100, no. 2 (2013): 396–401, doi.org/10.1016/j.fertnstert.2013.03.038.

300 **technically, in the United States:** Denmark has a five-year limit on cryopreservation storage of embryos. Switzerland, the United Kingdom, New Zealand, and some Australian states have enacted ten-year storage limits.

301n **increased health risks:** A few examples:

A 2019 study of more than one million children born in Denmark found that "the use of frozen embryo transfer, compared to children born to fertile women, was associated with a small but statistically significant increased risk of childhood cancer." Marie Hargreave, Allan Jensen, Merete Kjær Hansen, Christian Dehlendorff, Jeanette Falck Winther, Kjeld Schmiegelow, and Susanne K. Kjær, "Association Between Fertility Treatment and Cancer Risk in Children," *Journal of the American Medical Association* 322, no. 22 (2019): 2203–2210, doi.org/doi:10.1001/jama.2019.18037.

"The risks of heart defects, musculoskeletal and central nervous system malformations, preterm birth, and low birth weight are increased in children conceived by vitro fertilization (IVF)." Michael von Wolff and Thomas Haaf, "In Vitro Fertilization Technology and Child Health," *Deutsches Ärzteblatt International* 117, no. 3 (2020): 23–30, doi.org/10.3238/arztebl .2020.0023.

The main risks for these children are poorer perinatal outcome, birth defects, and epigenetic disorders. However, whether ART procedures or subfertility itself had led to these changes is still unresolved. The health situation for the next generation of ART-conceived children is an important question. In brief, there are still a number of unanswered questions, and well-designed studies on the topics described above are urgently needed. Yue-hong Lu, Ning Wang, and Fan Jin, "Long-Term Follow-up of Children Conceived Through Assisted Reproductive Technology," *Journal of Zhejiang University Science B* 14, no. 5 (2013): 359–371, doi.org/10.1631/jzus .B1200348.

301 **"A working knowledge of":** Noyes, Porcu, and Borini, "Over 900 Oocyte Cryopreservation Babies Born."

301 **considers whether:** Paul Kalanithi, *When Breath Becomes Air* (New York: Random House, 2016).

302 **Other limited guidance:** In its 2018 Ethics Committee opinion on egg freezing, ASRM says consent forms should include information about "potential and uncertain risks along with the limited safety and outcome data" and that "providers should disclose their own clinic-specific statistics, or lack thereof, for successful freeze-thaw and for live birth." See ASRM,

"Planned Oocyte Cryopreservation for Women Seeking to Preserve Future Reproductive Potential: An Ethics Committee Opinion," *Fertility and Sterility* 110, no. 6 (2018): 1022–1028, doi.org/10.1016/j.fertnstert.2018.08.027.

302 **more than 85 percent:** Pragati Kakkar, Joanna Geary, Tania Stockburger, Aida Kaffel, Julia Kopeika, and Tarek El-Toukhy, "Outcomes of Social Egg Freezing: A Cohort Study and a Comprehensive Literature Review," *Journal of Clinical Medicine* 12, no. 13 (2023): 4182, doi.org/10.3390/jcm12134182.

302 **not working:** A few examples:

A woman who thawed and fertilized ten eggs in 2020 learned none developed into viable embryos (*New York Times*, 2022). Gina Kolata, "'Sobering' Study Shows Challenges of Egg Freezing," *New York Times*, September 23, 2022, nytimes.com/2022/09/23/health/egg-freezing-age-pregnancy.html.

A woman in her early forties spent $50,000 on two cycles and ended up with no viable eggs (*Good Morning America*, 2019). Katie Kindelan, "When Freezing Your Eggs Does Not Work: What Women Should Know," *Good Morning America*, September 6, 2019, goodmorningamerica.com/wellness/story/freezing-eggs-work-women-65125606.

A thirty-five-year-old woman who also did two rounds and learned the same (*New York Times*, 2022). Alisha Haridasani Gupta and Dani Blum, "Hope, Regret, Uncertainty: 7 Women on Freezing Their Eggs," *New York Times*, December 23, 2022, nytimes.com/2022/12/23/well/family/egg-freezing-fertility.html.

302 **"I tried to have":** Lena Dunham, "False Labor: Giving Up on Motherhood," *Harper's Magazine*, December 2020, harpers.org/archive/2020/12/false-labor-lena-dunham-fertility/.

303n **Dayna:** She asked for her name to be changed because of her profession (lawyer) and because her legal case about her lost frozen eggs is not yet resolved.

CHAPTER 15

311 **39 percent increase:** Anne E. Martini, Samad Jahandideh, Ali Williams, Kate Devine, Eric A. Widra, Micah J. Hill, Alan H. DeCherney, and Jeanne E. O'Brien, "Trends in Elective Egg Freezing before and after the COVID-19 Pandemic," *Fertility and Sterility* 116, no. 3 (2021): e220, doi.org/10.1016/j.fertnstert.2021.07.596.

311 **a 95 percent increase:** Ali Williams, Shady Grove Fertility marketing team, email message to the author, December 3, 2021.

311 **Kindbody quadrupled:** Mary Pflum, "Egg Freezing Has Boomed during the Pandemic, as Women Opt to Wait Out Family Life," NBC News, April 24, 2021, nbcnews.com/business/business-news/egg-freezing-has-boomed-during-pandemic-women-opt-wait-out-n1264211.

311 **three times the number of women:** "Frozen Eggs More Efficient Option

Than In Vitro Fertilization for Women Starting Families Later," NYU Langone Health NewsHub, May 26, 2022, nyulangone.org/news/frozen-eggs-more-efficient-option-in-vitro-fertilization-women-starting-families-later.

311 **60 percent increase:** Human Fertilisation and Embryology Authority, "Fertility Treatment 2021: Preliminary Trends and Figures," 2023, hfea.gov.uk/about-us/publications/research-and-data/fertility-treatment-2021-preliminary-trends-and-figures/.

312 **Fatima:** She asked for her name to be changed because, she told me, for South Asian women it's often considered taboo to talk openly about topics like fertility and egg freezing. But she chose to share her story because she wants the subject to be talked about more.

314 **"When women come back":** Anna Louie Sussman, "The Promise and Perils of the New Fertility Entrepreneurs," *New Yorker*, May 19, 2021, newyorker.com/tech/annals-of-technology/the-promise-and-perils-of-the-new-fertility-entrepreneurs.

314n **tools to help people considering egg freezing:** Michelle Peate, Sherine Sandhu, Sabine Braat, Roger Hart, Robert Norman, Anna Parle, Raelia Lew, and Martha Hickey, "Randomized Control Trial of a Decision Aid for Women Considering Elective Egg Freezing: The Eggsurance Study Protocol," *Women's Health* 18 (2022), doi.org/10.1177/17455057221139673.

316 **monitor the safety:** Such as surveilling the environment inside the tank to see if the temperature is changing by even one degree, checking the tank's motion tilting, and monitoring the electric current in and out of the machine.

318 **too conservative:** David Sable, "White-Boarding the Future of IVF," *Medium*, January 30, 2021, dbsable.medium.com/healthcares-industry-in-waiting-white-boarding-the-future-of-ivf-9cecc150c3ba.

320 **"The ability to fertilize":** Rebecca Traister, *All the Single Ladies: Unmarried Women and the Rise of an Independent Nation* (New York: Simon & Schuster, 2016), 270.

320 **was removed in 2019:** American Society for Reproductive Medicine, "Fertility Preservation in Patients Undergoing Gonadotoxic Therapy or Gonadectomy: A Committee Opinion," *Fertility and Sterility* 112, no. 6 (2019): 1022–1033, fertstert.org/article/S0015-0282(19)32355-6/fulltext.

320 **hundreds of live births:** Angeliki Arapaki, Panagiotis Christopoulos, Emmanouil Kalampokas, Olga Triantafyllidou, Alkis Matsas, and Nikolaos F. Vlahos, "Ovarian Tissue Cryopreservation in Children and Adolescents," *Children* 9, no. 8 (2022): 1256, doi.org/10.3390/children9081256.

321 **"When I started":** Alexandra Sifferlin, "Exclusive: First U.S. Baby Born After a Uterus Transplant," *Time*, December 1, 2017, time.com/5044565/exclusive-first-u-s-baby-born-after-a-uterus-transplant/.

322 **successfully converting:** David Cyranoski, "Mouse Eggs Made from Skin Cells in a Dish," *Nature* 538, no. 301 (2016), doi.org/10.1038/nature.2016.20817.

322 **stem cells in mice:** Takashi Yoshino, Takahiro Suzuki, Go Nagamatsu, Haruka Yabukami, Mika Ikegaya, Mami Kishima, Haruka Kita, et al., "Generation of Ovarian Follicles from Mouse Pluripotent Stem Cells," *Science* 373, no. 6552 (2021): 282, doi.org/10.1126/science.abe0237.

323 **"is on the precipice":** Rob Stein, "Creating a Sperm or Egg from Any Cell? Reproduction Revolution on the Horizon," NPR, May 27, 2023, npr .org/sections/health-shots/2023/05/27/1177191913/sperm-or-egg-in-lab -breakthrough-in-reproduction-designer-babies-ivg.

323n **"We're really hopeful":** Emily Witt, "The Future of Fertility," *New Yorker,* April 17, 2023, newyorker.com/magazine/2023/04/24/the-future-of -fertility.

324 **"have it all":** "Why I Froze My Eggs," *Newsweek,* May 1, 2009, newsweek .com/why-i-froze-my-eggs-79867.

324n **"One of the central tensions":** Susan Burton, "The Outcomes," *The Retrievals* (podcast), produced by New York Times and Serial, August 3, 2023, nytimes.com/2023/08/03/podcasts/serial-the-retrievals-yale-fertility -clinic.html.

324 **Zoladex shots:** After she finished cancer treatment, Bridget's fertility doctor told her that "the jury is still really out" on whether or not Zoladex (the drug's chemical name is goserelin) is effective—which made Bridget feel lucky. "I certainly don't regret doing Zoladex, even if it turns out it did nothing," Bridget told me later, "because it made me *feel* like I was doing something to protect my fertility during a time that I was receiving, directly into my body, medication so toxic that the person administering it wore a hazmat suit." See Bo Yu and Nancy E. Davidson, "Gonadotropin-Releasing Hormone (GnRH) Agonists for Fertility Preservation: Is POEMS the Final Verse?," *Journal of the National Cancer Institute* 111, no. 2 (2019): 107–108, doi.org/10.1093/jnci/djy188.

326 **fallopian tubes and ovaries surgically removed:** Melissa Walker, Michelle Jacobson, and Mara Sobel, "Management of Ovarian Cancer Risk in Women with BRCA1/2 Pathogenic Variants," *Canadian Medical Association Journal* 191, no. 32 (2019): e886–e893, doi.org/10.1503/cmaj.190281.

326 **struggle to cobble together:** Marcia C. Inhorn, Daphna Birenbaum-Carmeli, Lynn M. Westphal, Joseph Doyle, Norbert Gleicher, Dror Meirow, Hila Raanani, Martha Dirnfeld, and Pasquale Patrizio, "Medical Egg Freezing: How Cost and Lack of Insurance Cover Impact Women and Their Families," *Reproductive Biomedicine and Society Online* 5 (2018): 82–92, doi.org/10.1016/j.rbms.2017.12.001.

328 **for intelligence:** "Genetic Test to Screen Embryos for Low Intelligence Developed in US," Progress Educational Trust, November 19, 2018, progress .org.uk/genetic-test-to-screen-embryos-for-low-intelligence-developed-in -us/.

328 **federal administrative agency:** Mary Ann Mason and Tom Ekman, *Babies*

of Technology: Assisted Reproduction and the Rights of the Child (New Haven, CT: Yale University Press, 2017), 198.

328 **"humans will begin":** Henry T. Greely, *The End of Sex and the Future of Human Reproduction* (Cambridge, MA: Harvard University Press, 2016), 2.

CHAPTER 16

331 **twenty-year clinical study:** Raffaella Fabbri, Rossella Vicenti, Valentina Magnani, Roberto Paradisi, Mario Lima, Lucia De Meis, Stefania Rossi, et al., "Ovarian Tissue Cryopreservation and Transplantation: 20 Years Experience in Bologna University," *Frontiers in Endocrinology* 13 (2022), doi .org/10.3389/fendo.2022.1035109.

339 **Thomas:** He asked for his name to be changed to protect the privacy of his and Remy's family.

Index

PGT (*see* preimplantation genetic testing)

PGT tests, 325, 325*n*, 326*n*, 328

Pill, the (*see* contraception)

Pincus, Gregory, 39*n*

pituitary gland, 69, 74

Pius XII, Pope, 215–16

placebo pills, 76

placenta, 174

planned egg freezing, 32–33*n*

Planned Parenthood, 38, 137, 144

Plants, Jeremy, 287, 288

Plants, Kate, 287–88

PMS (*see* premenstrual syndrome)

polycystic ovary syndrome (PCOS), 12, 93, 127, 132, 144, 215, 218

polyps, 132

pop culture, 142

Porcu, Elenora, 46–49, 330, 332–34

pornography, 142

Predictor pregnancy test, 124

pregnancies, 29, 55–56, 72–73

pregnancy prevention, 31, 114–15, 138, 201*n* (*see also* contraception)

pregnancy tests, 123–25, 131–33, 261

preimplantation genetic testing (PGT), 182

Prelude, 190–91, 254, 255, 291–92, 293*n*, 323

Prelude Method, 190

premature births, 173*n*

premenstrual syndrome (PMS), 76, 118, 217

Prestea, Ghana, 10

Princeton University, 185

privacy practices, 121–23, 151

PRL (*see* prolactin)

progesterone, 68, 69, 72–74, 110–11

synthetic, 75, 76

progestin, 75, 81

implants, 79,80

injection, 79, 80

Progyny, 183, 195, 260

Progyny Rx, 195

prolactin (PRL), 126

propofol, 65

prostate cancer, 219, 262

puberty, 28, 29, 68, 147, 219

Quartz, 215, 216

race, maternal and reproductive health and, 202–4

Radenkovic, Dina, 323*n*

radiation, 49, 50, 93, 261

radio frequency identification (RFID), 316

Ramirez, Leslie, 151–54

relationship dissolution, 97, 98, 100

religion

egg freezing and, 46, 47

sex education and, 25

reproductive longevity, 321–22

ABOUT THE AUTHOR

NATALIE LAMPERT is an award-winning journalist based in Boulder, Colorado. Her reporting focuses primarily on women's health and the fertility industry. A former Fulbright scholar, she has a master's degree in journalism from New York University and has written for *The New York Times*, *The New York Times Magazine*, *The Washington Post*, *The Atlantic*, *The Guardian*, *Slate*, *Marie Claire*, and *The New Republic*, among other publications. *The Big Freeze* is her first book.

natalielampert.com

Instagram: @natalie.lampert.writer

TikTok: @natalie.lampert

X: @natalielampert_

Threads: @natalie.lampert.writer

ABOUT THE TYPE

This book was set in Bembo, a typeface based on an old-style Roman face that was used for Cardinal Pietro Bembo's tract *De Aetna* in 1495. Bembo was cut by Francesco Griffo (1450–1518) in the early sixteenth century for Italian Renaissance printer and publisher Aldus Manutius (1449–1515). The Lanston Monotype Company of Philadelphia brought the well-proportioned letterforms of Bembo to the United States in the 1930s.